Research Methods in Community Medicine

D1388861

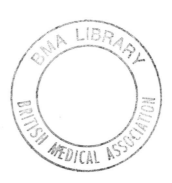

For Eleanor

Research Methods in Community Medicine

Surveys,
Epidemiological Research,
Programme Evaluation,
Clinical Trials

J. H. Abramson
Emeritus Professor of Social Medicine
The Hebrew University-Hadassah School of Public Health and
Community Medicine, Jerusalem

Z. H. Abramson, MD MPH
Beit Hakerem Community Clinic (Clalit Health Services)
and Department of Family Medicine,
The Hebrew University-Hadassah School of Medicine, Jerusalem

SIXTH EDITION

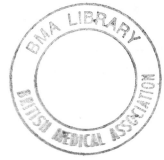

John Wiley & Sons, Ltd

First to fifth editions published by Churchill Livingstone, Edinburgh, as *Survey Methods in Community Medicine*

First edition 1974, Second edition 1979, Third edition, 1984, Fourth edition 1990, Fifth edition 1999
(reprinted 2004 and twice in 2005).

Translations: (Spanish) Ediciones Diaz de Santos, S.A., Madrid, 1990. (Indonesian) Gadjah Mada University
Press, Yogyakarta, 1991.

Other Wiley Editorial Offices

John Wiley & Sons Inc., 111 River Street, Hoboken, NJ 07030, USA

Jossey-Bass, 989 Market Street, San Francisco, CA 94103-1741, USA

Wiley-VCH Verlag GmbH, Boschstr. 12, D-69469 Weinheim, Germany

John Wiley & Sons Australia Ltd, 33 Park Road, Milton, Queensland 4064, Australia

John Wiley & Sons (Asia) Pte Ltd, 2 Clementi Loop #02-01, Jin Xing Distripark, Singapore 129809

John Wiley & Sons Canada Ltd, 6045 Freemont Blvd, Mississauga, Ontario, L5R 4J3

Wiley also publishes its books in a variety of electronic formats. Some content that appears in print may not
be available in electronic books.

Library of Congress Cataloging-in-Publication Data

British Library Cataloguing in Publication Data

A catalogue record for this book is available from the British Library

ISBN: 978-0-470-98661-5 (P/B)

Typeset in 10.5/12.5 Times by Thomson Digital, India
Printed and bound in Great Britain by Antony Rowe Ltd, Chippenham, Wiltshire.

Contents

Preface

The purpose of this book is to provide a simple and systematic guide to the planning and performance of investigations concerned with health and disease and with health care, whether they are designed to widen the horizons of scientific knowledge or to provide a basis for improved care in a specific community. It is not a compendium of detailed techniques of investigation or of statistical methods, but an ABC to the design, conduct and analysis of these studies. It is written for students and practitioners of community medicine and public health (epidemiologists, family physicians, nurses, health educators, administrators, and others) interested in the planning of health surveys, cohort and case-control studies, clinical and programme trials, studies of the use of health services, and other epidemiological and evaluative research. It may also be helpful to readers who wish only to enhance their capacity for the judicious appraisal of medical literature.

The book's change of name from 'Survey Methods' to 'Research Methods' reflects the fact that it deals with observational studies of all kinds, and clinical and programme trials, and not only with what are commonly regarded as surveys. Whatever its name, the book remains a simple introductory text, assuming little prior knowledge.

The book has been extensively revised and updated. A new chapter on the use of the Web for health research has been added, and so has an appendix that lists free computer programs that may be useful in the planning, performance, or analysis of studies. As in previous editions, copious endnotes and references are provided, for the benefit of readers who wish to go into things a little more deeply. These notes and references have also been revised and updated.

As before, there are references to Internet sites. As long as these sites remain accessible, they can be helpful as sources of accessory material

Making Sense of Data, our self-instruction manual on the interpretation of epidemiological data (3rd edition, Oxford University Press, 2001) and the *WinPepi* statistical programs for epidemiologists (described in Appendix C) may be regarded as companions to this volume.

J. H. Abramson

Z. H. Abramson

1

First Steps

The purpose of most investigations in community medicine, and in the health field generally, is the collection of information that will provide a basis for action, whether immediately or in the long run. The investigator perceives a problem that requires solution, decides that a particular study will contribute to this end, and embarks upon the study. Sound planning – and maybe a smile or two from Lady Luck – will ensure that the findings will be useful, and possibly even of wide scientific interest. Only if the problem has neither theoretical nor practical significance and the findings serve no end but self-gratification may sound planning be unnecessary.

Before planning can start, a problem must be identified. It has been said that 'if necessity is the mother of invention, the awareness of problems is the mother of research'.[1] The investigator's interest in the problem may arise from a concern with practical matters or from intellectual curiosity, from an intuitive 'hunch' or from careful reasoning, from personal experience or from that of others. Inspiration often comes from reading, not only about the topic in which the investigator is interested, but also about related topics. An idea for a study on alcoholism may arise from the results of studies on smoking (conceptually related to alcoholism, in that it is also an addiction) or delinquency (both it and alcoholism being, at least in certain cultures, forms of socially deviant behaviour).

While the main purpose is to collect information that will contribute to the solution of a problem, investigations may also have an educational function and may be carried out for this purpose. A survey can stimulate public interest in a particular topic (the interviewer is asked: 'Why are you asking me these questions?'), and can be a means of stimulating public action. A community self-survey, carried out by participant members of the community, may be set up as a means to community action; such a survey may collect useful information, although it is seldom very accurate or sophisticated.

This chapter deals with the purpose of the investigation, reviewing the literature, ethical aspects, and the formulation of the study topic.

First Steps

- Clarifying the purpose
- Reviewing the literature
- Ethical considerations
- Formulating the topic

Research Methods in Community Medicine: Surveys, Epidemiological Research, Programme Evaluation, Clinical Trials   J. H. Abramson and Z. H. Abramson   Copyright © 2008, John Wiley & Sons Ltd

Clarifying the Purpose

The first step then, before the study is planned, is to clarify its purpose: the 'why' of the study. (We are not speaking here of the researcher's psychological motivations – a quest for prestige, promotion, the gratifications of problem-solving, etc. – which may or may not be at a conscious level.) Is it 'pure' or 'basic' research with no immediate practical applications in health care, or is it 'applied' research? Is the purpose to obtain information that will be a basis for a decision on the utilization of resources, or is it to identify persons who are at special risk of contracting a specific disease in order that preventive action may be taken; or to add to existing knowledge by throwing light on (say) a specific aspect of aetiology; or to stimulate the public's interest in a topic of relevance to its health? If an evaluative study of health care is contemplated, is the motive a concern with the welfare of the people who are served by a specific practice, health centre or hospital, or is it to see whether a specific treatment or kind of health programme is good enough to be applied in other places also?

The reason for embarking on the study should be clear to the investigator. In most cases it will in fact be so from the outset, but sometimes the formulation of the problem to be solved may be less easy. In either instance, if an application is made for facilities or funds for the study it will be necessary to describe this purpose in some detail, so as to justify the performance of the study. The researcher will need to review previous work on the subject, describe the present state of knowledge, and explain the significance of the proposed investigation. This is the 'case for action'.

Preconceived ideas introduce a possibility of biased findings, and an honest self-examination is always desirable to clarify the purposes. If the reason for studying a health service is that the investigator thinks it is atrocious and wants to collect data that will condemn it, extra-special care should be taken to ensure objectivity in the collection and interpretation of information. In such a case, the researcher would be well advised to 'bend over backwards' and consciously set out to seek information to the credit of the service. Regrettably, not all evaluative studies are honest.[2]

To emphasize the importance of the study purpose, and maybe to make it clearer, let us restate it in the words of three other writers:

> The preliminary questions when planning a study are:
> 1. What is the question?
> 2. What will be done with the answer?[3]

> *Do not*: say that you will try to formulate a good subject.
> *Do*: tell what you want to accomplish with the subject.[4]

> Discover the 'latent objective' of a project. The latent objective is the meaning of the research for the researcher, and gives away his or her secret hopes of what (s)he will achieve. To detect this latent objective, it is often fruitful to 'begin at the end.' How will the world be changed after the research is published?[5]

Reviewing the Literature

The published experiences and thoughts of others may not only indicate the presence and nature of the research problem, but may be of great help in all aspects of planning and in the interpretation of the study findings. At the outset of the study the investigator should be or should become acquainted with the important relevant literature, and should continue with directed reading throughout. References should be filed in an organized way, manually or in a computerized database.[6] It is of limited use to wait until a report has to be written, and then read and cite (or only cite) a long list of publications to impress the reader with one's erudition – a procedure that may defeat its own ends, since it is often quite apparent that the papers and books listed in the extensive bibliography have had no impact on the investigation.

Papers should be read with a healthy scepticism; in Francis Bacon's words, 'Read not to contradict and confute, not to believe and take for granted … but to weigh and consider'.[7] Several guides to critical reading are available.[8] Remember that studies that have negative or uninteresting findings are less likely to be published than those with striking findings.[9]

If the title and abstract suggest that the paper may be of interest, then you should appraise the methods used in the study (which requires the kind of familiarity with research methods and their pitfalls that this book attempts to impart), assess the accuracy of the findings, judge whether the inferences are valid, and decide whether the study has relevance to your own needs and interests. Do not expect any study to be completely convincing, and do not reject a study because it is not completely convincing; avoid 'I am an epidemiologist' bias (repudiation of any study containing any flaw in its design, analysis or interpretation) and other forms of what has been called 'reader bias'.[10]

Search engines such as Google Scholar, and the increasing tendency to provide free access on the Internet to the full text of publications, have made it very much easier to find relevant literature. Google Scholar not only finds publications, it also finds subsequent publications that have cited them, and related publications, and it provides links to local library catalogues.

But, at the same time, the explosive growth in published material in recent years means that a computer search may find so many references (and so many of them irrelevant) that sifting them can be a demanding chore, to the extent that one may be misguidedly tempted to rely only on review articles, or on the abstracts provided by most databases, instead of tracking papers down and reading them.

Conducting a computer search in such a way that you get what you want – and don't get what you don't want – is not always easy. It is particularly difficult to get *all* of what you want. Investigators who wish to perform a systematic review of all previous published researches on a particular topic, for example, may be well advised to enlist the help of a librarian. A biomedical librarian advises the use of regular Google as well as Google Scholar if hard-to-find government or conference papers are sought, and also advises use of PubMed and other databases if the aim is an exhaustive search.[11] Most users find Google Scholar easy to use and very helpful – the answer to a maiden's prayer – but its coverage (in its present incarnation) is incomplete,[12] and in terms of accuracy, thoroughness, and up-to-dateness it falls short of PubMed, which provides access to over 16 million citations, mainly from MedLine, back to the 1950s. The way to use PubMed is explained on the website (http://?www.ncbi.nlm.nih.gov/entrez), and it is easy to use if requirements are simple; but otherwise, it has been said, 'If you enjoy puzzles, MedLine is great fun'.[13] A user-friendly simplified interface, SLIM, is now available.[14]

Ethical Considerations

Before embarking on a study the investigator should be convinced that it is ethically justifiable, and that it can be done in an ethical way. Ethical questions arise in both experimental and nonexperimental studies.

There is an obvious ethical problem whenever an experiment to test the benefits or hazards of a treatment is contemplated. However beneficial the trial may turn out to be for humanity at large, some subjects may be harmed either by the experimental treatment or by its being withheld. There is also an ethical problem in not performing a clinical trial, since this may lead to the introduction or continued use of an ineffective or hazardous treatment. 'Where the value of a treatment, new or old, is doubtful, there may be a higher moral obligation to test it critically than to continue to prescribe it year-in-year-out with the support merely of custom or wishful thinking.'[15] But, it has been pointed out, 'this ethical imperative can only be maintained if, and to the extent that, it is possible to conduct controlled trials in an ethically justifiable way'.[16] The heinous medical experiments conducted on helpless victims by Nazi physicians in the first part of the 20th century should never be forgotten.[17]

For an experimental study to be ethical, the subjects should be aware that they are to participate in an experiment, should know how their treatment will be decided and what the possible consequences are, should be told that they may withdraw from the trial at any time, and should freely give their informed consent. These requirements are not always easily accepted in clinical settings, and they are sometimes circumvented by medical investigators who feel that they have a right to decide their patient's treatment. Studies have shown that patients (especially poorly educated ones) who sign consent forms are often ignorant of the most basic facts. Special problems concerning consent may arise in cluster-randomized trials,[18] where clusters of people (e.g. the patients in different family practices) are randomly allocated to treatment or control groups (see p. 351), or where a total community is exposed to an experimental procedure or programme, or when experiments (such as trials of new vaccines) are performed in developing countries.[19]

Ethical objections to clinical trials are reduced if there is genuine uncertainty about the value of the treatment tested or the relative value of the treatments compared (*equipoise*) – for some investigators, it is sufficient that there is genuine uncertainty in the health profession as a whole, whatever their own views – and if controls are given the best established treatment. 'The essential feature of a controlled trial is that it must be ethically possible to give each patient any of the treatments involved'.[19]

Decisions on the ethicality of trials may not be simple.[20] Bradford Hill has said that there is only one Golden Rule, namely 'that one can make no generalization ... the problem must be faced afresh with every proposed trial'.

The goals of the research should always be secondary to the wellbeing of the participants. The Helsinki declaration states:

> Concern for the interests of the subject must always prevail over the interests of science and society ... every patient – including those of a control group, if any – should be assured of the best proven diagnostic and therapeutic method.

But researchers sometimes argue that obtaining an answer to the research question is the primary ethical obligation, so that they then 'find themselves slipping across a line that prohibits treating human subjects as means to an end. When that line is crossed, there is very little left to protect patients from a callous disregard of their welfare for the sake of research goals'.[21] This has raised debates about possible 'scientific imperialism', characterized by the performance of trials, sometimes with lowered ethical standards, in countries that are unlikely to benefit from the findings: 'Are poor people in developing countries being exploited in research for the benefit of patients in the developed world where subject recruitment to a randomized trial would be difficult?'[22]

In 1997, a furore was aroused at the disclosure that, in developing countries, controls were receiving placebos in trials, sponsored by the USA, of regimens to prevent the transmission of human immunodeficiency virus (HIV) from mothers to their unborn children, although there was an effective treatment that had been recommended for all HIV-infected pregnant women in the USA and some other countries. A debate ensued, the main issue being whether the Helsinki declaration's requirement that controls should be given the best current treatment was outweighed by the claims that a comparison with placebo was the best way of finding out whether the relatively cheap experimental regimens would be helpful in countries that cannot afford optimal care, and that the investigators were simply observing what would happen to the infants of the controls, who would anyway not have received treatment if there had been no study.

How well the trial is planned and performed is also important:

> Scientifically unsound studies are unethical. It may be accepted as a maxim that a poorly or improperly designed study involving human subjects – one that could not possibly yield scientific facts (that is, reproducible observations) relevant to the question under study – is by definition unethical. When a study is in itself scientifically invalid, all other ethical considerations become irrelevant. There is no point in obtaining 'informed consent' to perform a useless study.[23]

It is generally accepted that a study that is too small to provide clear results is *ipso facto* unethical. But it is has been argued that this is not necessarily so, since a larger sample size would impose the burden of participation on more subjects, without having a proportionate effect on the trial's capacity to yield clear results.[24]

Other ethical considerations may arise after the trial has started. If it is found to be in a subject's interest to stop or modify the treatment, or to start treating a control subject, then there should be no hesitation in doing so. If there is reason to think that continuation of the trial may be harmful, then it should be stopped forthwith. For example, the first randomized controlled trial of the protective effect against HIV infection of the performance of circumcision of young men, conducted in Orange Farm, a region close to Johannesburg in South Africa, was stopped as soon as an interim analysis revealed that the incidence of HIV infection was much higher in the controls than in the circumcised group.[25]

In nonexperimental studies[26] ethical problems are usually less acute, unless the study involves hazardous test procedures or intrusions on privacy. But here, too, there is a need for informed consent[27] if participants are required to answer questions, undergo tests that carry a risk (however small), or permit access to confidential records. The investigators should give an honest explanation of the purpose of the survey when enlisting subjects, and respondents should be told what their participation entails, and assured that they are free to refuse to answer questions or continue their participation. Pains should be taken to keep information confidential. Any promises made to participants, e.g. about anonymity or the provision of test results, should of course be kept.

Of particular importance is the question of what action should be taken if a survey reveals that participants would benefit from medical care or other intervention. In studies involving HIV antibody testing, subjects with positive results should obviously be notified, even if this affects the soundness of the study.[28]

The notorious Tuskegee study in Alabama is a horrible illustration of an unethical survey.[29] It began in 1932, with the aim of throwing light on the effects of untreated syphilis. Some 400 untreated Black syphilitics (mostly poor and uneducated) were identified and then followed up; their course was compared with that of apparently syphilis-free age-matched controls. Treatment of syphilis was withheld. By 1938–1939 it was found that a number of the men had received sporadic treatment with arsenic or mercury, and a very few had had more intensive treatment. In the interests of science 'fourteen young untreated syphilitics were added to the study to compensate for this'. Treatment was withheld even when penicillin was found to be effective and became easily available in the late 1940s and early 1950s. Participants received free benefits, such as free treatment (except for syphilis), free hot lunches, and free burial (after a free autopsy). By 1954 it was apparent that the life expectancy of the untreated men aged 25–50 was reduced by 17%. By 1963, 14 more men per 100 had died in the syphilitic group than in the control group. In 1972 there was a public outcry, and compensation payments were later made.

There are those who say that political decisions that may involve risk to human life, e.g. the raising of speed limits on interurban roads, without setting cut-off points for early termination in the case of adverse results, are unethical before–after experiments.[30]

In many countries informed consent is mandatory for studies of human subjects unless there are valid contraindications, such as qualms about alarming fatally ill patients with doubts about the efficacy of treatment. Many institutions have ethical committees that review and sanction proposed studies. Some investigators feel that this control is too permissive, but there are some who think it is too restrictive (it 'stops worthwhile research').[31] A fanciful account of the rise and fall of epidemiology between 1950 and 2000 (printed in 1981)[32] attributed the fall to ethical committees and regulations designed to protect the confidentiality of records.

At a different ethical level, consideration should be given to the justification for any proposed study in the light of the availability of resources and the alternative ways in which these might be used. Does the possible benefit warrant the required expenditure of time, manpower and money? Is it ethical to perform the study at the expense of other activities, especially those that might directly promote the community's health?

An honest endeavour to clarify the purpose of the study may lead to second thoughts: is the study really worth doing? A great deal of useless research is conducted. This wastes time and resources, and exposes the scientific method to ridicule.[33]

Formulating the Topic

When the purpose and moral justification of the study are clear, the investigator can formulate the topic he or she proposes to study, in general terms. In many cases this is easily done and almost tautological. For example, if the reason for setting up the study is that infant mortality is unduly high in a given population and there is insufficient information on its causes for the planning of an action programme, the topic of the study can be broadly stated as 'the causes of infant mortality in a defined population in a given time period'. If the reason for the investigation is that health education on smoking has been having little effect, and that it is considered that certain new methods may be more effective, the investigation will be a comparative study of defined educational techniques for the reduction of smoking.

In other instances the formulation of the topic may be less easy, since the researcher may have difficulty in deciding precisely what study is needed to solve the research problem, taking account of practical limitations. As an illustration, a problem arose in a tuberculosis programme; the extent of public participation in X-ray screening activities fell short of what was desired, and there were indications that the tuberculosis rate was higher among people who did not come for screening. It was decided to seek information that would help to improve the situation, but considerable thought was required before a study topic could be formulated. The alternative topics were the reasons for nonparticipation and those for participation. For a variety of reasons, it was decided that the latter approach would be more useful.[34]

As another example, a researcher interested in a possible association between eating fish and coronary heart disease has several alternative approaches. One, for example, is to study the previous dietary habits of people with and without coronary heart disease; another is to follow up groups of people whose diets differ, and determine the occurrence of the disease during a defined period; and a third is to examine statistics on the disease rates and average fish consumption of different countries. The decision will be based both on the ease with which the required information can be obtained and on the probability of obtaining convincing evidence, one way or the other.

At this early stage, the formulation of the topic of study may be regarded as a provisional one. The feasibility of a valid study still has to be determined. When planning and the pretesting of methods get under way, it frequently happens that unpredicted difficulties come to light, requiring a modification of the topic or even leading to a decision that there is no practicable way of solving the research problem.

Notes and References

1. Geitgey DA, Metz EA. Nursing Research 1969; 18: 339.
2. A dishonest evaluation of health care may be *eyewash* (an appraisal limited to aspects that look good), *whitewash* (covering up failure by avoiding objectivity, e.g. by soliciting testimonials), *submarine* (aimed at torpedoing a programme, regardless of its worth), a *postponement ploy* (noting the need to seek facts, in the hope that the crisis will be over by the time the facts are available), etc. Providers of care who evaluate services that they themselves provide should take pains to confute the criticism that this is like 'letting the fox guard the chicken house' (Spiegel AD, Hyman HH. Basic health planning methods. Aspen Systems; 1978).
3. Feinstein A. Clinical epidemiology: the architecture of clinical research. Philadelphia: W.B. Saunders; 1985. Cited by Vandenbroucke JP. Alvan Feinstein and the art of consulting: how to define a research question. Journal of Clinical Epidemiology 2002; 55: 1176.
4. Verschuren PJM. De probleemstelling van een ondersoek. Utrecht: Aula; 1986. Extract translated and cited by Vandenbroucke JP (2002; see note 3).
5. Vandenbroucke JP (2002; see note 3).
6. Numerous computer programs for *storing and managing references* are available. Google Scholar and other programs can automatically add citations to databases. For free reference managers, see Appendix C.

    For investigators loath to use computers, a card index is a substitute (one reference per card), with full bibliographic details (names of all authors, first and last page numbers, etc.) to avoid another hunt when a bibliography is prepared for the report.

    If printouts, photocopies, reprints or tear-out copies of articles or abstracts are collected, then they should be filed and indexed in an orderly way. The planning of a filing system is described in detail by Haynes RB, McKibbon KA, Fitzgerald D, Guyatt GH, Walker CJ, Sackett DL (How to keep up with the medical literature. Annals of Internal Medicine 1986; 105: 149, 309, 574, 636, 810, 978).
7. Bacon F. 1620 Novum organum. English translation. Open Court Publishing; 1994.
8. *Guides to critical reading* include: (a) Greenhalgh T (How to read a paper: the basics of evidence based medicine, 2nd edn. London: BMJ Books; 2001). Ten excerpts from a previous version that appeared in successive issues of the British Medical Journal [vol 315] from 19 July 1997 are available on the Internet at http://www.bmj.com/collections/read.dtl. (b) Sackett DL, Straus SE, Glasziou P, Richardson WS, Rosenberg W, Haynes RB (Evidence-based medicine: how to practice and teach EBM, 3rd edn. New York: Churchill Livingstone; 2005. pp. 81–117). (c) A series of 'Users' Guides to the Medical Literature' occasionally published in the Journal of the American Medical Association between 3 November 1993 and 13 September 2000.

    Also, see Crombie IK (A pocket guide to critical appraisal, 2nd edn. Blackwell Publishing; 2007) and Abramson JH, Abramson ZH (Making sense of data: a self-instruction manual on the interpretation of epidemiologic data, 3rd edn. New York: Oxford University Press; 2001).
9. *Publication bias* is an established fact in the health field: negative or inconclusive studies are often 'tucked away in desk drawers' or rejected; e.g. see: Easterbrook PJ, Berlin JA, Gopalan R, Matthews DR (Publication bias in clinical research. Lancet 1991; 337: 867), Dickersin K, Min YI (Publication bias: the problem that won't go away. Annals of the New York Academy of Sciences 1993; 703: 135), Stern JM, Simes RJ (Publication bias: evidence of delayed publication in a cohort study of clinical research projects. British Medical Journal 1997; 315: 640).

'Health journals are … interested in news – they will always want to report the earthquake that happened and not all the places without earthquakes', (Lawlor DA. Editorial: Quality in epidemiological research: should we be submitting papers before we have the results and submitting more hypothesis-generating research? International Journal of Epidemiology 2007; 36: 940).

Investigators who conduct meta-analyses that combine the findings of different studies often appraise the validity of their conclusions by computing a *fail-safe N*, i.e. the number of unpublished negative studies that would be needed to render the overall finding nonsignificant or trivial (for software, see Appendix C). A number of registers of clinical trials have been set up, in the hope that this will permit unpublished results to be sought and taken into account.

10. Forms of *reader bias* include *rivalry bias* (pooh-poohing a study published by a rival), *personal habit bias* (overrating or underrating a study to justify the reader's habits, e.g. a jogger favouring a study showing the health benefits of running), *prestigious journal bias* (overrating results because the journal has an illustrious name), and *pro-technology* and *anti-technology* bias (overrating or underrating a study owing to the reader's enchantment or disenchantment with medical technology). (Owen R. Reader bias. Journal of the American Medical Association 1982; 247: 2533.)

11. Giustini D. How Google is changing medicine. British Medical Journal 2005; 331: 1487.

Advanced search techniques for use with Google Scholar are described by Noruza A (Google Scholar: the new generation of citation indexes. Libri 2005; 55: 170).

12. Burright M. Database reviews and reports: Google Scholar – science & technology. 2006. Available at http://www.istl.org/06-winter/databases2.html.

13. Sackett *et al.* (2005; see note 8). For a simple guide to the use of Medline, see Greenhalgh T (How to read a paper: the Medline database. British Medical Journal 1997; 315: 180).

Finding a specific article, or a few articles on a specific topic, is easy. But an exhaustive search is another story. According to the Cochrane Handbook, an exhaustive PubMed hunt for randomized controlled trials (for a meta-analysis) requires 26 search terms over and above those specifying the topic of the trials (Higgins JPT, Green S (eds), Cochrane handbook for systematic reviews of interventions [updated September 2006], appendix 5b.3. Available at http://www.cochrane.org/resources/handbook/hbook.htm).

14. SLIM (Slider Interface for MedLine/PubMed Searches), is available at http://pmi.nlm.nih.gov/slim.

15. Green FHK, cited by Hill (1997; see note 20).

16. Roy DJ. Controlled clinical trials: an ethical imperative. Journal of Chronic Diseases 1986; 39: 159.

17. Seidelman WE (Mengele Medicus: medicine's Nazi heritage. Milbank Quarterly 1988; 66: 221) cites the horrors committed by Mengele and other Nazi physicians as warnings against 'ethical compromise where human life and dignity become secondary to personal, professional, scientific, and political goals'. Also, see Seidelman WE (Nuremberg lamentation: for the forgotten victims of medical science. British Medical Journal 1996; 313: 1463) and Annas GJ, Grodin MA (eds) (The Nazi doctors and the Nuremberg Code: human rights in human experimentation. New York: Oxford University Press; 1995).

Experiments on prisoners in the USA are described by Hornblum AM (They were cheap and available: prisoners as research subjects in twentieth century America. British Medical Journal 1997; 315: 1437).

18. In *cluster-randomized trials*, e.g. those in which communities or general practices are randomly assigned to treatment or control groups, it is generally impracticable to obtain informed consent for inclusion in the trial from every individual subject before assignment.

However, in cluster-randomized trials in which intervention is targeted at individuals (e.g. if vitamin or placebo capsules are administered), subjects may be given the option of leaving the trial (after assignment) and choosing an alternative, e.g. routine care. And in studies where outcomes are measured at an individual level, subjects may be required to give their assent to measurements or access to their medical records; this may be regarded as less important if outcomes are studied only at a group level (e.g. changes in hypertension prevalence).

Opinions differ on the importance of informed consent in cluster-randomized trials, especially in control groups receiving conventional care. However, especially if intervention or nonintervention carries risks, informed consent should probably always be requested from the groups' 'gatekeepers' (who can provide access to their members) – or, preferably, 'guardians' (who can be expected to protect the groups' interests), such as head teachers, community leaders, or local health or political authorities. Because of possible conflicts of guardians' interests, particularly if the guardians are health authorities, approval should always be obtained from an ethics committee.

For fuller discussions of ethical considerations in cluster-randomized studies, see Donner A, Klar N (Pitfalls of and controversies in cluster randomization trials. American Journal of Public Health 2004; 94: 416), Hutton JL (Are distinctive ethical principles required for cluster randomised clinical trials? Statistics in Medicine 2001; 20: 473), and Edwards SJL, Braunholtz DA, Lilford RJ, Stevens AJ (Ethical issues in the design and conduct of cluster randomised controlled trials. British Medical Journal 1999; 318: 1407).

The 1991 CIOMS International Guidelines for Ethical Review of Epidemiological Studies state: 'When it is not possible to request informed consent from every individual to be studied, the agreement of a representative of a community or group may be sought, but the representative should be chosen according to the nature, traditions and political philosophy of the community or group. Approval given by a community representative should be consistent with general ethical principles. When investigators work with communities, they will consider communal rights and protection as they would individual rights and protection. For communities in which collective decision-making is customary, communal leaders can express the collective will. However, the refusal of individuals to participate in a study has to be respected: a leader may express agreement on behalf of a community, but an individual's refusal of personal participation is binding.'(cited by Donner and Klar 2004, *op. cit.*)

19. Regarding *research in developing countries*, international guidelines state: 'Rural communities in developing countries may not be conversant with the concepts and techniques of experimental medicine … Where individual members of a community do not have the necessary awareness of the implications of participation in an experiment to give adequately informed consent directly to the investigators, it is desirable that the decision whether or not to participate should be elicited through the intermediary of a trusted community leader. The intermediary should make it clear that participation is entirely voluntary, and that any participant is free to abstain or withdraw at any time from the experiment'. (Proposed International Ethical Guidelines for Biomedical Research Involving Human Subjects published by the World Health Organization and the Council for International Organizations of Medical Sciences. Cited by Hutton JL (Ethics on medical research in developing countries: the role of international codes of conduct. Statistical Methods in Medical Research 2000; 9: 185)).

It may also be practicable to obtain the subjects' informed consent as a second stage, after consent has been received from a community leader, as demonstrated in a vaccine trial in Senegal (Preziosi M-P, Yam A, Ndiaye M, Simaga A, Simondon F, Wassilak SGF. Practical experiences in obtaining informed consent for a vaccine trial in rural Africa. New England Journal of Medicine 1997; 336: 370).

Ethical considerations in field trials in developing countries are reviewed by Smith PG, Morrow RH, (eds) (Methods for field trials of interventions against tropical diseases: a 'toolbox'. Oxford: Oxford University Press; 1991. pp. 71–94).

20. The *ethical aspects of clinical trials* were emphasized by Sir Austin Bradford Hill 1977 (A short textbook of medical statistics. London: Hodder and Stoughton. p. 223), who on his election to the Royal Society was recognized as 'the leader in the development in medicine of the precise experimental methods now used nationally and internationally'.

The basic principle is neatly summarized in the following exchange: 'Mr Ederer: "If you could give only one bit of advice to a clinician planning a clinical trial, what would you tell him?" Dr Davis: "A one-word answer might be 'don't'. If you are determined to do it, my advice would be from the beginning put yourself in the patient's position and develop the protocol so you would be happy to be one of the subjects. If you cannot do that, you'd better not start."' (Davis MD. American Journal of Ophthalmology 1975; 79: 779).

See the *Helsinki declaration*, available at http://www.wma.net/e/policy/b3.htm.

21. Angell M. Editorial: The ethics of clinical research in the Third World. New England Journal of Medicine 1997; 337: 847.

22. Wilmshurst P. Editorial: Scientific imperialism. British Medical Journal 1997; 314: 840. Other extracts: 'Should research be conducted in a country where the people are unlikely to benefit from the findings because most of the population is too poor to buy effective treatment? … Drug companies have performed research on children and adults in countries such as Thailand and the Philippines that do not conform to the Declaration of Helsinki and could not be conducted in the developed world. Reasons quoted for conducting research in Africa rather than developed countries are lower costs, lower risk of litigation, less stringent ethical review, the availability of populations prepared to give unquestioning consent, anticipated underreporting of side effects because of lower consumer awareness … In some experiments in developing countries it is difficult for patients to refuse to participate … participation in a trial may be the only chance of receiving any treatment'.

23. Rutstein DD. In: Freund FA (ed), Experimentation with human subjects. London: George Allen & Unwin; 1972.

24. Bacchetti P, Wolf LE, Segal MR, McCulloch CE. Ethics and sample size. American Journal of Epidemiology 2005; 161: 105.

25. Auvert B, Taljaard D, Lagarde E, Sobngwi-Tambekou J, Sitta R, Puren A. Randomized, controlled intervention trial of male circumcision for reduction of HIV infection risk: the ANRS 1265 trial. PloS Medicine 2005; 2: 1112.

26. For *ethical aspects of epidemiological research*, see: Coughlin SS (Ethical issues in epidemiologic research and public health practice. Emerging Themes in Epidemiology 2006; 3: 16) and Susser M, Stein Z, Kline J (Ethics in epidemiology. Annals of the American Academy of Political and Social Science 1978; 437: 128 [reprinted in Susser M. Epidemiology, health and society: selected papers. New York: Oxford University Press; 1987. pp. 13–22]).

27. A specimen 'informed consent' form for use in an interview survey is provided by Stolley PD, Schlesselman JJ (Planning and conducting a study. In: Schlesselman JJ (ed), Case-control studies: design, conduct, analysis. New York: Oxford University Press; 1982. pp. 69–104).

28. The 'To tell or not to tell' dilemma in studies involving HIV testing, and possible solutions, are discussed by Avins A, Lo B (To tell or not to tell: the ethical dilemmas of HIV test notification in epidemiologic research. American Journal of Public Health 1989; 79: 1544), Kegeles S, Coates TJ, Lo B, Catania J (Mandatory reporting of HIV testing would deter men from being tested. Journal of the American Medical Association 1989; 261: 1989), and Avins A, Woods W, Lo B, Hulley S (A novel use of the link-file system for longitudinal studies of HIV infection: practical solution to an ethical dilemma. AIDS 1993; 7: 109).

29. Thomas SB, Quinn SC. The Tuskegee syphilis study, 1932 to 1972: implications for HIV education and AIDS risk education programs in the Black community. American Journal of Public Health 1991; 81: 1498.

30. Richter E, Barach P, Herman T, Ben-David G, Weinberger Z. Extending the boundaries of the Declaration of Helsinki: a case study of an unethical experiment in a non-medical setting. Journal of Medical Ethics 2001; 27: 126.

31. Waters WE. Ethics and epidemiological research. International Journal of Epidemiology 1985; 14: 48.

32. Rothman KJ. The rise and fall of epidemiology, 1950–2000 A.D. New England Journal of Medicine 1981; 304: 600.

33. 'Time, talent, and money are sometimes squandered on the measurement of the trivial, the irrelevant, and the obvious … A friend of mine who has a gift for felicitous expression has distinguished between "ideas" research on the one hand and "occupational therapy for the university staff" on the other, and once referred to a research project as "squeezing the last drop of blood out of a foregone conclusion"' (Lord Platt. Medical science: master or servant. British Medical Journal 1967; 2: 439).

See an amusing compilation by Hartston W (The drunken goldfish: a celebration of irrelevant research. Unwin Hyman; 1988) of actual research results (Do rats prefer tennis balls to other rats? Can pigeons tell Bach from Hindemith? Does holy water affect the growth of radishes?) that serves 'to drop a gentle hint that there might be too much research going on, and much of that is taken far too seriously'.

Useless research is satirized in the Journal of Irreproducible Results (for details and a sample of contents, visit www.jir.com on the Internet).

34. Rosenstock IM, Hochbaum GM. Some principles of research design in public health. American Journal of Public Health 1961; 51: 266.

2

Types of Investigation

Before discussing the detailed planning of a study, we will consider the types of investigation and their nomenclature. The primary distinction is between surveys (or observational studies) and experiments (trials). The various types of epidemiological and evaluative studies will be reviewed in this chapter.

Surveys and Experiments

Since a survey is most easily defined negatively, as a nonexperimental investigation, we will start by defining an experiment.

An *experiment* is an investigation in which the researcher, wishing to study the effects of exposure to, or deprivation of, a defined factor, decides which subjects (persons, animals, towns, etc.) will be exposed to, or deprived of, the factor. Experiments are studies of deliberate intervention by the investigators. If the investigator compares subjects exposed to the factor with subjects not exposed to it, this is a *controlled experiment*; the more care that is taken to ensure that the two groups are as similar as possible in other respects, the better controlled is the experiment. In a controlled experiment on the effect of vitamin supplements, for example, it is the investigator who decides who will and who will not receive such supplements; in a survey, by contrast, people who happen to be taking vitamin supplements are compared with people who are not.

A study is a true experiment only if decisions about exposure to the factor under consideration (e.g. to whom will vitamin supplements be offered) are made by the experimenter. A researcher who wants to conduct an experiment does not always have full control over the situation, and may be unable to make such decisions. It may be possible, however, to construct a study that resembles an experiment, although in this respect it falls short of being a true one. For example, it may be feasible to make observations before and after some intervention not under the investigator's control (medical treatment, exposure to a health education programme, etc.) and to make parallel observations in an unexposed group. The study may then be called a *quasi-experiment*[1] (although some experts prefer to regard such studies as nonexperimental). This term is also sometimes used if the allocation to experimental and control groups (even if under the experimenter's control) is not random (see *randomization*, p. 328).

Research Methods in Community Medicine: Surveys, Epidemiological Research, Programme Evaluation, Clinical Trials   J. H. Abramson and Z. H. Abramson   Copyright © 2008, John Wiley & Sons Ltd

Although quasi-experiments are sometimes given the unflattering appellation of 'pseudo-experiments', they are often well worth doing when a true experiment is not feasible (see pp. 347 and 349); but their findings must be interpreted with caution – it may be difficult to be sure that the outcome is, in fact, attributable to the intervention.

The term *natural experiment* is often applied to circumstances where, as a result of 'naturally' occurring changes or differences, it is easy to observe the effects of a specific factor. A famine may permit a study of the effects of starvation. A recent example is the demonstration of a raised schizophrenia rate in the offspring of mothers who were exposed to a famine at the time of conception or early pregnancy.[2] Snow's classic comparison of cholera rates in homes with different water sources, some more contaminated than others, in London in the middle of the 19th century,[3] may also be termed a 'natural experiment' or 'experiment of opportunity'. 'Natural experiments' are surveys or, at most, quasi-experiments (if they examine the effects of man-made changes not planned as experiments, as in the demonstration that the incidence of myocardial infarction in a community in Montana was lower during the operation of a smoking ban in public places than before or after the enforcement of the ban).[4]

Manipulations of animals or human beings are not synonymous with experiments. An investigator who studies bacteriuria in pregnancy by needling the bladders of pregnant women through their abdominal walls in order to collect urine for examination is conducting a survey, not an experiment. An experiment is always a study of change.

A *survey* (or *observational study*)[5] is an investigation in which information is systematically collected, but the experimental method is not used; that is, there is no active intervention by the investigators. In this book, 'survey' is used in a broad sense to mean a nonexperimental study of any kind and does not have the narrow connotations sometimes associated with the term, such as a public opinion survey, a questionnaire survey, a descriptive study of population characteristics, a field survey, or a household survey. Surveys are not necessarily brief operations; they may involve long-term surveillance (see p. 25) or repeated interviews or examinations.

Descriptive and Analytic Studies

Studies may be *descriptive* or *analytic*.

A *descriptive* study sets out to describe a situation, e.g. the distribution of a disease in a population in relation to age, sex, region, etc. An *analytic* (or *explanatory*) study tries to find explanations or examine causal processes (Why does the disease occur in these people? Why do certain people fail to make use of health services? Can the decreased incidence of the disease be attributed to the introduction of preventive measures? Does treatment reduce the risk of complications?). This is done by formulating and testing hypotheses, which may have various sources,[6] including the findings of previous descriptive studies.

An analytic study may be used to explain a local situation in a specific population in which the investigator is interested, or to obtain results of a more general applicability, e.g. new knowledge about the aetiology of a disease.

All descriptive studies are surveys, but surveys can also be analytic; experiments are obviously analytic. The distinction between a descriptive and an analytic survey is not always clear, and many surveys combine both purposes.

Cross-sectional and Longitudinal Studies

Studies, whether descriptive, analytic or both, can be usefully categorized as cross-sectional or longitudinal, depending on the time period covered by the observations. A *cross-sectional* study (an 'instantaneous', 'simultaneous', or 'prevalence' study) provides information about the situation that exists at a single time, whereas a *longitudinal* ('time-span') study provides data about events or changes during a period of time.

A survey in which children are measured in order to determine the distribution of their weights and heights, or to compare heights at different ages, is cross-sectional; the children are examined once, at about the same time (not necessarily on the same day). A survey in which the same children are examined repeatedly in order to appraise their growth is longitudinal. If the influence on child growth of parents' smoking habits is investigated in any of these surveys, the study is an analytic one. Most experiments are longitudinal studies that follow up different groups to measure events or changes; some only compare the status of the groups after the experimental exposure ('postmeasure only' trials), without measuring their initial status.

Any longitudinal survey in which a group (or 'cohort') of individuals (however selected) is followed up for some time may be called a cohort ('follow-up', 'panel') study; but the term 'cohort study' is generally used more restrictively, to refer to an analytic longitudinal study (see p. 20). 'Cohort study' should not be confused with 'cohort analysis'.[7] A study of the occurrence of new cases of a disease is an *incidence* study, and a follow-up study of persons born in a defined period is a *birth-cohort* study.

Note that the distinction between cross-sectional and longitudinal studies depends only on whether the information collected refers to a particular time. The *timing* of the study – *when* it is conducted, i.e. at the same time as the events studied (a *concurrent* study) or afterwards (a *historical* study) – is not relevant. Nor does it matter whether the study uses previously recorded data, or data collected after the start of the study; these two kinds of data are best termed *retrolective* and *prolective* respectively (from the Latin root of the word 'collect')[8] rather than 'retrospective' and 'prospective', to avoid confusion with other meanings of the latter terms. Note also that the term 'cross-sectional' is sometimes used in other senses, e.g. for studies of total populations or representative samples ('cross-sections') of them.

In some studies, data that refer to the present time are treated as if they referred to the past. Reported disease in the subject's relatives, for example, may be taken as evidence of prior exposure to genetic or other familial factors; or in a study of the association between lead poisoning and behavioural problems in school, the lead content of milk teeth may be used as an indicator of lead poisoning in early childhood.[9] It has been suggested that such studies should be called *pseudolongitudinal*.

Epidemiological Studies

Epidemiology is the study of the distribution and determinants of health-related states or events in specified populations, and the application of this study to control of health problems.[10]

Epidemiological studies have three main uses. First, they serve a diagnostic purpose. Just as a diagnosis of the patient's state of health is a prerequisite for good clinical care, so a *community diagnosis* (see Chapter 34) or *group diagnosis*, leading to a *needs assessment*,[11] provides a basis for the care of a specific community (or other defined group). Epidemiological studies – descriptive and analytic – provide the required information about health status and the determinants of health in a specific community or group. Second, epidemiological studies (mainly analytic surveys) can throw light on aetiology, prognostic factors, the natural history of disease, and growth and development. Such knowledge is of general interest and has a wide applicability, in addition to the help it provides in specific local situations. Third, epidemiological studies (surveys and experiments) can contribute to the evaluation of health care both in specific local situations (how well an accident prevention programme is working) and in general (whether this vaccine prevents disease). Surveys of population health, it has been said, 'can be both the *alpha* and *omega* of health care by being the vehicle for both the discovery of need and the evaluation of the outcome of care and treatment'.[12]

The role of epidemiological studies in community-oriented primary care, which integrates the care of individuals with the care of the community as a whole, will be described in Chapter 34.

A schematic classification of epidemiological studies is shown on the next page.

Descriptive epidemiological surveys may be cross-sectional (how many blind people there are in the population) or longitudinal. Longitudinal surveys investigate change, e.g. studies of child growth and development, or a changing suicide rate, or the 'natural history' of disease (what the course of events after infection with HIV is), or the occurrence of new cases of disease or deaths in the population. They include clinical studies that describe the features or progress of a series of patients. Descriptive epidemiological surveys do not aim to find explanations, but their findings are often presented by age, sex, region, and other demographic variables. If the associations with the latter variables are explored in detail, then the survey can be regarded as both descriptive and analytic.

Analytic epidemiological surveys and *experiments and quasi-experiments* may be group-based, individual-based, or multilevel.

Group-based analytic surveys

A *group-based* analytic survey[13] is a comparison of groups or populations. It is a study of a group of groups, not a group of individuals. Such studies are sometimes termed *ecological* or *correlation* studies. As an example, a group of countries could be compared with respect to their death rates from cirrhosis of the liver, on the one hand, and the average consumption of alcohol and various nutrients on the other hand.[14] Or

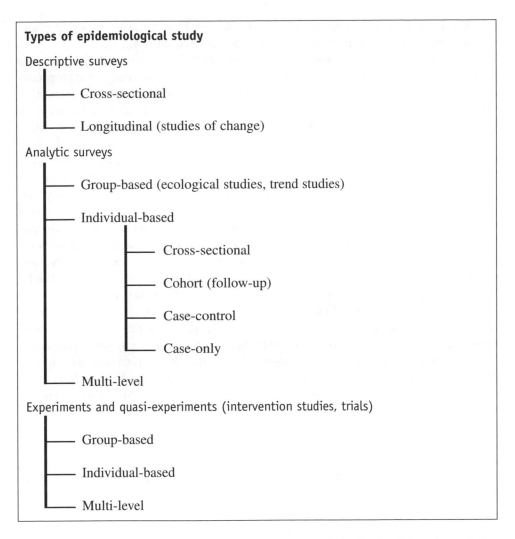

Types of epidemiological study

Descriptive surveys

— Cross-sectional

— Longitudinal (studies of change)

Analytic surveys

— Group-based (ecological studies, trend studies)

— Individual-based

— Cross-sectional

— Cohort (follow-up)

— Case-control

— Case-only

— Multi-level

Experiments and quasi-experiments (intervention studies, trials)

— Group-based

— Individual-based

— Multi-level

general practices could be compared, as in a recent study in England that showed that statins (lipid-lowering drugs) were prescribed more in practices serving deprived communities, irrespective of the prevalence of coronary heart disease and diabetes and the proportion of ethnic minorities and elderly patients.[15]

We could also conduct a *trend or time-series* study[16] by comparing the findings of descriptive studies performed in the same group at different times, e.g. by analysing the changing mortality rate from a disease in relation to changes in average fat intake and per capita tobacco consumption.[17] Such studies often produce results of considerable interest, like the doubling of the rate of fractures of the proximal femur in Oxford over a 27-year period.[18] Comparisons of trends in different populations may be instructive: a study of liver cirrhosis mortality in 25 European countries between 1970 and 1989 showed different trends in different regions, but the rates declined in all regions a few years after a decrease in per capita alcohol consumption; there was also evidence of a birth-cohort effect,[5] portending a future decrease in mortality in western and southern Europe, and an increase in eastern and northern Europe.[19]

Group-based studies are sometimes denigrated, on two main grounds. First, because they sometimes yield misleading results as a result of the inaccuracy, inappropriateness or unavailability of data, often obtained from national statistical offices or other official sources. But even then, they may serve to draw attention to differences or trends meriting further investigation. The strong positive correlation between infant mortality and the number of doctors per 10,000 population demonstrated in 1978 in a comparison of 18 developed countries in Europe and North America did not necessarily mean that infants should be kept away from doctors, but it raised important questions, even if the correlation was a reflection of other (then unknown, and now partly known) factors for which data were not available.[20] Doll and Peto have pointed out that although the striking correlations between colon cancer and meat consumption and between breast cancer and fat consumption, observed in international comparisons, may not mean that eating meat or fat is a major aetiological factor, they certainly show that the large international differences in the rates of these neoplasms are not chiefly genetic in origin, and suggest that these cancers are largely avoidable.[21]

Second, it may be misleading to apply the findings of a group-based study at an individual level; this has been termed the *ecologic fallacy*, a type of *cross-level bias*. Death rates from road accidents may be higher in richer countries, but within countries they may be higher in poorer people. If we find that populations with a high consumption of beer tend to have a high death rate from cancer of the rectum,[22] this does not necessarily mean that *individuals* who drink more beer are prone to develop this tumour; this should be tested in an individual-based survey, or maybe in a rather pleasant experiment.

The term 'ecologic fallacy' has unfortunately tended to throw ecologic studies into disrepute. But the findings of group-based studies can be important in their own right, and there is no reason to expect that their findings will necessarily be valid at an individual level[22] (or, conversely, that findings at an individual level will necessarily be valid at a group level, which has been called the *'atomistic fallacy'*).[23] A comparison of villages in Mexico showed a strong association between dengue infection (the presence of antibodies) and exposure to *Aedes aegyptii* mosquitoes; this was a useful finding, although no such association existed at an individual level.[24] Similarly, the observation that after floods in Bangladesh there was an increase in the proportions of children who manifested aggressive behaviour and enuresis is of interest, although the behaviour of individual children did not vary according to the danger of drowning they personally experienced.[25]

Group-based studies are sometimes the only appropriate study design, e.g. in comparisons of groups exposed to different environmental influences[26] or differing with respect to processes of intra-group transmission or interaction, and sometimes they facilitate the study of relationships with environmental exposures that are difficult to measure at an individual level. Group-based studies have assumed greater importance with the resurgence of interest in the influence of societal and other group processes on health, and in the determinants of the health status of human populations.[27]

Individual-based analytic surveys

Individual-based analytic surveys are, of course (like all epidemiological studies), studies of groups, but they utilize information about each individual in the group. In their simplest form, such surveys are performed to test a hypothesis that a specific causal factor is a determinant of a specific disease (or other outcome), by measuring each individual's exposure to the postulated causal factor and the presence of the disease in each individual.

Most individual-based analytic surveys can be categorized as cross-sectional, cohort or case-control studies, or as combinations of these types.

An analytic *cross-sectional study* examines the associations that exist in a group or population (or a sample of a group or population) at a given time. The study may be based on retrolective i.e., (previously recorded) or prolective data.

A *cohort study* is an analytic *follow-up* or *prospective* study in which people who are (respectively) exposed and not exposed to the postulated causal factor(s), or who have different degrees of exposure, are compared with respect to the subsequent development of the disease (or other outcome under study); the people who are followed up are referred to as the cohort. If the disease is one that cannot be contracted twice, then people who have it at the outset (before the follow up) are generally excluded from the comparison.

Note two sources of possible terminological confusion: the term 'cohort study' is sometimes used for a descriptive (nonanalytic) follow-up study, and the term 'prospective' is often used to indicate the collection of data after the start of a study (prolective data; see p. 15), rather than a cohort-study design.

A cohort study resembles an experiment, except that exposure or nonexposure is not controlled by the investigator. Specific subjects may be chosen for follow-up because of their exposure or nonexposure to the causal factor, or a cohort may be selected in some other way (say, because of residence in a specific neighbourhood), characterized with respect to exposure status, and followed up. As an example, baseline information about drinking habits and other characteristics was obtained for a population sample of Finnish beer-drinkers; after a 7-year follow up, a comparison of men who initially had different drinking habits showed that mortality was three times as high among men who had beer binges (six or more bottles per session) than among those who usually drank less than three bottles each time (allowing for differences in age, smoking, total alcohol consumption, and other factors that might affect mortality).[28]

Previously collected (retrolective) and historical data are often used in cohort studies. An extreme example is a comparison of the mortality of obese and nonobese persons, the data being their weight when they originally took out life insurance policies (before the study) and their survival from then until the time of the study. This may be called a *historical prospective study* (among other terms).[29] As another example, a cohort study that started in 1976, in which 121,700 nurses were followed up by postal questionnaire every 2 years, was able to demonstrate that their weight at birth had a strong inverse relationship with the occurrence of coronary heart disease between 1976 and 1992, using birth weights reported in the 1992 questionnaire; the authors describe their design as 'retrospective self report of birth weight in an ongoing longitudinal cohort of nurses'.[30]

In a typical *case-control study* to examine the relationship between a suspected causal factor and a disease (or other outcome), prior exposure to the causal factor is compared in people with the disease and in controls who are representative of the population 'base' from which the cases came.[31] Ideally, the controls are people who would have become cases in the study if they had developed the disease. This condition is most easily met in a case-control study performed within a defined population. It can also be easily satisfied if the case-control study is performed in the framework of a cohort study, so that the experience of new cases identified in the study cohort can be compared with that of controls from the same cohort. This is a *nested case-control study*, where the controls are selected from cohort members who were free of the disease at the time the corresponding case developed it. If a case-control study is performed in a defined cohort, a *case-base* or *case-cohort* design can be used, by selecting controls who represent the total cohort, regardless of their future disease status.

There are two main types of case-control study: *classic*, *cumulative* or *cumulative-incidence* case-control studies, in which the controls are selected after the risk of becoming a case has passed (e.g. at the end of an epidemic); and *density* or *incidence-density* case-control studies, in which cases and controls are sampled throughout the period of the study (the cases at the time they develop the illness, and the controls from people free of the illness at the time the cases develop it).

The selection of cases and controls for a case-control study will be considered in more detail in Chapter 9.

As a simple example of a case-control study, women students who acquired their first urinary tract infection were compared with sexually active women without a history of urinary tract infection, drawn from a random sample of all students at the same university. Questions about condom use in the previous fortnight indicated that use of an unlubricated condom strongly increased the risk of urinary tract infection (compared with no birth control method); the increased risk was much smaller if the condom was lubricated or spermicide-coated.[32]

Two examples of nested case-control studies are:

1. Men killed in road accidents during a 15-year cohort study of steelworkers were compared with control workers drawn from the same cohort. One of the findings was that exposure to high levels of noise at work was associated with an approximately doubled risk of being killed in a road accident.[33]
2. Participants in the cohort study of 121,700 nurses were asked in 1982 to submit toenail clippings (and 68,213 did so) in order to permit use of the concentrations of iron, arsenic, zinc and other trace elements in the clippings as measures of the intake of these elements. The toenail trace element levels of new cases of breast cancer identified between 1982 and 1986 were then compared with those of 459 individually matched controls. A simple cohort design would have required assays of clippings from 68,213 nurses, instead of about 900.[34]

Most case-control studies are 'time-span' (longitudinal) studies in which the measurements of cause and outcome refer, or are believed to refer (pseudolongitudinal studies – see p. 15) to different points in time. The data may be obtained retrolectively or prolectively.

In some case-control studies, however, no assumption can be made that the measurements can be attributed to different times, or (especially if the postulated causal factor and the postulated outcome may both have been present for some time before the study) there may be no certainty as to which came first (the 'cart-or-horse' problem); a study of the relationship between obesity and physical inactivity (measured at the same time) is an example. Also, it may not be conceptually clear that one of the variables can be considered a cause of the other.

A comparison of cases and controls that is based on associations existing at a single time should, for practical purposes, be classified as a case-control study rather than a cross-sectional one, since it is subject to the same considerations as other case-control studies with regard to (for example) the selection of subjects and how they may affect the analysis and interpretation of findings. For example, a study of 70-year-old snorers who are compared with non-snorers from the same sample in order to determine whether snoring is related to atherosclerotic manifestations[35] can be regarded as a case-control study in which the requirement that case and controls should be drawn from the same population base is well met.

It may be noted that not all case-control comparisons are case-control studies, i.e. studies in which cases of an outcome condition are compared with controls in order to investigate causal hypotheses. For example, a comparison of the birth weights of children born to samples of women who bleed during pregnancy (cases) and those who do not (controls) is a cohort study – the cases and controls are the subjects who are, respectively, exposed and not exposed to the postulated causal factor; this is a form of clinical follow-up study. Other case-control comparisons have nothing to do with the testing of an aetiological hypothesis (e.g. in evaluative studies of screening or diagnostic tests).

Combinations of the above three study types (hybrid designs) can be used.

Each of the above study designs has its advantages and disadvantages.[36] Case-control studies generally require less time than cohort studies and are relatively simple to perform, since (like cross-sectional studies) they avoid the difficult task of following up the subjects, and they usually require fewer subjects. But the fact that information about exposure to the 'cause' is generally obtained when the disease is already present may produce various kinds of bias. There may, for example, be recall bias (cases may be more likely to report exposure than controls, or vice versa) or exposure suspicion bias (the investigator's knowledge that the illness is present may stimulate an especially intensive search for evidence of exposure).[37] Appropriate controls are often difficult to find, and the use of inappropriate controls may distort the findings.

Cohort studies are preferable in many ways. They generally leave less doubt about the time relationships between exposure and the disease, and can more easily provide information about the degree of risk associated with exposure, about the natural history of the disease, and about other effects of the exposure. But losses to follow-up are frequent, and may skew the results. Moreover, a cohort study may be impracticable if the disease is rare or if it develops very long after exposure to the cause. For example, an association between severe diarrhoea and the development of cataract many years later has been demonstrated in case-control studies, not in cohort studies, in four populations.[38]

Case-only studies are not descriptive studies of series of patients, but analytic studies in which the cases act as their own controls. They have several variants.[39] They aim to assess the effect of a suspected trigger event (a transient exposure), e.g. vaccination, cocaine use, heavy physical exertion, or sexual activity, on the onset of a disease or disease episodes (e.g. relapses of multiple sclerosis, exacerbations of asthma, autism, intussusception, stroke, myocardial infarction). They are easy to do, although their analysis is not simple. *Case-crossover studies*, which are akin to case-control studies, are based on a comparison of trigger events in a defined period prior to the onset, and in earlier 'control' periods of the same duration, on the assumption that there are no systematic changes in extrinsic factors other than age, which is controlled in the analysis. The *self-controlled case series method* is essentially a comparison of the incidence in specified periods after exposure with the incidence in the absence of exposure.

Case-control studies can sometimes offer an opportunity for useful 'add-on' studies,[40] such as follow-up studies of the cases or controls, a cross-sectional analytical study of the epidemiology of the disease (if the cases are representative of all cases in a defined population), and case-only studies.

Multilevel surveys

Multilevel analytical surveys[41] are both individual based and group based. They utilize information both about the individuals and about the group (or groups) to which the individuals belong (or the context in which they live), and explore relationships between attributes at the one level (the group or context) and the other (the individual level). They do not merely classify the individuals according to their group membership or context (which family, which school, which community, etc.) – this is an attribute of the individual, and it could be included in an individual-based study. They also use relevant information about the attributes of the group or context, i.e. *ecologic variables* (or *contextual variables*). These may be *aggregate variables* (also called *derived variables*), which are derived from the attributes of individuals (e.g. mean income, the proportion who smoke, the prevalence of a disease, the suicide rate, or the level of herd immunity), or *global variables* (also called *primary variables*), which are not (e.g. environment pollutants, the weather, antismoking legislation, the pattern of relationships between the members of the group, the number of organizations in the community, etc.). In the analysis, account can also be taken of any *clustering* within the groups, i.e. the tendency for the individuals in a group to have similar characteristics.

A multilevel study might find, for example, that higher rates of depression in immigrants (which might be attributed to the effect of immigration or to ethnic factors) occur only among immigrants living in communities in which they are a small minority, pointing to the importance of the context. In their classic studies of pellagra, Goldberger *et al.* found that the risk of the disease was related to the availability of fresh fruits and vegetables in the village, independently of individuals' incomes, and that the protective effect of a high income against pellagra was lower in villages where the availability of these foodstuffs was poor.[42] In the Philippines, maternal education was found to protect against the risk of infant diarrhoea in wealthier communities but not in poorer ones.[43] In Scotland, diastolic blood pressure, cholesterol levels, and alcohol consumption were found to differ in different districts, even after controlling for social class and other variables measured at the individual level.[44] In Wales, residents of localities where more people received unemployment, disability and other welfare benefits were found to have poorer mental health, after controlling for their own employment status and other characteristics associated with mental health; this contextual effect was strongest in residents who were themselves disabled.[45] In China, residence in villages with a higher mean income was associated with higher fasting blood sugar levels, after adjustment for household income, education, and other individual characteristics.[46]

Multilevel studies might include other levels too, besides the group and individual levels, with expansion upwards to broader groups and contexts (children in which class, in which school, in which city, etc.) or downwards, even reaching the cellular or molecular level (see p. 280). As not very obvious examples, studies of the effects of both systemic and local factors might regard patients as contexts for their eyes, teeth, or warts.[47]

Experiments and quasi-experiments

Epidemiological experiments that are designed to test cause–effect hypotheses may be termed *intervention studies*.[48] They can be performed only if it is feasible and ethically justified to manipulate the postulated cause. ('The bearing of children, exposure to hazards, or personality type, are not normally subject to experiment'.)[49] Experiments and quasi-experiments conducted to appraise the value of treatments, preventive procedures and health-care programmes are generally termed *trials* – *clinical trials* (see Chapter 32) or *programme trials* (see Chapter 33).

Like surveys, intervention studies may be group based, individual based, or multilevel. When the effect of fluoride on dental caries was investigated by fluoridating the water supplies of some towns and the subsequent occurrence of dental caries in these towns compared with that in control towns, this was a group-based experiment; the outcome variable was an aggregate variable. On the other hand, when the hypothesis that the administration of oxygen to premature infants caused retrolental fibroplasia (a blinding disease) was tested by administering oxygen continuously to some babies and not to others,[50] this was an individual-based experiment.

Trials that compare clusters of subjects who are randomly allocated to treatment and control groups are usually called *cluster-randomized* or *group-randomized* trials (see p. 349). Cluster-randomized trials, in which an intervention is applied in some randomly selected clusters (e.g. general practices) and not in others, and outcomes are measured at an individual level, may be regarded as multilevel trials. Multicentre trials in which individuals are randomized to treatment and control groups need not be regarded as multilevel trials, unless it is wished to appraise the effects of characteristics of the various centres, i.e. of contextual variables.

Evaluative studies

Evaluative studies[51] are those that appraise the value of health care – they set out to measure how 'good' care is. (The criteria used will be discussed in Chapter 5.)

Evaluative studies are of two main types. These may be termed *reviews* and *trials*, and are distinguished by their different purposes.

Types of evaluative study

1. Programme reviews
2. Trials
   (i) Of care given to groups and populations:
        Programme trials
   (ii) Of care given to individuals:
        Clinical trials (of curative or preventive care)
        Trials of screening and diagnostic tests

A *programme review* is motivated by concern with the welfare of the specific patients, community or population to whom care is given, and it evaluates the care given to them. It may evaluate a particular programme that operates in a defined setting with well-defined aims, such as case-finding, immunization, the control of hypertension, fluoridation of water supplies, etc. (A *programme* may be defined as 'any enterprise organized to eliminate or reduce one or more problems').[52] It may also evaluate a specific health service (a national or regional service, a health centre, a group practice, a hospital, etc.), a part or aspect of a service, or even the work of an individual practitioner, and may be called a *service review.*

An essential feature of a *programme review* is that the findings should be helpful to whoever makes decisions about the specific programme or service. It follows that the evaluation can be conducted within the framework of the assumptions accepted by the decision maker or makers, e.g. the assumption that the performance of certain procedures will have beneficial effects. These assumptions, on which the programme is based, are not necessarily questioned or tested. The evaluation results can be useful without necessarily being found convincing by those who doubt the validity of the assumptions on which the programme is founded. Programme and service reviews are akin to a physician's periodic reviews of the treatment given to a specific patient, which permit a decision as to whether to continue, modify or stop therapy. These assessments are an indispensable part of the clinical process, although the clinician can seldom obtain convincing evidence of the extent to which changes in the patient's condition can be attributed to the treatment. Programme reviews are generally descriptive surveys, sometimes with an analytic component.

A *programme trial*, by contrast, sets out to obtain generalizable knowledge, which can be applied in other settings, about the value of a *type* of health care provided for a group or population. To meet its purpose a trial must yield conclusions that are well enough substantiated to be generally convincing. It is not enough merely to demonstrate a beneficial effect, but there must be evidence that the effect can be attributed to the care given. To this end, pains must be taken to eliminate or allow for the possible influence of other factors. Programme trials may be experiments or quasi-experiments.

It is important to distinguish between programme reviews and programme trials, since the questions they ask and the methods they use are different. In a review, basic assumptions are not in question and definitive tests of cause–effect hypotheses are not required; it is wasteful and may be self-defeating to use excessively rigorous study techniques. A trial, on the other hand, may be inconclusive if methods are insufficiently rigorous. There are other differences as well, which also have implications for the planning of the study. To be useful, a review must usually be rapid and (if possible) ongoing, i.e. performed in real time. Changes in circumstances, personnel and policy lead to frequent changes in the procedures used in a service, and there may be little practical benefit in evaluating a programme as it used to be some years previously. If appraisal is rapid, it can give early warning of inadequacies and provide an up-to-date factual basis for decisions. Speed is less important in a trial. Further, a review is carried out in a service-oriented setting – this is the review's *raison d'être*. Evaluation may not be seen as an important element, and little time and resources may be available for special information-collecting procedures. A trial, on the other hand, is more likely to be conducted as a specific investigative procedure. Not infrequently, the programme is set up specially, as a test or demonstration.

An evaluation of a programme may be of a hybrid type, e.g. when a programme trial is conducted in the context of a service review. This may happen if there is a call for the appraisal of an innovative feature of the service, or if certain of the assumptions on which the service is based are questioned, or if there is a wish to generalize from the experience of the service. In such instances there will be a need for the demanding methods of study that are appropriate to a trial, as well as for the less rigorous ones needed for a review of other aspects of the service. Difficulties often arise when a programme trial is conducted in the setting of an established service, since evaluation and service may make competing demands.

A *clinical trial* appraises the worth of a form of care (preventive, curative, educational, etc.) given to individuals, rather than to a group or population; it may be an experiment or a quasi-experiment.

Trials may also be conducted to evaluate screening and diagnostic tests (see pp. 171–173).

While programme and clinical trials require separate consideration (see Chapters 32 and 33), there is a degree of overlap between them, as some programme trials are based on a comparison of individuals who are exposed and not exposed to the programme under study. Individual-based programme trials of this sort do not differ in their design from other clinical trials.

Some trials have double objectives: when testing a new form of treatment, the aim may be both to appraise its value for individuals and to evaluate the programme whereby it is provided to the public.

The use of case-control studies for the evaluation of preventive and therapeutic procedures is discussed on page 320.

The term *inbuilt evaluation* may be used if the evaluation is planned in advance and the requisite information is collected in a systematic way as an integral part of the provision of a service.

Medical audit is a technique used mainly in service reviews, whereby the quality of a service is evaluated by appraising the quality of the care given to individuals. It will be discussed in more detail in Chapter 21.

Surveillance

Surveillance[53] denotes the maintenance of an ongoing watch over the status of a group or community. It yields information about new and changing needs, and provides a basis for appraising the effects of health care. A watch may be kept on health status – in terms of mortality, morbidity, nutritional status, child growth and development, or other indices – and on environmental hazards, health practices, and other factors that may affect health.

There is considerable confusion about the use of the terms 'surveillance' and 'monitoring', and they are often used interchangeably. Monitoring is probably best used to refer to the maintenance of an ongoing watch over the activities of a health service, e.g. the provision of answers to questions such as 'What are we doing at the present moment?' or 'What does it cost in resources to do what for whom?'[54]

Surveillance of the occurrence of diseases, especially infectious diseases, may be based on ongoing or periodic examination of data collected by clinical care services, or on reporting (sometimes required by law) by clinicians or laboratories. In some instances, sentinel networks of services are set up for this purpose. The term *inbuilt surveillance* may be applied if a health service has set up routine surveillance procedures. Outbreaks of 'new' diseases (such as Lyme disease, legionella disease, AIDS, and severe acute respiratory syndromes) have generally come to light not as a result of routine surveillance, but as a result of observations by astute individuals who reported their suspicions to a public health agency.[55]

Because of concern about possible bioterrorist attacks, there has been increased interest in *syndromic surveillance* – 'surveillance using health-related data that precede diagnosis and signal a sufficient probability of a case or an outbreak to warrant further public health response'.[56] This is called 'syndromic' because it aims to detect clustering in space and time of a syndrome, not a specific disease. It uses nonspecific indicators, such as an increase in over-the-counter sales of antidiarrhoeal drugs, or complaints of diarrhoea or other specified symptoms, or absenteeism. Simulations suggest that it may be most effective for diseases with a narrow distribution of incubation periods (before signs or symptoms appear), a long prodromal period (of early signs and symptoms) and a steep epidemic curve. The efficacy of syndromic surveillance is not proved.[57]

In the context of community-oriented primary care, surveillance is usually based on periodic analysis of records designed for the easy retrieval of information about risk factors and diagnoses relevant to the practice's ongoing community programs. *Demographic surveillance*[58] of the community – ongoing measurement of the size of the population, its age and sex composition, and other demographic characteristics – which (apart from other purposes) provides the denominator data without which rates and other meaningful measures of group health cannot be calculated, may require routine procedures for the ascertainment and recording of births, deaths and movements.

The surveillance of environmental hazards requires appraisal not only of the presence, degree, and potential effects of hazards, but also of the likely amount of exposure to them, and is hence beset with uncertainties.[59]

Other Terms

The term *exploratory study* is often applied to a descriptive survey designed to increase the investigator's familiarity with the problem he or she wishes to study. The aim may be to formulate a problem for more precise investigation, to develop hypotheses, to clarify concepts, or to make the investigator more familiar with the phenomenon he or she wishes to investigate or with the setting in which it will be studied. It is not always necessary to use quantitative methods in a survey of this sort; at this stage, it may be sufficient, for example, to build up a simple list of the foodstuffs or dishes eaten in a community (with no numerical information) as a basis for the design of a questionnaire for use in the study proper. An exploratory study of this sort is sometimes called a *pilot study*; however, this term is better confined to another connotation, namely a dress rehearsal of an investigation performed in order to identify defects in the study design.

A descriptive survey in which a very large number of characteristics are studied, i.e. in which the net is thrown wide, performed in the hope that the results will select hypotheses for subsequent testing, is sometimes unflatteringly referred to as a *fishing expedition*.

A *methodological study* is one performed with the purpose of collecting information on the feasibility or accuracy of a research method (see Chapters 16 and 17). In community medicine, the aim of such a study is usually the evaluation of an investigative procedure for use in community diagnosis.

A *morbidity survey* is a study, usually descriptive, of the occurrence and distribution of a disease or diseases in a population. It may be a *prevalence study*, concerned with all cases of the disease present in the population at a given point in time or during the period of the survey, or an *incidence study*, concerned only with new cases (new patients, or episodes of illness) occurring or diagnosed during a given period. A *two-stage morbidity study* is one in which screening tests (see p. 171) are used to identify persons who may have the disease, and the presence of the disease is then determined by more exact tests.

The term *household survey* usually refers to a descriptive survey of illnesses or disability, performed by interviewing persons in their own homes, often by questioning a single informant about other members of the household.

KAP studies are studies of knowledge, attitudes and practices.

Outbreak investigations,[60] or epidemiological *field investigations*, are surveys that aim to determine the causes of an outbreak in order to control its spread. They may be descriptive, analytic or both.

Health practice research (*health services research, operational research*) is concerned with organizational problems – with the planning, management, logistics and delivery of health-care services. It deals with manpower, organization, the utilization of facilities, the quality of health-care, cost, the relationship between need and demand, patient satisfaction with services, and other topics. It makes use of systems analysis, computer simulation, and other sophisticated techniques of operations research.[61]

Clinical trials of new drugs may be classified as phase I, II, III or IV trials. Phase I trials assess the effects and safety of the drug in healthy volunteers, phase II trials assess efficacy and safety in small groups of patients, and full-blown trials of the kind we will discuss in Chapter 32 may be called phase III trials (if the drug has not yet been licensed for distribution) or phase IV trials (after the drug has been launched).[62]

Notes and References

1. *Quasi-experiments* are often used in evaluative studies. They compare groups, or compare observations made at different times ('time-series design'), or both ('multiple-group time-series design').

    Quasi-experimental designs are described by Trochim W (ed) (Advances in quasi-experimental design and analysis. New Directions for Program Evaluation Series, Number 31. San Francisco, CA: Jossey-Bass; 1986), Campbell DT, Stanley JC (Experimental and quasi-experimental designs for research. Chicago, IL: Rand McNally; 1966), Campbell DT (Factors relevant to the validity of experiments in social settings. In: Schulberg HC, Sheldon A, Baker F, eds. Program evaluation in the health fields. New York, NY: Behavioral Publications; 1969), Cook TD, Campbell DT (Quasi-experimentation: design and analysis issues for field settings. Chicago, IL: Rand McNally; 1979), and Kleinbaum DG, Kupper LL, Morgenstern H (Epidemiologic research: principles and quantitative methods. Belmont, CA: Lifetime Learning Publications; 1982. pp. 44–47).

    Quasi-experimental designs used in studies of measures to control infectious diseases are discussed by Harris AD, Bradham DD, Baumgarten M, Zuckerman IH, Fink JC, Perencevich EN (The use and interpretation of quasi-experimental studies in infectious diseases. Antimicrobial Resistance 2004; 38: 1586).
2. The relationship between schizophrenia and prenatal exposure to the famine that occurred in the western Netherlands in 1944–1945 is described by Susser E, Neugebauer R, Hok HW, Brown AS, Lin S, Labovitz D, Gorman JM (Schizophrenia after prenatal famine: further evidence. Archives of General Psychiatry 1996; 53: 25). The association was confirmed in a study of the aftermath of the Chinese famine of 1959–1961 (St Clair D, Xu M, Wang P, Yu Y, Fang Y, Zhang F, Zheng X, Gu N, Feng G, Sham P, He L. Rates of adult schizophrenia following prenatal exposure to the Chinese famine of 1959–61. Journal of the Aerican Medical Association 2006; 294: 557).
3. Snow J. On the mode of communication of cholera. Churchill; London; 1855 (facsimile edition: New York, NY: Hafner; 1965).

4. Sargent RP, Shepard RM, Glantz SA. Reduced incidence of admissions for myocardial infarction associated with public smoking ban: before and after study. British Medical Journal 2004; 328: 977.
5. The term *observational study* does not imply that methods other than observation (e.g. questionnaires and documentary sources) are not used. Another term used for nonexperimental studies is 'naturalistic'.
6. How hypotheses about a possible cause are generated 'is little understood. They are products of their times, what is in the air, of what is known and being thought important, and of the prepared mind and individual imagination. .. Where epidemiological hypotheses come from is also interesting: they emerge-from everywhere. .. and from nowhere in particular' (Morris JN. Uses of epidemiology, 3rd edn. Edinburgh: Churchill Livingstone; 1975. pp. 233–249).
7. *Cohort analysis* refers to the investigation of data concerning people born in various specific time periods (e.g. 1970–1979) in order to learn about the morbidity, mortality, etc. of each birth cohort or its various subgroups, and compare people born in different periods. This may reveal a *cohort effect*, i.e. there may be differences in morbidity, mortality, etc. when people of the same age in different birth cohorts are compared, as a result of differences in the experience of different cohorts. In a cross-sectional survey, 50-year-olds may be shorter and have a lower mean IQ than 30-year-olds, not because they are older, but because they belong to different cohorts with different prior experiences. In New York, women born in the 'baby boom' years following World War II tend to rate themselves as less healthy, and to decline in health more rapidly as they age, than women of the same ages born in earlier years (Chen H, Cohen P, Kasen S. Cohort differences in self-rated health: evidence from a three-decade, community-based, longitudinal study of women. American Journal of Epidemiology 2007; 166: 439).
8. Feinstein AR. Clinical biostatistics: LVII. A glossary of neologisms in quantitative clinical science. Clinical Pharmacology and Therapeutics 1981; 30: 564.
9. Needleman HL, Gunnoe C, Leviton A, Reed R, Peresie H, Maher C, Barrett P. Deficits in psychologic and classroom performance of children with elevated dentine lead levels. New England Journal of Medicine 1979; 300: 689.
10. Last JM. A dictionary of epidemiology, 4th edn. New York, NY: Oxford University Press; 2001. (A simpler definition: 'Epidemiology is what epidemiologists do'.)
11. Needs appraisal is reviewed by Mooney G, Jan S, Wiseman V (Measuring health needs. In: Detels R, McEwen J, Beaglehole R, Tanaka H (eds), Oxford textbook of public health, 4th edn, vol 3. The practice of public health. New York, NY: Oxford University Press; 2002. pp. 1765–1772) and Wright W (ed) (Health needs assessment in practice. London: BMJ Publishing Group, 1998. Six excerpts appeared in successive issues of the British Medical Journal [vol 316] from 25 April 1998).
12. Acheson RM, Hall DJ. In: Acheson RM, Hall D, Aird L (eds), Seminars in community medicine, vol 2: health information, planning, and monitoring. London: Oxford University Press, 1976. pp. 145–164.
13. *Group-based (ecologic) studies* are discussed in depth by (among others) Susser M (The logic in ecological: I. The logic of analysis. American Journal of Public Health 1994; 84: 825), Susser M (The logic in ecological: II. The logic of design. American Journal of Public Health 1994; 84: 830), and Morgenstern H (Ecologic studies. In: Rothman K J, Greenland S (eds), Modern epidemiology, 2nd edn. Philadelphia, PA: Lippincott-Raven; 1998. pp. 459–480).
    Biases in ecologic studies are discussed by Diez-Roux AV (Bringing context back into epidemiology: variables and fallacies in multilevel analysis. American Journal of Public Health 1998; 88: 216) and Greenland S, Robins J (Invited commentary: Ecologic studies – biases, misconceptions, and counterexamples. American Journal of Epidemiology 1994; 139: 747) and in the commentaries that follow the latter paper. Cross-level bias may have various causes; for example, if risk to an individual is caused only by very high exposures to a causal factor (a threshold effect), the average exposure of a group of people may not reflect the average risk of its members.
14. Qiao Z-K, Halliday ML, Coates RA, Rankij J G (Relationship between liver cirrhosis death rate and nutritional factors in 38 countries. International Journal of Epidemiology 1988; 17: 414).

The authors found that a higher average intake of protein, vitamins A and B2 and calcium (none of which was related to average alcohol consumption) was associated with a lower mortality from liver cirrhosis. They concluded that these relationships were not necessarily causal, but indicated a need for further studies.

15. This comparison of 8,576 general practices, which was based on national Quality and Outcomes Framework (QOF) data, national Prescribing Analyses and CosT (PACT) data, information about practice characteristics, and national census data, also suggested underprescribing of statins to the elderly and possibly to ethnic minorities. The authors point out the shortcomings of their data (Ashworth M, Lloyd D, Smith RS, Wagner A, Rowlands G. Social deprivation and statin prescribing: a cross-sectional analysis using data from the new UK general practitioner 'Quality and Outcomes Framework'. Journal of Public Health 2007; 29: 40).

16. *Time trend analysis* requires special statistical methods (for software, see Appendix C) because consecutive values may be correlated with each other. See Zeger SL, Irizarry R, Peng RD (On time series analysis of public health and biomedical data. Annual Review of Public Health 2006; 27: 57).

17. After analysing trends in New Zealand during a 12-year period, for example, Jackson R, Beaglehole R (Trends in dietary fat and cigarette smoking and the decline in coronary heart disease in New Zealand. International Journal of Epidemiology 1987; 16: 377) concluded that changes in fat and tobacco consumption provided a biologically plausible explanation for at least part of the decline in coronary mortality.

18. Boyce WJ, Vessey MP. Rising incidence of fracture of the proximal femur. Lancet 1985; i: 150. A later study showed an increase in hospital admissions for fractured femur between 1968 and 1986 in England as a whole, as well as in Oxford. The findings suggested a cohort effect (Evans JG, Seagroatt V, Goldacre MJ. Secular trends in proximal femoral fracture, Oxford record linkage study area and England 1968–86. Journal of Epidemiology and Community Health 1997; 51: 424). The rate continued to rise until 1991–1992, and then stabilized (Balasegaram S, Majeed A, Fitz-Clarence H. Trends in hospital admissions for fractures of the hip and femur in England, 1989–1990 to 1997–1998. Journal of Public Health Medicine 2001; 23: 11).

19. Corrao G, Ferrari P, Zambon A, Torchio P, Arico S, Decarli A. Trends of liver cirrhosis mortality in Europe, 1970–1989: age–period–cohort analysis and changing alcohol consumption. International Journal of Epidemiology 1997; 26: 100.

20. The *Cochrane anomaly*: the authors of the paper describing a positive correlation between the number of doctors and infant mortality were not able to find an explanation: 'we must admit defeat and leave it to others to extricate doctors from their unhappy position' (Cochrane AL, St Leger AS, Moore F. Health service 'input' and mortality 'output' in developed countries. Journal of Epidemiology and Community Health 1978; 32: 200; reprinted in Journal of Epidemiology and Community Health 1997; 51: 344). McPherson K (Health services and mortality in developed countries: a comment. Journal of Epidemiology and Community Health 1997; 51: 349) pointed out the value of the study in 'raising questions whose importance might not otherwise have been appreciated'.

An explanation was subsequently offered by Young FW (An explanation of the persistent doctor-mortality association. Journal of Epidemiology and Community Health 2001; 55: 80), who reported that expanding urban–industrial regions attract an oversupply of doctors, and that, independently, rural people migrate to these areas, where they experience an increase in death rates, and found that the positive association between mortality and doctors disappeared when he inserted an appropriate test variable – a measure of migration to industrializing regions – in the equation.

But this adjustment did not lead to a negative association between the number of doctors and mortality, so that, at most, 'doctors may be off the hook to some extent' (St Leger S. The anomaly that finally went away? Journal of Epidemiology and Community Health 2001; 55: 79).

21. Doll R, Peto R. The causes of cancer. Oxford: Oxford University Press; 1981. pp. 1204–1205.
22. Breslow NE, Enstrom JE. Geographic correlations between cancer mortality rates and alcohol–tobacco consumption in the United States. Journal of the National Cancer Institute 1974; 53: 531. Individual-based studies yield conflicting findings on this issue.
23. Schwartz S. The fallacy of the ecological fallacy: the potential misuse of a concept and the consequences. American Journal of Public Health 1994; 84: 819. The converse fallacy is termed *atomistic* by Diez-Roux AV (1998; see note 13). It has also been called the 'individualistic' fallacy.
24. Koopman JS, Longini IM Jr. The ecological effects of individual exposures and nonlinear disease dynamics in populations. American Journal of Public Health 1994; 84: 836.
25. Durkin MS, Kahn N, Davidson LL, Zaman SS, Stein ZA. The effects of a natural disaster on child behavior: evidence for posttraumatic stress. American Journal of Public Health 1993; 83: 1549.
26. For example, Katsouyanni K, Touloumi G, Spix C, Schwartz J, Balducci F, Medina S, Rossi G, Wojtyniak B, Sunyer J, Bacharova L, Schouten J P, Ponka A, Anderson HR (Short term effects of ambient sulphur dioxide and particulate matter on mortality in 12 European cities: results from time series data from the APHEA project. British Medical Journal 1997; 314: 1658).
27. The importance of *social and ecological processes* is stressed by (among others) Susser M, Susser E (Choosing a future for epidemiology: II. From black box to Chinese boxes and eco-epidemiology. American Journal of Public Health 1996; 86: 674), Krieger N (Epidemiology and the web of causation: has anyone seen the spider? Social Science and Medicine 1994; 39: 887), and Diez-Roux AV (1998; see note 13).
28. Kauhanen K, Kaplan GA, Goldberg DE, Salonen JT. Beer binging and mortality: results from the Kuopio ischaemic heart disease risk factor study, a prospective population based study. British Medical Journal 1997; 315: 846. Beer binging was strongly associated with fatal myocardial infarction, as well as with fatal injuries and other external causes. The effects of differences in age, smoking, total alcohol consumption, and other factors that might affect mortality were taken into account.
29. A *historical prospective study* may be called a nonconcurrent prospective study, a retrospective cohort study, a prospective study in retrospect, or a retrospective design with forward directionality (all this in the interest of greater clarity!).
30. Rich-Edwards JW, Stampfer MJ, Manson JE *et al.* Birth weight and risk of cardiovascular disease in a cohort of women followed up since 1976. British Medical Journal 1997; 315: 837. For references to numerous other studies demonstrating that fetal malnutrition may affect health in adult life, see Scrimshaw NS (Editorial: The relation between fetal malnutrition and chronic disease in later life. British Medical Journal 1997; 315: 825).
31. An essential principle of *case-control studies* is that cases and controls should be drawn from the same population 'base': 'If a case-control study enrols cases and controls from the same underlying population at risk of the outcome and can measure exposure status validly in them, the results obtained will be identical to those from a properly performed cohort study' (Weiss NS. Case-control studies. In: Detels R *et al.* 2002, pp. 543–551; see note 11). 'The case-control design can be considered a more efficient form of the follow-up study, in which the cases are those that would be included in a follow-up study and the controls provide a fast and inexpensive means of inferring the person-time experience according to exposure in the population that gave rise to the cases' (Rothman KJ. Modern epidemiology. Boston, MA: Little, Brown; 1986. p. 64). (The 'person-time' concept is explained in note 4 in Chapter 10).

    Case-cohort and nested case-control methods are compared by Langholz B, Thomas DC (Nested case-control and case-cohort methods of sampling from a cohort: a critical comparison. American Journal of Epidemiology 1990; 131: 169).

    If the effect under study is not the occurrence of a disease, but the level of some measurement, use can be made of *outcome-dependent sampling*, which is a case-control-like procedure adapted for continuous outcomes – an overall random sample is supplemented by random samples of (say) subjects with particularly high and particularly low levels. The planning and analysis of such studies require special procedures (Zhou H, Chen J, Rissanen TH, Korrick SA, Hu H, Salonen JT, Longnecker MP. Outcome-dependent sampling: an efficient sampling and inference procedure for studies with a continuous outcome. Epidemiology 2007; 18: 461).

32. Foxman B, Marsh J, Gillespie B, Rubin N, Koopman JS, Spear S. Condom use and first-time urinary tract infection. Epidemiology 1997; 8: 637.

33. Barreto SM, Swerdlow AJ, Smith PG, Higgins CD. Risk of death from motor-vehicle injury in Brazilian steelworkers: a nested case-control study. International Journal of Epidemiology 1997; 26: 814.

34. Garland M, Morris JS, Colditz GA *et al*. Toenail trace element levels and breast cancer: a prospective study. American Journal of Epidemiology 1996; 144: 653. Note the description of this case-control study as 'prospective'. The results provided no evidence of an important effect of arsenic, copper, chromium, iron or zinc on breast cancer risk.

35. Snoring was not found to be associated with atherosclerotic manifestations (Jennum P, Schultz-Larsen K, Christensen NJ. Snoring and atherosclerotic manifestations in a 70-year-old population. European Journal of Epidemiology 1996; 12: 285). Other good news for snorers is that snoring in pregnancy does not endanger the fetus, according to a cohort study (Loube D, Poceta JS, Morales MC, Peacock MD, Mitler MM. Self-reported snoring in pregnancy: association with fetal outcome. Chest 1996; 109: 885).

36. *Cohort, case-control* and *cross-sectional studies* are discussed in all textbooks of epidemiology. Their uses and limitations are described in Detels R *et al*. 2002 (see note 11), in the chapters by Feinleib M, Breslow NE (Cohort studies; pp. 553–567), Weiss NS (Case-control studies; pp. 543–551), and Abramson J (Cross-sectional studies; pp. 509–528). The pros and cons of numerous study designs, including hybrid ones, are discussed by Kleinbaum *et al*. 1982 (see note 1).

   For classic examples of cohort and case-control studies, see pp. 584–725 and pp. 458–583 respectively of Buck C, Llopis A, Najera E, Terris M (eds) (The challenge of epidemiology. Washington, DC: Pan American Health Organization; 1988).

   Case-control studies are discussed in detail in a symposium edited by Armenian HK (Applications of the case-control method. Epidemiologic Reviews 1994; 16: 1), which includes papers on applications in genetic epidemiology, demography, occupational health and other fields. See also Schlesselman JJ (Case-control studies: design, conduct, analysis. New York, NY: Oxford University Press; 1982), Ibrahim MA (ed) (The case-control study: consensus and controversy. Journal of Chronic Diseases 1979; 32: 1), and Breslow N (Design and analysis of case-control studies. Annual Review of Public Health 1982; 3: 29).

37. Sackett DL Bias in analytic research. Journal of Chronic Diseases 1979; 32: 51.

38. An association between severe diarrhoea and cataract, attributed to the lasting effect of severe dehydration, has been shown by four case-control studies – three in populations in India and one in Oxfordshire, England: Minassian DC, Mehra V, Jones BR (Dehydrational crises from severe diarrhoea or heatstroke and risk of cataract. Lancet 1984; i: 751), Minassian DC, Mehra V, Verrey JD (Dehydrational crises: a major risk factor in blinding cataract. British Journal of Ophthalmology 1989; 73: 100), Ughade SN, Zodpey S, Khanolkar V, Kulkarni H (Risk factors of cataract: a case control study. Journal of Clinical Epidemiology 1997; 50(Suppl 1): S10), and Harding JJ, Harding JS, Egerton M (Risk factors for cataract in Oxfordshire: diabetes, peripheral neuropathy, myopia, glaucoma and diarrhoea. Acta Ophthalmologica 1989; 67: 510).

   This association, although strong (one of the Indian studies suggested that 38% of blinding cataract might be attributable to repeated dehydrational crises resulting from severe life-threatening diarrhoeal disease and/or heatstroke), may be an artefact resulting from information bias.

39. *Case-only studies* are described by Farrington CP (Control without separate controls: evaluation of vaccine safety using case-only methods. Vaccine 2004; 22: 2064) and Whitaker HJ, Farrington CP, Spiessene B, Musonda P (Tutorial in biostatistics: the self-controlled case series methods. Statistics in Medicine 2006; 25: 1768).

   Macros for use with commercial statistical programs, for analysing self-controlled case series studies, are available at http://statistics.open.ac.uk/sccs/.

40. Stang A, Jöckel K-H. Appending epidemiological studies to conventional case-control studies (hybrid case-control studies). European Journal of Epidemiology 2004; 19: 527.

41. *Multilevel analytical surveys* are explained at greater length by Blakely TA, Woodward AJ (Ecological effects in multi-level studies. Journal of Epidemiology and Community Health 2006; 54: 367), Diez-Rouz AV (Bringing context back into epidemiology: variables and fallacies in multilevel analysis. American Journal of Public Health 1998; 88: 216), and Diez-Roux AV, Schwartz S, Susser E (Ecological variables, ecological studies, and multilevel studies in public health research. In: Detels R *et al.* (2002, vol. 2, pp. 493–507; see note 11).

42. Goldberger J, Wheeler GA, Sydenstrycker E. A study of the relation of family income and other economic factors to pellagra incidence in seven cotton mill villages of South Carolina in 1916. Public Health Reports 1920; 35: 2673.

43. Dargent-Molina P, James SA, Strogatz DS, Savitz DA. Association between maternal education and infant diarrhea in different household and community environments of Cebu, Philippines. Social Science and Medicine 1994; 38: 343.

44. Hart C, Ecob R, Smith GD. People, places and coronary heart disease risk factors: a multilevel analysis of the Scottish Heart Health Study archive. Social Science and Medicine 1997; 45: 893.

45. This apparent effect of the context on mental health might be partly due to a tendency for people to move into poorer neighbourhoods as a result of unemployment or disability (Fone DL, Lloyd K, Dunstan FD. Measuring the neighbourhood using UK benefits data: a multilevel analysis of mental health status. BMC Public Health 2007; 7: 69).

46. Cai L, Chongsuvivatwong V, Geater A. Contextual socioeconomic determinants of cardiovascular risk factors in rural south-west China: a multilevel analysis. BMC Public Health 2007; 7: 72).

47. Altman DG. Commentary: systematic reviewers face challenges from varied study designs. British Medical Journal 2002; 325: 467.

48. For classic examples of epidemiological experiments, see Buck C *et al.* (1988, pp. 726–806; see note 36).

49. Susser M, Stein Z, Kline J. Ethics in epidemiology. Annals of the American Academy of Political and Social Science 1978; 437: 128.

50. Kinsey VE, Hemphill FM. Etiology of retrolental fibroplasia: preliminary report of a cooperative study of retrolental fibroplasia. American Journal of Ophthalmology 1955; 40: 166.

51. Texts on *evaluative studies* include: Fink A (Evaluating fundamentals: guiding health programs, research, and policy. Beverly Hills, CA: Sage Publications; 1993) and St Leger AS, Schnieden H, Walsworth-Bell JP (eds) (Evaluating health services' effectiveness: a guide for health professionals, service managers, and policy makers. Open University; 1991).

52. Kane RL, Henson R, Deniston OL. In: Kane RL (ed.). The challenges of community medicine. New York, NY: Springer, 1974. pp 213–233.

53. *Surveillance.* See Berkelman RL, Stroup DF, Buehler JW (Public health surveillance. In: Detels R *et al.* 2002, pp.759–778; see note 11) and Buehler JW 1998 (Surveillance. In: Rothman KJ, Greenland S 1998, pp. 435–457; see note 11).

   Data mining techniques (see note 2, Chapter 4) may be used for the early detection of a cluster of cases, e.g. see Niu MT, Erwin DE, Braun NM (Data mining in the US Vaccine Adverse Event Reporting System (VAERS): early detection of intussusception and other events after rotavirus vaccination. Vaccine 2001; 19: 4627).

54. The meanings of the terms *surveillance* and *monitoring* are discussed by Acheson RM, Hall DJ (1976, p. 126; see note 12). 'Monitoring' often denotes not only watching, but also using the observations as a basis for continual modification of goals, plans or activities; Knox EG (ed) Epidemiology in health care planning. Oxford: Oxford University Press; 1979. pp. 18–19, 127–129.

55. *The role of the astute observers.* Two mothers in Lyme, Connecticut, reported that the number of juvenile rheumatoid arthritis cases in their community seemed too high to be due to chance. An American Legion official reported that in the past week he had gone to eight funerals of veterans who had recently attended a convention. A physician sent an e-mail asking about a rumour transmitted through a chat room about people dying in Guangzhou, China (of what was later called SARS). Researchers in San Francisco reported an extraordinarily high rate of CMV infection, a drug technician noted an increase in pentamidine requests, and physicians noted increases in *Pneumocystis carinii* pneumonia and Kaposi's sarcoma cases; HIV was identified 3 years later (Dato V, Wagner MM, Fapohunda A. How outbreaks of infectious disease are detected: a review of surveillance systems and outbreaks. Public Health Reports 2004; 119: 464).

56. Centers for Disease Control. Syndromic surveillance: an applied approach to outbreak detection. Available at http://www.cdc.gov/epo/dphsi/syndromic.htm. The website offers syndrome definitions for diseases associated with bioterrorism-associated agents.

57. Berger M, Shiau R, Weintraub JM. Review of syndromic surveillance: implications for waterborne disease detection. Journal of Epidemiology and Community Health 2006; 60: 543.
    Accurate information on the size and composition of a population is seldom easy to obtain. See p. 361.

59. A recent textbook on risk assessment in public health starts with the joke 'Why did God invent risk assessment? To give astrologers credibility' (Robson MG, Toscano WA. Risk assessment for environmental health. Jossey Bass; 2007).

60. *Outbreak investigations.* See Ungchusak K (The principles of an epidemic field investigation. In: Detels R *et al.* 2002, pp. 529–541; see note 11) and Dwyer DM, Strickler H, Goodman RA, Armenian HK (Use of case-control studies in outbreak investigations. Epidemiologic Reviews 1994; 16: 109). For descriptions of classic studies of epidemics, see Buck C *et al.* (1988, pp. 415–557; see note 36).

61. *Health services research methods* are described by (among others) Crombie IK, Davies HTO (Research in health care: design, conduct and interpretation of health services research. Chichester: Wiley; 1996) and Shi L (Health services research methods [Delmar series in health services administration]. Delmar Publications; 1996).
    For a treasure-house of papers on health services research (concepts, methods and implications for health policy), see White KL, Frenk J, Ordonez C, Paganini JM, Starfield B (eds) (Health services research: an anthology. Washington, DC: Pan American Health Organization; 1992). A number of classic studies are collected in Buck C *et al.* (1988, pp. 809–964; see note 36).

62. Rang HP, Dale MM, Ritter JM, Flower RJ. Rang & Dale's pharmacology, 6th edn. Edinburgh: Churchill Livingstone; 2007. p. 784.

3

Stages of an Investigation

1. Preliminary steps; see Chapter 1
   (a) Clarifying the purpose
   (b) Reviewing the literature
   (c) Ethical considerations
   (d) Formulating the topic
2. Planning; see Chapters 2–23
3. Preparing for data collection; see Chapter 24
4. Collecting the data; see Chapter 25
5. Statistical analysis; see Chapter 26
6. Interpreting the results; see Chapters 27–29
7. Writing a report; see Chapter 30

The stages of an investigation may be listed in a logical sequence, in which each phase is dependent on the preceding one. After the investigator has clarified the purpose of the study and formulated its topic in general terms, a detailed plan can be prepared. Preparations for data collection can then be made by testing the methods and making practical arrangements. The data are then collected and processed. The researcher can then sit down to make sense of the findings and decide on their theoretical and practical implications; and, finally, the world can be told.

In practice, this scheme is seldom followed rigidly, even by the most obsessional of researchers. There are two main reasons for this. First, it may be convenient for certain stages to overlap. For example, some of the preparations for the collection of data may be made before the study plan is complete, or it may be possible to collect and even analyse some types of information before other aspects have been fully planned. Second, and more important, the various phases may be influenced not only by the preceding phases, but also by subsequent ones. As one example, unforeseen snags may appear when the methods are tested, or even after data collection has commenced, sending the investigator 'back to the drawing board'. As another example, in the above scheme the interpretation of findings follows their processing, which seems logical; but a basic element of the scientific method is that inferences are drawn from facts, and these inferences are then tested by obtaining further facts; this means that, usually, except in the simplest of investigations, the researcher interprets the data that have been processed, decides

Research Methods in Community Medicine: Surveys, Epidemiological Research, Programme Evaluation, Clinical Trials   J. H. Abramson and Z. H. Abramson   Copyright © 2008, John Wiley & Sons Ltd

what further analyses are needed, interprets the new facts, and so on; processing and interpretation have a two-way influence on each other, and usually proceed hand in hand.

Although 'reviewing the literature' is shown as a preliminary step in the above scheme, directed reading usually continues throughout the study. The published experiences and thoughts of others may not only indicate the presence and nature of the research problem, but may be of great help in all aspects of planning and in the interpretation of the findings.

Needless to say, the value of any investigation depends on sound planning, which may necessitate a considerable amount of effort. The closer the attention to detail is, the better the prospects of a fruitful study are. The planning phase may take more of the investigator's time, or even of the total duration of the investigation, than any other phase of the study.

A dilemma frequently faced by investigators seeking research funds is that the success of the application may depend on the quality of the study plan, so that a considerable investment of time is required for planning, without any assurance that the study will actually be performed.

The Planning Phase

1. Formulation of study objectives; see Chapters 4 and 5
2. Planning of methods
   (a) The study population (whom?); see Chapters 6–9
       Selection and definition
       Sampling
       Size
   (b) Variables (what to measure?); see Chapters 10–14
       Selection
       Definition
       Scales of measurement
   (c) Methods of collecting data; see Chapters 15–21
   (d) Methods of recording and processing; see Chapters 22 and 23

The first step in planning is to formulate the objectives of the investigation. The investigator already knows why the study is being undertaken, and has formulated the topic in general terms (see Chapter 1). The detailed study objectives must now be formulated: what knowledge is the study designed to yield? (Note that the term 'objective' is sometimes used to indicate what we have called the 'purpose' of the study on p. 2; we are specifically excluding this connotation.) This decision determines the further planning of the investigation, and the methods of the study can be judged by their appropriateness to these study objectives.

The second step is to plan the methods. Consideration must be given to:

1. *The study population* (see Chapters 6–9). Whom is it proposed to study? Will a sample or samples be used? How will sampling be done? What will be the sample size?
2. *The variables to be studied* (Chapters 10–14). What characteristics will be measured? How will the variables be defined? What scales of measurement will be used?

3. *Methods of data collection* (Chapters 15–21). Will data be collected by direct observation, from documentary sources, or by interviews or self-administered questionnaires? What are the detailed procedures and questions to be used?
4. *Methods of recording and processing* (Chapters 22 and 23). How will the data be recorded? What data-processing techniques will be used? What is the analysis plan?

The various elements of planning are interdependent; they should be regarded as different aspects on which attention must be focused, rather than as discrete entities. A decision on the characteristics to be measured, for example, may depend not only on the study objectives, but on the nature of the study population and on the practicability of various methods of data collection; and a detailed consideration of the methods required to satisfy the study objectives may lead to a reformulation of the objectives.

Some investigators see their main planning task as the design of a 'form' – a schedule on which findings will be recorded, or a questionnaire – and make this their first (and sometimes only) planning activity. This approach cannot be recommended.

It is usually helpful to commit the study plan to writing, whether briefly or in detail, since human memory is fallible. The study objectives and an outline of the methods will in any case have to be described in the report of the study. If an application is made for research funds, then the objectives and methods may have to be stated in a detailed study protocol.

It may not be frivolous to suggest that, as the plan of the study begins to take form and a clearer picture emerges of the effort and cost involved, the investigator should consider whether the investigation is still seen as worthwhile: Is its performance warranted by the importance of the problem that was its starting point? It is better to scrap a study at the outset than to decide afterwards that it was not worth doing.

Must a Study be Perfect?

In the pages that follow, a great deal of attention will be paid to various aspects of sound planning: the careful choice of definitions, the use of standardized and accurate methods of collecting information, etc. The better the techniques of investigation, the greater are the prospects of producing useful findings, and the more certain the researcher can be that the findings will be reproducible. However, there are very few perfect studies. Almost invariably, practical difficulties, oversights and accidents produce methodological imperfections. What is important is that the investigator should be aware of these imperfections, examine their impact, and take them into account in interpreting the findings; if this is done, the study will still be a sound and possibly a useful one. The investigator should strive for perfection, even if it is unattainable (in the words of the poet Robert Browning, 'Ah, but a man's reach should exceed his grasp, or what's a Heaven for?'), but must be prepared to make compromises with reality. In fact, an undue insistence on impeccable techniques at all costs may well ruin a study. There is much truth in the statement that 'in science as in love a concentration on technique is quite likely to lead to impotence'.[1]

Reference

1. Berger PL. Invitation to sociology: a humanistic perspective. Harmondsworth: Penguin Books, 1969. p. 24.

4

Formulating the Objectives

In a fable, three princes of Serendip 'were always making discoveries, by accidents and sagacity, of things which they were not in quest of'. Accidental discoveries in the health field are more common than some researchers may care to admit,[1] but we cannot rely on serendipity. Even *data mining*,[2] which is computerized serendipity (the use of a computer to dig through data in order to find previously unknown patterns or relationships), requires decisions by the investigator as to what kinds of information the computer should hunt for.

Having decided *what* to study and *why* (i.e. the study's topic and purpose), the investigator can now formulate the study objectives: What knowledge should the study yield? *What questions* should it answer? Serendipity apart, one is likely to learn only (at best) what one sets out to learn.

The explicit formulation of study objectives is an essential step in the planning of a study. It may be an exaggeration to say that 'a question well-stated is a question half-answered',[3] but a question that is poorly stated or unstated is unlikely to be answered at all. The specification of objectives determines the whole subsequent planning of the study. 'If you don't know where you're going, it is difficult to select a suitable means for getting there'.[4] In fact, 'if you're not sure where you're going, you're liable to end up someplace else'.[4]

Objectives of Descriptive Surveys

The objectives of a descriptive survey of a specific group or population – a survey carried out with a diagnostic purpose – are usually easy to formulate. The investigator needs only to state the characteristics he or she wants to measure. These may be diseases, deaths, or other 'disagreeable Ds' (disabilities, discomforts, dissatisfactions, deviations from statistical or social norms); they may be positive aspects of health (e.g. physical fitness, mental ability,[5] life expectancy, quality of life); or they may be somatic or psychological characteristics (body weight, biological markers,[6] behaviour patterns, left-handedness,[7] etc.) that are not necessarily negative or positive, but are seen as elements of health status or expressions of health. There are numerous

Research Methods in Community Medicine: Surveys, Epidemiological Research, Programme Evaluation, Clinical Trials   J. H. Abramson and Z. H. Abramson   Copyright © 2008, John Wiley & Sons Ltd

health indicators and health indices, serving different ends and appropriate in different circumstances.[8] The investigator may also want to study other characteristics of the group (demographic, biological, behavioural, social or cultural), or environmental features. There may also be interest in the health services provided for the population, or in their use.

Such objectives are easily stated, e.g. 'to determine the infant mortality rate in population Y during period Z', 'to measure the incidence of rabies', 'the prevalence of scabies', 'the case fatality rate of tabes', 'the distribution of head circumference in babies', 'the seasonality of stings by stray bees', etc.

Objectives may be stated in general terms, e.g. 'to measure the prevalence of disability (in population Y at time Z)', or more specifically, e.g. in terms of mobility, capacity to work, ability to perform activities of daily living, or other selected functions. The more specifically the objectives are stated, the more helpful they will be in the further planning of the study. A formulation that is too general, e.g. 'to study the health status of …' will not be helpful at all. If general objectives are stated, then more specific ones should be listed as well. Careful thinking about specific objectives may help to ensure that the study meets its purposes.

Even in a simple descriptive survey there is usually interest in obtaining separate information for different groups – for specific age groups, for the two sexes, for ethnic groups or parts of a city, etc. The objective might be stated as 'to measure X in population Y by age, sex (etc.)'. In a survey of the 'community diagnosis' type, findings may provide pointers to the different health needs of different parts of the population. If alcoholics are concentrated in one neighbourhood, that neighbourhood may need a special programme.

Not uncommonly, a descriptive survey centres not on the characteristic (say, disease D) in which interest actually lies, but on something that is known to be associated with this characteristic. The main circumstances in which the study may focus on an associated characteristic or characteristics (C) are as follows:

1. If it is easy to obtain information about C and difficult to obtain information about D, C may be used as a *proxy measure* of D. As an example, an investigator may be interested in the occurrence of prostatic hypertrophy in a community; if examinations to establish the diagnosis are not feasible, the proxy may be a specific symptom pattern that is believed to be associated with the disease. It may be possible to estimate the prevalence of D from the prevalence of C.[9]
2. The presence of C may be of use as a *screening test*, i.e. to discriminate between people who are likely and those who are unlikely to have D. Once people who have C (say a high casual blood pressure measurement) have been identified, they can be invited to be examined more fully in order to determine whether D (hypertensive disease) is present. To warrant such use of the association, C must be easier to study than D; C and D must be present at the same time; and certain other conditions (see pp. 172–173) must be met. The study objective might be stated at a group level as 'to measure the prevalence rate of C', or at an individual level as 'to identify people with positive screening tests for D'.

3. If C precedes D in time, then it may be of use as a *risk marker*, i.e. to distinguish between people who are likely and those who are unlikely to develop D in the future. The presence of C identifies vulnerable individuals or groups (*at-risk* or *high-risk* groups) who are especially likely to develop the disorder, and who hence have a special need for preventive care. C points to the increased risk; it does not necessarily cause it. It may be a cause, or it may be a precursor or early manifestation of the disorder, or it may be an effect or correlate of whatever factor increases the risk. Bald men have an increased risk of dying of coronary heart disease,[10] and elderly men with impaired memories have an increased risk of dying in the next 5 years.[11] But these are certainly not causal relationships – any special preventive care given to these high-risk men would not include prescribing a toupee or a course of memory training. In one study, elderly subjects who did not respond to a postal questionnaire had a more than twofold risk of dying in the next year – not, presumably, cause and effect.[12] On the other hand, a high diastolic blood pressure, another risk marker for mortality in elderly men,[11] is presumably also a risk *maker*, i.e. one reason for the high risk. Whether a risk marker affects risk is often unclear.[13] And whether the risk marker is a useful one is quite another question (see p. 173). In a descriptive study, the stated objective might be to 'determine the prevalence of a (specified) risk marker' or 'to identify people who are at special risk of a (specified) disorder'. *Health risk appraisal*[14] is a particular instance of the use of risk markers.

4. C may also be of interest because it is a *cause* of D, i.e. its presence or degree influences the risk of developing D. If C is amenable to change, and if a change in C will reduce the risk of D, then there may be a case for intervention directed at C. In such instances C is possibly best termed a *modifiable risk factor* (the adjective 'modifiable' refers both to the factor and to the risk). The unqualified term '*risk factor*' is generally used, but this unfortunately has more than one meaning; it is also often used to denote any cause of a disorder (modifiable or not), and sometimes to denote a risk marker. A causal factor may or may not be of use as a risk marker; it may or may not be possible to modify it, and modifying it may or may not modify the risk – often, in the words of the American humorist Will Rogers, 'We know lots of things we used to dident know but we don't know any way to prevent em happening'.[15] The general objective of a descriptive study of modifiable risk factors might be formulated as 'to determine the prevalence of' or 'to identify people who have' specified factors.

Objectives of Analytic Studies

Experiments and analytic surveys seek information about associations between variables, i.e. about whether and how different characteristics 'hang together'. The aim may be to explain the health status of a specific group or population, to seek new knowledge about factors affecting health and disease, or to test the value of tools used in health care, e.g. screening or diagnostic tests or risk markers, etc.

Analytic surveys commonly have a descriptive as well as an analytic element. A survey of elderly people with foot problems, for example, aimed to discover the extent to which they used chiropody services – useful descriptive information in its own right – and also whether their use was related to age, sex, living alone, the number and type of foot problems, etc.[16]

Possible formulations of the study objective, when an association is to be investigated, include 'to examine the association between infant mortality rates and region', 'to determine whether there is a difference between the rates in regions A and B', and 'to test the hypothesis that the rates in regions A and B differ'. *Hypotheses* are suppositions that are tested by collecting facts that lead to their acceptance or rejection. They are *not* assumptions that are to be taken for granted, neither are they beliefs that the investigator sets out to prove. They are 'refutable predictions' (TH Huxley wrote of 'the great tragedy of Science – the slaying of a beautiful hypothesis by an ugly fact').

A hypothesis may be stated as a positive declaration (sometimes called the *research hypothesis*, *study hypothesis*, or *substantive hypothesis*), e.g. 'the infant mortality rates in regions A and B are different' or 'the rate is higher in region A than in region B', or as a negative declaration (*null hypothesis*), e.g. 'there is no difference between the rates' or 'the rate is not higher in region A than in region B'. Statistical testing of an association requires the formulation of a null hypothesis, which is tested against a specific *alternative*;[17] this alternative ('that there is a difference between the two regions', or 'that the rate is higher in region A') is the 'research hypothesis'. If statistical testing is intended, then it is advisable to make the hypotheses as specific as possible at this stage, and not to leave them implicit (as in 'to study the association between mortality and region').

In a case-control study designed to examine a possible causal relationship between smoking and a disease, typical specific hypotheses might be that the proportion of smokers is higher among cases than among controls, that the proportion of heavy smokers is higher among cases than among controls, that the average age at starting smoking is earlier among cases than among controls, etc. In a cohort study set up for the same purpose, the hypotheses would relate to the relative incidence of the disease among persons with different smoking habits. The value of epidemiological hypotheses is enhanced if they deal not only with the combined occurrence of the postulated cause and effect (i.e. when one is present, does the other tend to be present?), but also with the quantitative *dose–response* relationship between cause and effect (e.g. when there is more intensive exposure to the cause, is the disease more frequent, more severe, earlier in its onset, etc.?) or with the *time–response* relationship (the relationship to the time interval since exposure).

As will be seen in Chapter 28, if we want to know *why* there is an association between two variables, we will usually need analyses that take account of the way the association is influenced by other characteristics. The selection of these other variables will be discussed on pp. 101–104. If the investigator wishes, they may be mentioned when the study objectives are formulated, e.g. by saying that the association will be tested 'holding sex and ethnic group constant' or 'controlling for' these variables, or that the hypothesis will be tested separately in each sex and ethnic group, or by listing the 'modifying' and 'confounding' variables that will be taken into account (these terms will become clearer later).

Remember, there is still lots of time for these decisions; the planning of the study is still in its early stages, and study objectives can be rethought and reformulated as often as we wish.

Spelling Out the Objectives

It is usually helpful to formulate the study objectives explicitly in writing, as a guide to the planning of appropriate study methods. They may or may not be published in the ultimate study report.

For convenience, the objectives are often first stated in fairly general terms, followed by a more detailed statement of the relevant specific objectives. In a study whose general objective is to determine the incidence of cancer by occupation in New Zealand,[18] a specific objective might be 'to determine the incidence rates of cancer (separate and combined sites) in occupational categories and selected specific occupations, controlling for age and socioeconomic status'. In a study with a general objective of examining the association between the mental health status of mothers and the nutritional status of their children,[19] specific objectives might be 'to compare the mental health status of mothers of malnourished children and mothers of well-nourished children, controlling for mother's age, education and number of children, income, and the child's birthweight' and 'to test the hypothesis that educational status affects the association between mother's mental health and child's nutritional status'.

The stated objectives should satisfy three requirements. First, they must meet the requirements of the study. This is usually easily achieved in a descriptive survey, but in planning an analytic survey or experiment there may be considerable difficulty in the formulation of a hypothesis; this is where the creative researcher comes into their own. Second, the objectives should be phrased clearly – unambiguously and very

---

Requirements of study objectives
1. They must meet the purposes of the study
2. They should be formulated clearly
3. They should be expressed in measurable terms

---

specifically – leaving no doubt as to precisely what has to be measured. Third, they should be phrased in measurable terms. That is, the objectives should be realistic (answerable questions, testable hypotheses) and formulated in operational terms, which can be applied in practice. 'Any fool can ask a question; the trick is to ask one that can be answered.'[20]

A few imaginary and actual examples follow.

1. To improve the community's health' and 'to plan a programme for improving the community's health' are not appropriate study objectives for a community health survey. They explain *why* the study is being conducted (the *purpose* of the study), but do not stipulate what knowledge the study is designed to yield. 'To determine the community's health needs' might be an appropriate general objective, but a much

more detailed formulation is required. Does the researcher propose, for example, to determine the community's perceived needs, or to examine the availability or use of health services, or to determine the incidence of specified disorders or the prevalence of specified disorders or risk factors?

2. A survey of diabetes was conducted in an English community.[21] Its first objective was '(1). To establish exactly the number of diabetics'. This is a clear statement; but the formulation is incomplete, since the investigators also measured the prevalence rate of diabetes and established the age and sex distribution of cases. The second objective was '(2). To discover the undiagnosed cases of diabetes'. This is not a complete statement, as the investigators also wanted to answer questions about the hitherto unknown cases. It should go on: 'and to compare their age and sex distribution with that of known cases'. The next objective was '(3). To investigate the possible hereditary factors'. This is far too nonspecific to be helpful as a blueprint in planning the study. Did the investigators intend to examine familial clustering among the people they examined? Did they want to see if prevalence was higher among the offspring of consanguineous marriages? Did they want to look for an association with the occurrence of diabetes-related genes? Or (as was actually the case) did they want to compare the frequency of positive family histories of diabetes among known diabetics, newly discovered diabetics, and nondiabetics, controlling for age and sex? One last example from this study: '(6). To repeat the whole survey at a future date'. This is hardly a study objective.

3. A report on a national study of cerebral palsy in adolescence and adulthood[22] states: 'The primary objectives of the study were: (1). To learn about the extent and nature [of the problem] and the specific needs of cerebral palsied youngsters and adults through a sociomedical study. (2). To collect epidemiological data on the cerebral palsied'. These formulations may be useful as starting points in planning a study, or as summary statements in a report, but would not be very useful as blueprints. Much further detail is needed for this purpose. (The study itself is a good one, and it is clear that the investigators actually did have specific and well thought out objectives.) Another stated objective, 'To evoke the interest of local communities and public agencies in the problems and needs of the cerebral palsied', is a laudable purpose for a study, but not what we have called a study objective. It might be stated as an objective of an action programme, not of a study.

4. The objective of a study was stated to be 'to study the effects of vaccination against measles'. This formulation is completely nonspecific, and could have given the investigator little help in planning the study. Was the investigator interested in the development of serological changes, or in differences in antibody titre between groups of vaccinated and nonvaccinated children, or in differences in the subsequent incidence of measles? The study turned out to be a descriptive survey of the incidence of fever, pain at the injection site, and other manifestations immediately after vaccination.

5. A hypothesis including the word 'cause', such as one that the habitual drinking of coffee is a cause of cancer of the bladder, must be made more specific before it can be tested. Is it proposed to determine whether the incidence rate of the disease in

different countries or at different times is correlated with the average consumption of coffee per head (group-based analytic surveys), or to determine whether patients drink more coffee than controls (a cross-sectional or case-control study), or to determine whether the incidence of new cases is higher among persons who drink much coffee than among those who take less coffee, and lowest among those who drink no coffee at all (a prospective survey or a rather unlikely experiment)? 'Controlling for age, sex, smoking habits (etc.)' would probably be specified in the hypothesis.

6. The hypothesis that the occurrence of a disease 'is associated with diet' is not sufficiently specific. The investigator may aim to compare the dietary histories of cases and controls, or compare incidence rates in vegetarians and others, or seek correlations between national disease rates and food consumption data. Nor is it stated in operational terms. In what aspect of diet is the investigator interested? – in the average daily intake of calories, proteins, fats and other specific nutrients, or in the average amounts consumed of milk, meat, and other specific foodstuffs, or in the number of days a week that meat, fish, etc. are usually eaten, or in the average number of meals taken per day? It may be felt that such decisions can be postponed until later in the planning phase. There is no great harm in this, but it is arguable that since these decisions may be very close to the nub of the research problem, they should be made at an early stage of planning. They are of a different order of importance from decisions on various methods of measurement, such as the choice of a technique for measuring the daily caloric intake (questioning, self-maintained dietary records, weighing of dishes and leftovers, etc.). Similar considerations arise when other vague terms are used, such as 'nutritional status', 'disability', 'emotional health', or 'stress'.

Notes and References

1. *Serendipity*: 'One sometimes finds what one is not looking for', said Sir Alexander Fleming, the serendipitous discoverer of penicillin (see Henderson JW. The yellow brick road to penicillin: a story of serendipity. Mayo Clinic Proceedings 1997; 72: 683). Other discoveries based on unplanned 'chance' observations (immunization with attenuated pathogens, anaphylaxis, the connection between the pancreas and diabetes, etc.) are listed by Comroe JH Jr (Roast pig and scientific discovery: parts I and II. American Review of Respiratory Disease 1997; 115: 853 and 1035) and Beveridge WIB (The art of scientific investigation, 3rd edn. New York: Vintage Books; 1957). The latter book, which stresses that 'the most important instrument in research must always be the mind of man', concentrates on the 'mental skills' of scientific investigation, such as the ability to recognize the importance of a chance or unexpected observation, to interpret the clue and develop a hypothesis, and to follow up the initial finding in a systematic way.

    'The most exciting phrase to hear in science, the one that heralds new discoveries, is not "Eureka!" but "That's funny..."' (attributed to Isaac Asimov; but one contributor to a spirited discussion, in a blog, of whether he actually said it and what he actually said, and if so where, remarked 'I thought the most exciting phrase in science was "The grant has been approved"').

2. *Data mining* uses a wide variety of advanced statistical methods, and sometimes employs artificial intelligence (AI) or neural network techniques, in order to detect, interpret, and predict

qualitative or quantitative patterns in data (Ramakrishnan N, Grama AY. Data mining: from serendipity to science. Computer 1999; 32(8): 34). The investigator decides which techniques, models (e.g. for classification, clustering, or associations), and variables will be used.

'The use of data mining has been advocated in epidemiological studies, e.g. to find clustering or relationships with diseases or to predict outcomes. But the findings may be spurious (fortuitous) ones. Flouris AD, Duffy J (European Journal of Epidemiology 2006; 21: 167) point out that 'an important limitation of AI systems is that, being – essentially – *post hoc* analyses, they may be capitalizing on a chance pattern of error in the data set. Cross-validation … can moderate this risk but in the end the result has held up over only two sets of data'. However, 'the discovery of a potentially robust pattern is a worthy finding and can be used to direct future research'.

See *data dredging* (note 1, Chapter 27).

3. Isaac S, Michael WB. Handbook in research and evaluation for education and the behavioural sciences. San Diego: EdITS; 1977. p. 2.

4. Mager RF. Preparing instructional objectives, 3rd edn. Jaico; 2005.

5. Methods of testing *intelligence*, and their use in epidemiological studies, are described by Deary IJ, Batty GD (Glossary: cognitive epidemiology. Journal of Epidemiology and Community Health 2007; 61: 378), who say 'Intelligence is here taken to mean psychometric intelligence, as tested by standardised mental tests'. (In other words, intelligence is defined as what is measured by intelligence tests.) A high IQ in the first two decades of life is predictive of lower rates of mortality in middle to late adulthood (Batty GD, Deary IJ, Gottfredson L. Premorbid (early life) IQ and later mortality risk: systematic review. Annals of Epidemiology 2007; 17: 278).

6. *Biological markers*, or *biomarkers*, are biochemical, molecular, genetic, immunological or other indicators (often quantitative) of past exposure, biological changes, disease processes, or predisposition to disease. Examples: lead content of blood, creatinine clearance, human leucocyte antigens, alpha-fetoprotein, antibody titres. See, for example, Perera FP (Molecular epidemiology: on the path to prevention? Journal of the National Cancer Institute 2000; 92: 602).

7. *Left-handedness* is mentioned in the text as a reminder of the wide gamut of questions that surveys may ask. Not that left-handedness is necessarily trivial – it may increase the risk of hand injuries, fractures, injuries in general, and kyphosis (Taras JS, Behrman MJ, Degnan GG. Left-hand dominance and hand trauma. Journal of Hand Surgery 1995; 20: 1043. Stellman SD, Wynder EL, DeRose DJ, Muscat JE. The epidemiology of left-handedness in a hospital population. Annals of Epidemiology 1997; 7: 167. Wright P, Williams J, Currie C, Beattie T. Left-handedness increases injury risk in adolescent girls. Perceptual and Motor Skills 1996; 82: 855. Nissinen M, Heliovaara M, Seitsamo J, Poussa M. Left handedness and risk of thoracic hyperkyphosis in prepubertal schoolchildren. International Journal of Epidemiology 1995; 24: 1178).

Left-handedness may also be a risk marker, although not a useful one, for premenopausal breast cancer (Ramadhani MK, Elias SG, van Noord PAH, Grobbee DE, Peeters PHM, Uiterwaal CSPM. Innate left-handedness and risk of breast cancer: case-cohort study. British Medical Journal 2006; 331: 882). Readers' responses to this paper are a salutary demonstration of the confusion between risk markers and risk factors (http://www.bmj.com/cgi/eletters/331/7521/882).

And left-handed women apparently have an increased risk of dying of colorectal cancer and stroke (Ramadhani MK, Elias SG, van Noord PAH, Grobbee DE, Peeters PHM, Uiterwaal SPM. Innate handedness and disease-specific mortality in women. Epidemiology 2007; 18: 208).

8. *Health indicators* for use with adults are reviewed by McHorney CA (Health status assessment methods for adults: past accomplishments and future challenges. Annual Review of Public Health 1999; 20: 309).

Indicators that are useful for comparing populations or individuals are not always suitable for detecting changes; see 'responsiveness', p. 196.

'*Health index*' may be a synonym for 'health indicator', or may refer to a numerical index based on two or more indicators, such as the Health Problem Index ('Q value') devised by the Division of Indian Health in the United States. This is based mainly on the mortality rate, the average age at death, and the numbers of outpatient visits and hospital days per head; see Haynes MA (In: Reinke WA (ed.), Health planning: qualitative aspects and quantitative techniques. Baltimore, MD: Johns Hopkins University; 1972. p. 158).

9. For methods of estimating the confidence limits of the prevalence of a disease in a population from the prevalence of a proxy attribute in the population or a sample, see Peritz E (Estimating the ratio of two marginal probabilities in a contingency table. Biometrics 1971; 27: 223 (correction note: 1971; 27: 1104)) and Rogan WJ, Gladen B (Estimating prevalence from the results of a screening test. American Journal of Epidemiology 1978; 107: 71).

10. Ford ES, Freedman DS, Byers T. Baldness and ischemic heart disease in a national sample of men. American Journal of Epidemiology 1996; 143: 651.

11. Abramson JH, Gofin R, Peritz E. Risk markers for mortality among elderly men: a community study in Jerusalem. Journal of Chronic Diseases 1982; 35: 565.

    A cohort study in Holland showed a similar association (Gussekloo J, Westendorp RGJ, Remarque EJ, Lagaay AM, Heeren TJ, Knook DL. Impact of mild cognitive impairment on survival in very elderly people: cohort study. British Medical Journal 1997; 315: 1053).

12. Hebert R, Bravo G, Korner-Bitensky N, Voyer L. Refusal and information bias associated with postal questionnaires and face-to-face interviews in very elderly subjects. Journal of Clinical Epidemiology 1996; 49: 373.

    A similar association was found in an 11-year follow-up of adolescents who were asked to complete mailed health questionnaires – nonrespondents had a twofold risk of death (Mattila V M, Parkkari J, Rimpela A. Adolescent survey non-response and later risk of death – a prospective cohort study of 78,609 persons with 11-year follow-up. BMC Public Health 2007; 7: 87). Could this be used as a ploy to encourage response? ('Fill in the questionnaire and LIVE!')

13. Cohort studies of elderly men have found that little walking, despite ability to walk, was predictive of more future physical disability and earlier death. Do these findings express a protective effect, as the researchers suggest, or is 'little walking' only a risk marker? (Clark DO. The effect of walking on lower body disability among older Blacks and Whites. American Journal of Public Health 1996; 86: 57. Hakim AA, Petrovitch H, Burchfiel CM *et al*. Effects of walking on mortality among nonsmoking retired men. New England Journal of Medicine 1998; 338: 94).

14. *Health risk appraisal* is the use of a battery of information on health-related behaviour, exposure to environmental hazards and personal characteristics in order to estimate an individual's chances of acquiring specific diseases, of dying, etc. It has mainly been used to enable individuals to identify hazards and to motivate them to lessen them. The technique offers promise as a tool for use in community medicine, both for identifying high-risk individuals and as a way of gauging a group or population's risk of preventable diseases and other outcomes. Many programmes overreach existing scientific knowledge in order to accomplish the former aim. An important criticism is that the message generated for the client is based on the sometimes questionable assumption that changes made by the individual will necessarily change the risk, i.e. that risk markers are modifiable risk factors. Health risk appraisal may be offered as an incentive to make participation in a health survey attractive.

    Health hazard appraisal usually refers to environmental exposures.

15. Cohen JM, Cohen MJ. The Penguin dictionary of modern quotations. Harmondsworth: Penguin Books; 1976. p. 194.

16. Harvey I, Frankel S, Marks R, Shalom D, Morgan M. Foot morbidity and exposure to chiropody: population based study. British Medical Journal 1997; 315: 1054.

17. See note 10, Chapter 28.
18. Firth HM, Cooke KR, Herbison GP. Male cancer incidence by occupation: New Zealand, 1972–1984. International Journal of Epidemiology 1996; 25: 14.
19. De Miranda CT, Turecki G, Mari JDJ *et al*. Mental health of the mothers of malnourished children. International Journal of Epidemiology 1996; 25: 128.
20. Lemkau PV, Pasamanick B. Problems in evaluation of mental health programs. American Journal of Orthopsychiatry 1957; 27: 55.
21. Walker JB, Kerridge D. Diabetes in an English community: a study of its incidence and natural history. Leicester: Leicester University Press; 1961.
22. Margulec I (ed.). Cerebral palsy in adolescence and adulthood: a rehabilitation study. Tel Aviv: Jerusalem Academic Press, 1966. p. 8.

5

The Objectives
of Evaluative Studies

When we evaluate a treatment or other health-care procedure we are making a value judgement. To reduce the subjective element in this judgement we should base the appraisal on facts and use explicit criteria. An evaluative study sets out to collect these facts, and the facts to be collected should be specified in the study objectives.

Evaluative studies may be descriptive, analytic, or both, and their objectives should be formulated accordingly, along the lines suggested in Chapter 4. This chapter will review the basic questions commonly asked in evaluative studies of all kinds, and will then discuss their application to programme reviews. Consideration will be given in later chapters to their application to other evaluative studies – to clinical and pro-gramme trials (Chapters 32 and 33) and to evaluations of screening and diagnostic tests (pp. 171–173) and risk markers (p. 173).

The need for objective data should be reflected in the wording of the specific study objectives. The challenge faced by the evaluator is to translate a 'How satisfactory is ...?' question into a set of study objectives that are free of terms requiring value judgements. In an evaluation of routine medical examinations of schoolchildren, for example, the specific objectives might be to determine the prevalence of previously undiagnosed chronic disorders, or the number of children treated, or successfully treated, as a consequence of the routine examinations. Words like 'good', 'bad', 'should' and 'ought' have no place here.

The basic questions that are commonly asked in evaluative studies are listed on the next page. These questions specify the dimensions of care that are commonly appraised, whether as separate issues or as components of global appraisals. They pro-vide a framework for the formulation of specific study objectives. In these questions, 'care' refers to whatever procedure is being evaluated – care directed at individuals or populations, screening and other diagnostic activities, or environmental health programmes.

We will discuss each basic question separately and consider its role as a basis for the formulation of clear-cut study objectives.

Research Methods in Community Medicine: Surveys, Epidemiological Research, Programme Evaluation, Clinical Trials   J. H. Abramson and Z. H. Abramson   Copyright © 2008, John Wiley & Sons Ltd

> **The basic questions of evaluative studies**
>
> 1. *Requisiteness*
>   To what extent is care needed?
> 2. *Quality*
>   (a) How satisfactory is the *outcome*?
>   Attainment of desirable effects *(effectiveness)*?
>   Absence of undesirable effects *(harmlessness)*?
>   (b) How satisfactory is the *process*?
>   *Performance of activities* by the providers of care?
>   *Compliance* and the *utilization of services* by the recipients of care?
>   (c) How satisfactory are the facilities and setting *(structure)*?
> 3. *Efficiency*
>   How efficiently are resources used?
> 4. *Satisfaction*
>   How satisfied are the people concerned?
> 5. *Differential value*
>   How do the above features differ in different categories or groups or in different circumstances?

Requisiteness

The first question concerns the *requisiteness* ('appropriateness', 'relevance') of care. To what extent is care *needed*?[1] It can hardly be of value if there is no need for it. This question may be asked in reviews of all established programmes and services, which may have outlived their need. It is not asked in trials; the need for care is a precondition for a trial rather than a question the trial sets out to answer.

The appraisal by health professionals of the need for care generally requires, *inter alia*, facts about the nature, extent and severity of the problem or problems that the programme aims to solve, and of other problems that compete for the available resources, as well as facts about the availability of resources. Account may also be taken of *perceived need* (as stated by patients or public) and *expressed demand* (e.g. requests for care, as reflected by the use of services, waiting lists for treatment, etc.). When formulating study objectives, thought should be given to the specific facts required for these purposes.[1]

Quality

The quality of health care may be judged from information about effects (*outcome evaluation*), about the performance of activities (*process evaluation*), or about facilities and settings (*structure evaluation*). In each instance, the question asked is 'How satisfactory?', and the evaluative study aims to yield the objective facts required to answer this question.

Numerous schemes of evaluation have been proposed, and it may not greatly matter which is used. Beware of schemes that focus only on an appraisal of the structural and organizational context within which health care is provided, while neglecting the actual care given and its effects. Appraisals of such attributes as the availability, accessibility, comprehensiveness and coordination of services, continuity of care, and accountability – if based on hard facts rather than impressions – may indicate whether the setting is conducive to a satisfactory quality of care. But (unless inadequacies are striking) firm conclusions about the quality of care generally require evaluation of the process and outcome of care as well.

Outcome

Both desirable and undesirable effects should always be measured, since a full appraisal of outcome depends on the balance between these – a judgement that may not be easy, since it requires decisions on the relative weight to be given to qualitatively different outcomes (effects on mortality, morbidity, working capacity, the quality of life, etc.). The popular term *risk/benefit ratio*[2] should be avoided, unless desirable and undesirable effects can be measured on the same scale, as in a comparison of the numbers of deaths that might be caused and prevented by a new treatment (a ratio is one number divided by another).

Effectiveness refers to the degree of achievement of desirable effects. These may be expressed at the individual level (recovery from disease, restoration of function, etc.) or at the group or community level (changes in mortality and morbidity rates, changes in a community's knowledge or practices, environmental changes, etc.).

Effectiveness is generally distinguished from *efficacy*. While definitions vary, 'efficacy' may be used to refer to the benefits observed when a procedure is applied as it 'should' be, and with full compliance by all concerned, i.e. 'under ideal conditions'. The term is usually reserved for benefits at the individual level, as measured by a clinical trial. 'Effectiveness' then refers to the benefits observed at the population level, or among people to whom the procedure or service is offered. 'Efficacy' answers the question, 'can the procedure or service work?', whereas 'effectiveness' answers the question, 'does it work?'[3] A programme for the control of hypertension in a community would use drugs known to be efficacious; the community programme might or might not be effective. In Gambia, trials of insecticide-treated bed-nets (to reduce malaria) showed that, under ideal conditions, these could prevent 63% of child mortality, but in a practical community programme context the reduction was only 25%.[3]

Clear-cut explicit criteria of effectiveness (or efficacy) are readily available if the activities under evaluation have well-defined predetermined goals, i.e. situations or conditions whose attainment was set up as an aim. (We will refer to these as 'goals' rather than 'objectives', so as not to confuse them with study objectives; some authors distinguish between the 'goals' and 'objectives' of health-care programmes.)[4] The extent of accomplishment of these aims is a realistic measure of effectiveness. With this method of evaluation in mind, effectiveness is sometimes defined as the extent to which pre-established goals are attained as a result of the activity.

This 'goal attainment' approach (which will be further discussed on p. 346) can be used only if predetermined goals are known or can be inferred, and if it is possible to measure their attainment. For the latter purpose, they must be expressed in clear and specific terms. It is not easy to appraise the effectiveness of an antenatal programme if its goal is expressed in such general terms as 'to promote the health of the mother and baby'. If the goals are 'to reduce the stillbirth rate', 'to reduce the number of babies born with Down's syndrome', etc., evaluation is easier. It is especially easy if precise quantitative targets are stated, e.g. 'to reduce the stillbirth rate to 15 per 1000 births'.

If the goal attainment model cannot be used, the investigator will need to formulate his or her own criteria, or to use standards[5] or criteria formulated by experts. The need for such (additional) criteria should be considered even when the goal attainment model is used, so as to avoid the danger of 'tunnel vision' – an investigator who concentrates only on the preset goals may not see beneficial outcomes that were not specified as goals, and may be blind to adverse effects.

When possible, *end results* – i.e. effects on health status – should be used as criteria of effectiveness, even if the production of these effects is not a direct aim of the procedure or programme under evaluation. A highly 'successful' case-finding programme may merit a negative evaluation if the detection of new cases resulted in no improvement in health status. The ultimate criterion of effectiveness is the extent to which the underlying problem is alleviated or prevented. This is sometimes referred to as the *adequacy* of the intervention. A programme that deals with only a small part of a large problem may be regarded as inadequate, however well it works.

Adverse effects[6] may be missed unless they are sought. These include not only side-effects of medication ('The children crippled by thalidomide are on their slow procession through the special schools for the handicapped, following those made deaf by streptomycin who succeeded the infants blinded by oxygen'[7]), but overdependence, anxiety, and other less obvious effects. An editorial entitled 'The menace of mass screening' in a public health journal points to the morbidity caused among children with innocent heart murmurs who falsely perceive themselves as having heart disease, and the disability caused to children as a result of being identified as carriers of the sickle-cell trait.[8] Being labelled as hypertensive may produce symptoms of depression,[9] and being told that one is 'at risk' (especially with the current expansion of genetic testing) may have far-reaching consequences.[10]

Process

An appraisal of the *performance of activities* requires information on the services provided – what kinds, and how much? First, if there is a programme plan that lays down what activities *should* be performed, then these requirements provide ready-made yardsticks. If the stated intention was to make contact with every known blind person at least once a year, or to examine the developmental status of all year-old children, or to X-ray the chests of all patients with pneumonia after their treatment, to what extent were these things done? Second, in some programmes, *coverage*[11] may be a useful criterion – what proportion of the people who can or should receive a service (the target population) actually receive it? A third approach, especially in studies of the quality of medical care, is to prepare a detailed formulation of the activities that it is believed should be carried out, usually in relation to a specific diagnosis or other medical problem, and to compare actual performance with this set of standards (see 'Medical audit' in Chapter 21).

A further basis for evaluation is provided by information on the activities of patients or public – the *utilization of services* (what services, and how much?), the degree of *compliance* with advice or instructions (taking of medicines, keeping of appointments, dietary changes, etc.) and the degree of *community participation* in the programme. Clear-cut criteria are not usually available. The appraisal of activities (by providers and recipients of care) may be extended to studies of knowledge and attitudes that may influence overt behaviour, and of relationships and communication between providers and recipients.

Structure

Finally, information on *facilities and settings* also provides a basis for the appraisal of quality. Are equipment, accommodation, suitably qualified personnel, laboratory facilities, etc. available? Recommended norms[5] are sometimes used as criteria, e.g. for numbers of hospital beds. How accessible are services to those who need them? (What are the organizational and fiscal arrangements? Transport facilities? Are there language barriers? etc.) Is the service accountable, and to whom? Are there organizational arrangements to permit continuity of care, teamwork and coordinated functioning, coordination and cooperation with other agencies (including arrangements for patient referrals and information transfer), and community participation?

Efficiency

Efficiency[12] (or *economic efficiency*) refers to the cost in resources that is incurred in achieving results. It is determined by the balance between what is put in (in time, manpower, equipment, etc., or their monetary equivalent) and what is got out. Collecting the required facts on inputs and outputs is a major task of a study of efficiency. The burgeoning of managed care,[13] a term used for 'a variety of methods of financing and organizing the delivery of comprehensive health care in which an attempt is made to control costs by controlling the provision of services', has led to an intensified interest in economic evaluation.

Studies of economic efficiency require special expertise, unless cost is measured in nonmonetary terms, e.g. as the number of nurses, hours of work, hospitalization days, hospital beds, or waiting-time required for a particular purpose, or the number of screening tests required to identify one case.

Studies of economic efficiency are of three main types: cost–benefit analysis, cost-effectiveness analysis, and cost–utility analysis.

Cost–benefit analysis, which requires both costs and benefits to be measured in monetary terms, so that inputs and outputs are measured on the same scale, is concerned with *allocative efficiency* – it aims to answer questions about the allocation of resources to different programmes. Account should be taken of the cost of providing the service and the cost of not providing it, taking account of all known outcomes, both desirable and undesirable. The collection of adequate data and the conversion of benefits to monetary units present considerable theoretical and practical difficulty.[14] Over half the so-called cost–benefit studies reported in the health-care literature do not meet the above definition of a cost–benefit study; most of the studies are cost comparisons, with no accounting of benefits.[15]

Cost-effectiveness analysis, which does not require the benefits to be converted to money terms, deals with the *technical efficiency* of different methods of care in producing a specified effect on health. It compares the costs of alternative ways of achieving a similar effect, or compares the benefits that may be obtained at the same cost by different means. It may simply compare the costs of different ways of achieving an equivalent effect (*cost-minimization analysis*). Or it may compare *cost-effectiveness ratios* (costs per unit of effect), e.g. by calculating the average cost per unit of care (cost per test, per day in hospital, per patient treated, per year of life saved, etc.) for comparison with other programmes or recommended standards. A limitation of cost-effectiveness analyses is that only a single outcome (the principal objective of the programme) is taken into account. Studies that report costs and effects separately, but not their relationship, are sometimes called cost-consequence analyses. Detailed recommendations for the performance and reporting of cost-effectiveness analyses have been made by an expert panel.[16]

As an example, consider the comparison of three ways of reducing heart disease by controlling cholesterol levels in children: population-wide intervention centred on health education (A), universal screening (B), and selective screening for children with a family history of coronary heart disease (C). The comparison indicated that A would cost 2.6 times as much per year as B, and 17.5 times as much as C. But A would save 6.8 times as many years of life as B, and 32.6 times as many as C. A was thus the most cost effective: its cost per year of life saved would be about a third of that of B and about half of that of C.[17] As another example, different studies of smoking interventions have found wide variations in their cost per year of life saved: nicotine gum, $8,481 to $13,331 (for men); nicotine patches, $1,796 to $2,949 (men); physician counselling, $1,454 to $4,244; nurse counselling, $241[18] – a cheap method can be more cost effective, without necessarily being more effective (might economists and managed-care professionals be more concerned with the cost of saving a year of life than with the number of years of life saved?).

Cost–utility analysis, which 'lies somewhere between cost–benefit and cost-effectiveness analysis',[19] measures the different effects that a programme has on life expectancy and the quality of life and combines them, using weights that may take account of the individual's or community's views, into a number of 'healthy years'. One scale that is widely used for this purpose is the Euroqol EQ-5D scale, whose dimensions are mobility, self-care, usual activities, pain/discomfort, and anxiety/depression.[20]

The 'healthy year' measures that are commonly used[12,21] are quality-adjusted life-years (QALYs), healthy year equivalents (HYEs), and disability-adjusted life-years (DALYs), all of which convert years of unhealthy life to healthy years (only arithmetically, alas). The programmes can then be compared with respect to their costs per QALY, HYE, or DALY. A cost–utility analysis thus permits an assessment both of technical efficiency and (by enabling programmes to be compared without converting their effects into monetary terms) of allocative efficiency. Non-health benefits and losses (such as gains or losses in production) and non-health-care costs are not taken into account.

Satisfaction

If patients or public are satisfied with their health care, this does not necessarily mean that their care is of high quality. Satisfaction does, however, enhance the prospects of compliance and the continued utilization of services, and it is also an important additional end result in its own right, whether for altruistic reasons, because of an interest in consumerism, or, in a world where users of health care are seen as customers,[22] because of its implications for financial support or profitability.

The measurement of satisfaction[23] requires a survey of attitudes or of overt acts or experiences from which attitudes can be inferred, such as changes of physician or the lodging of complaints. Patients may be unwilling to report dissatisfaction, but may be prepared to give information about specific features of care and the importance they attach to them. In one survey, for example, 95% of patients said they were 'fully satisfied', but 28% reported that their consultation had not been conducted in private (ranked first in importance among the nonmedical factors) and 65% said the facility could be cleaner (ranked second in importance).[24]

Attention may also be paid to the satisfaction of health professionals. Although the gratification of health workers can hardly be regarded as a central purpose of health care, 'it is reasonable to assume that the best technical care cannot be maintained if the persons who provide it are unhappy with the work they do and the conditions under which it is done'.[25]

Differential Value

The value of a procedure or programme may differ for different patients or population groups, or in different circumstances. This possible nonuniformity appears as a separate item in our list (Question 5) because of its importance and the frequency with which it is forgotten. This question could actually be asked as an extension of each of the other questions: To what extent is care needed by various groups of the population? How do effectiveness and safety vary in different categories of patients or population groups? Are services equally available to all parts of the population? Equality or (more importantly) *equity* may be among the touchstones in evaluating a programme.[26] Why was the rate of hysterectomies during a 20-year period consistently twice as high among young women in the southern United States as it was in the northeastern states?[27] Are the people who use a service the ones who need it? Women with a low risk of cancer of the cervix may participate in a screening programme, while high-risk groups may stay away; this tendency for people in most need of care to be those least likely to receive it has been called the 'inverse care law'.[28] Who is more compliant, who is less compliant? And so on. If such questions are to be asked, they must be formulated as study objectives.

Objectives of Programme Reviews

A programme review (see p. 23) aims to provide a feedback that will be helpful to whoever makes decisions about the programme. To be useful, the findings must be provided rapidly, and in real time if possible. Since measurement of outcomes would often be relatively protracted or difficult, interest generally centres on the process rather than the outcome of care, and on requisiteness (especially in long-established programmes), the availability of equipment and other facilities, the public's satisfaction, and differences between population groups or categories in their need for care, use of services, and coverage. Programme reviews differ in this respect from programme trials, in which the central issue is usually the outcome (see Chapter 33).

The assumption (on which the programme is based) that the planned activities of the programme are beneficial is generally not in question. If it is, then the more rigorous methods of a programme trial are required. The issue is whether these activities are conducted as planned; their performance can thus be used as a criterion of the quality of care. Data on activities can usually be obtained far more readily and rapidly than data on outcome, often as a by-product of routine work, i.e. from inbuilt monitoring procedures. If there is no record of what activities were planned – as is often the case in a clinical service – then arbitrary standards may be applied, e.g. by using medical audit techniques (see p. 212).

This emphasis on measures of 'process' and 'structure' does not mean that measures of outcome have no place in a programme review. On the contrary, information on outcomes may be valuable even without rigorous evidence that they are actually consequences of the programme. It is usually assumed that changes (or their absence) are, at least to some extent, reflections of the effectiveness of the programme. Hence, they are often used as a basis for decisions on the need for continuation or modification of the programme. At the very least, they may indicate whether there is a need for more detailed evaluative study.

Short-term outcomes are usually the easiest to measure. Measurement of long-term outcomes may require information about members of the target population with whom there is no routine contact, or with whom contact has ceased. It may also involve a long-term follow-up, with its attendant difficulty and delay. However, if surveillance procedures are available to provide data on relevant end results, such as mortality rates, case fatality rates, or changes in the health status of patients or the population, then this information is often especially helpful. If the programme has predetermined outcome goals, then information on their accomplishment is, of course, particularly meaningful.

In a programme review, the appraisal of efficiency, like that of quality, has special features. Although detailed studies of inputs may be undertaken, emphasis is often put on simple observations that can be used as a basis for decisions aimed at enhancing efficiency. Such observations relate especially to evidence of wasteful operation: the avoidable use of expensive or ineffective drugs, overstaffing, delays, the underexploitation of expensive equipment, superfluous activities, unnecessary hospitalization, unduly long institutional care, etc. Use is not necessarily made of explicit standards in appraising these observations. If cost-effectiveness studies are undertaken, then cost is usually balanced against estimates or subjective appraisals of effectiveness, or against the performance of assumedly beneficial activities (used as a proxy measure of effectiveness).

The formulation of study objectives usually presents no difficulties in a simple programme review. If cause–effect hypotheses are to be tested (are the outcomes attributable to the programme?), then the methods of a programme trial (Chapter 33) must be used.

Notes and References

1. 'Program directors are concerned with *appropriateness* when they ask, "Are our program objectives worthwhile and do they have a higher priority than other possible objectives of this or other programs?"' (Deniston OL, Rosenstock IM, Getting VA. Evaluation of program effectiveness. Public Health Reports 1968; 83: 323. Reprinted in Schulberg HC, Sheldon A, Baker F (eds) (Program evaluation in the health fields. New York, NY: Behavioural Publications; 1969. pp. 219–239)).

   For references to *needs appraisal*, see note 11, Chapter 2. Needs appraisal in the context of community-oriented primary care is discussed in Chapter 34.
2. 'Risk–benefit ratio or risk–benefit nonsense' is the title of a report describing a Medline search that found many papers that used the term 'risk–benefit ratio' without explaining its meaning (Ernst E, Resch KL. Journal of Clinical Epidemiology 1996; 49: 1203).
3. Lengeler C, Snow RW. From efficacy to effectiveness: insecticide-treated bednets in Africa. Bulletin of the World Health Association 1996; 74: 325.
4. Dictionary definitions: *objective*, 'the precisely stated end to which efforts are directed, specifying the population outcome, variable(s) to be measured, etc.'; *target*, 'an aspired outcome that is specifically stated, e.g. what a health promotion program will achieve by a specified date, for example, reduced unwanted pregnancy rates, lower teenage smoking rates, enhanced QALYs [quality-adjusted life years]. Usually expressed in quantitative terms' (Last JM. A dictionary of epidemiology, 4th edn. New York, NY: Oxford University Press, 2001.)

   But 'terms such as goals, objectives, targets and aims are often used interchangeably, and there are no exact agreed definitions. Where more than one is used in a single context a hierarchy of specificities may be implied. Thus, a general goal is translated into a set of more precise objectives, and these into even more specific targets or aims'. (Knox EG (ed.). Epidemiology in health care planning. Oxford: Oxford University Press; 1979. p.15).
5. *Norms* and *standards* prescribed by an authority as 'what is desirable' may be used as criteria for evaluating facilities, performance, outcome, and cost. A distinction is sometimes made between norms and standards. Definitions of 'norms', 'standards' and 'criteria' are discussed by Donabedian A (Criteria, norms and standards of quality: what do they mean? American

Journal of Public Health 1981; 71: 409). Standards may be normative or empirical (see p. 212). They may specify a 'minimum' (minimum acceptable), an 'ideal' level, the 'desired achievable' level, or a 'maximum'.

6. Methods of studying adverse reactions to therapy are briefly reviewed by Sartwell PE (Iatrogenic disease: an epidemiologic perspective. International Journal of Health Services 1974; 4: 89). The 'current iatrogenic pandemic' is described and copiously documented by Illich I (Limits to medicine: medical nemesis: the expropriation of health. Harmondsworth: Penguin Books; 1977). A lecture, 'Medical nemesis', based on the book, was published in the Lancet in 1974 and reprinted in 2003 (Lancet 2003; 57: 919).

7. Morris JN. Uses of epidemiology, 3rd edn. Edinburgh: Churchill Livingstone; 1975. p. 92.

8. Bergman AB. American Journal of Public Health 1977; 67: 601.

9. A community survey in California identified people who were normotensive and not receiving medical care for hypertension, but had previously been told they were hypertensive. These 'mislabelled' people had more symptoms of depression and reported being in poorer health than other normotensives, controlling for possible confounding by age, sex, education, marital status, ethnicity, and the presence of other disorders. The mislabelled hypertensives had as many symptoms of depression as correctly labelled hypertensives (Bloom JR, Monterossa S. Hypertension labeling and sense of well-being. American Journal of Public Health 1981; 71: 1228).

    A study of a US national sample yielded similar findings: normotensives whose doctors had told them they had high blood pressure had lower 'general wellbeing' scores than other normotensives, as did 'correctly labelled' hypertensives, whether under treatment or not (Monk M. Psychologic status and hypertension. American Journal of Epidemiology 1980; 112: 200).

10. Kenen RH. The at-risk health status and technology: a diagnostic invitation and the 'gift' of knowing. Social Science and Medicine 1996; 42: 1545. Reprinted in Sidell M, Jones L, Katz J, Peberdy A (Debates and dilemmas in promoting health: a reader. Houndmills: MacMillan Press; 1997. pp. 306–313).

11. The evaluation of health service *coverage* is discussed by Tanahashi T (Health service coverage and its evaluation. Bulletin of the World Health Organization 1978; 56: 295). The importance of 'measuring what we do not do – the gap between what is done and what could and should be done', and the potential for such studies in general practices with stable populations is stressed by Hart JT (Measurement and omission. British Medical Journal 1982; 284: 1686).

    See also: Soucat A, Levine R, Wagstaff A, Yazbeck A, Griffin C C, Johnston T, Hutchinson P, Knippenberg R. Assessing the performance of health services in reaching the poor. In: Shah A (ed.), Measuring government performance in the delivery of public services, vol. 2 of Handbook on public sector performance reviews. Washington, DC: The World Bank; 2003 (http://www1.worldbank.org/wbiep/decentralization/library1/Measuring%20Government%20Performance_Vol%202_chapter6.pdf).

12. Economic evaluation of health care: see Auld MC, Donaldson C, Mitton C, Shackley P (Health economics and public health) and Jamison DT (Cost-effectiveness analysis: concepts and applications), both in Detels R, McEwen J, Beaglehole R, Detels R, McEwen J, Beaglehole R, Tanaka H (eds). Oxford textbook of public health, 4th edn, vol 2. The practice of public health. New York, NY: Oxford University Press; 2002. pp. 877–901 and 903–919 respectively.

    The above chapters describe quality-adjusted life-years (QALYs), healthy year equivalents (HYEs), and disability-adjusted life-years (DALYs).

13. The definition of *managed care* is cited from Inglehart JK (Physicians and the growth of managed care: health policy report. New England Journal of Medicine 1994; 331: 1167). Despite the potential benefits of managed care, many clinicians and other health professionals are concerned by the negative consequences of an overemphasis on economic factors (see Silver G. Editorial: The road from managed care. American Journal of Public Health 1997; 87: 8).

According to a probably fictional report, Hippocrates turned down an appointment in a health maintenance organization on ethical grounds: 'a medical system that has minimal concern for ethics … and is run by financial people instead of doctors, nurses, or anyone else who cares for the patients' (Pruchnicki A. First, do no harm [pending prior approval]. New England Journal of Medicine 1997; 337: 1627).

14. The less tangible costs of illness (i.e. other than impaired productivity) are seldom taken into account in cost–benefit studies, and estimates of the effects of preventive programmes are often speculative because of the paucity of epidemiological evidence (Drummond MF. Survey of cost-effectiveness and cost–benefit studies in industrialized countries. World Health Statistics Quarterly 1985; 38: 383).

An analysis of economic evaluation studies revealed that in only 14% was uncertainty taken into account satisfactorily; in another 25%, the handling of uncertainty was 'adequate' (Briggs A, Sculpher M. Sensitivity analysis in economic evaluation: a review of published studies. Health Economics 1995; 4: 35f).

A sceptical reader may find that the methods of estimation used in some cost–benefit studies are reminiscent of the method of weighing a pig attributed to John Burns: find a plank that is absolutely straight, balance it at dead centre so that it is absolutely level, place the pig on one end, and pile stones on the other end until the plank is exactly level again. Then carefully guess the weight of the stones. This is the weight of the pig.

15. Zarnke KB, Levine MAH, O'Brien BJ. Cost–benefit analyses in the health-care literature: don't judge a study by its label. Journal of Clinical Epidemiology 1997; 50: 813. 'Every Tom, Dick, and Harry is named "John"' (attributed to Sam Goldwyn).

16. The consensus statement of the Panel on Cost-Effectiveness in Health and Medicine is described in three reports: Russell LB, Gold MR, Siegel JE, Daniels N, Weinstein MC (The role of cost-effectiveness analysis in health and medicine. Journal of the American Medical Association 1996; 276: 1172); Weinstein MC, Siegel JE, Gold MR, Kamlet MS, Russell LB (Recommendations of the Panel on Cost-effectiveness in Health and Medicine. Journal of the American Medical Association 1996; 276: 1253); Siegel JE, Weinstein MC, Russell LB, Gold MR (Recommendations for reporting cost-effectiveness analyses. Journal of the American Medical Association 1996; 276: 1339).

Also, see Drummond MF, Sculpher MJ, Torrance GL, O'Brien, BJ, Stoddart GL (Methods for the economic evaluation of health care programmes, 3rd edn. Oxford University Press; 2003).

17. The study of options for controlling children's cholesterol levels made extensive use of sensitivity analysis, by seeing how results would be affected by different estimates of the risk associated with cholesterol level, the stability of cholesterol level, the degree of compliance, the change of cholesterol with diet, and the costs of screening and dietary intervention. These variations did not affect the ranking of the three programmes (Berwick DM, Cretin S, Keeler E. Cholesterol, children, and heart disease: an analysis of alternatives. Pediatrics 1985; 68: 721).

18. Cheung AM, Tsevat J. Commentary: economic evaluations of smoking interventions. Preventive Medicine 1997; 26: 271.

19. Auld et al. (2002; see note 12).

20. Rabon R, de Charro F. EQ-5D: a measure of health status from the EuroQol Group. Annals of Medicine 2001; 33: 337.

21. For a comparison of the pros and cons of HYEs and QALYs, see Johannesson M, Pliskin JS, Weinstein MC (Are healthy-years equivalents an improvement over quality-adjusted life years? Medical Decision Making 1993; 13: 281).

22. Hudak PL, McKeever P, Wright JG. The metaphor of patients as customers: implications for measuring satisfaction. Journal of Clinical Epidemiology 2003; 56: 103.

23. *Patient satisfaction*. See Carr-Hill RA. (The measurement of patient satisfaction. Journal of Public Health Medicine 1992; 14: 236). Issues and concepts are reviewed in detail by Sitzia J, Wood N (Patient satisfaction: a review of issues and concepts. Social Science and Medicine 1997; 45: 1829), who point out that very few patients express dissatisfaction, and that maybe a report of satisfaction 'should not be interpreted as indicating that care was "good" but simply that nothing "extremely bad" occurred'.

Nine methods of measuring patient satisfaction are compared by Ford RC, Bach SA, Fottler MD (Methods of measuring patient satisfaction in health care organizations. Health Care Management Review 1997; 22: 74).

24. Bernhart MH, Wiadnyana IG, Wihardjo H, Pohan I. Patient satisfaction in developing countries. Social Science and Medicine 1999; 48: 989.

25. Donabedian A. Evaluating the quality of medical care. Milbank Memorial Fund Quarterly 1966; 44(3, part 2): 166.

26. *Equity* is discussed by Lucas AO (Health policies in developing counties. In: Detels R, McEwen J, Beaglehole R, Tanaka H (eds), Oxford textbook of public health, 4th edn, vol 1. The scope of public health. New York, NY: Oxford University Press; 2002. pp. 281–295).

27. Pokras R, Hufnagel VG. Hysterectomies in the United States, 1965–84. Vital and Health Statistics series 13 no. 92; 1987.

28. Hart JT. The inverse-care law. Lancet 1971; i: 495.

6

The Study Population

The *study population* is the group that is studied, either *in toto* or by selecting a sample of its members. The units in the group may be persons, families, medical records, certificates, nursery schools, specimens of milk, house-flies, or dustbins. In the following discussion, emphasis will be placed on human study populations. If a sample is chosen, the study population from which it is selected may be called the *sampled population* or the *parent population*.

There may be more than one study population, e.g. in a group-based epidemiological study that compares countries, or an evaluative study that compares health-care organizations. A cohort study may be performed in a single population, or in more than one. In a case-control study, cases and controls should ideally be drawn from the same study population (the selection of subjects for a case-control study will be discussed in Chapter 9).

At an early stage in the planning of any study, a number of issues concerning the study population (or populations) may require consideration.

Study population and selection of subjects

1. What study population? What are its characteristics?
2. Does the study population represent a broader reference population?
3. Will sampling be used (see Chapter 8)?
4. Will controls be used (see Chapter 7)?

Selecting the Study Population

Often, the investigator will have implicitly chosen the study population when defining the topic of the investigation, because of interest in a specific community, a specific health programme, or the testing of a treatment for a specific category of patient. In other instances it may be necessary to make a purposeful choice of a study population, taking account of appropriateness and practicability.

The *appropriateness* of the study population refers mainly to its suitability for the attainment of the objectives of the study. If the hypothesis is that cancer is related to the consumption of carrots or cucumbers, is the population one where

Research Methods in Community Medicine: Surveys, Epidemiological Research, Programme Evaluation, Clinical Trials   J. H. Abramson and Z. H. Abramson   Copyright © 2008, John Wiley & Sons Ltd

it can be expected that there will be sufficient variation in carrot or cucumber intake to permit the hypothesis to be tested? On the other hand, there may be too much variation in a population, and the objectives may be such that they can be best met by restricting the study to a selected category, such as one sex or a single age group or families of a standard size and composition, in order to avoid the effects of characteristics that may confuse the issue. Maybe the study would best be performed in a very special kind of population – among vegetarians or monks – or in an occupational group subjected to seasonal emotional stress. The choice of a suitable study population is one of the factors making for originality in research. Paradoxically, some aetiological processes may best be investigated in a population where the disease under study is rare; it would be difficult to study the possibility that asymptomatic urinary tract infection may be an occasional cause of anaemia in a population with a high prevalence of anaemia caused by hookworm disease or dietary iron deficiency.

A specific study population may also be chosen because it is believed to be typical of a broader reference population to which the investigator wishes to generalize the findings. If a trial is restricted to a small subgroup of patients, say patients with severe disease, its results may be applicable only to people with severe disease. If the screening test under study is intended for use in a general practice, there is little point in testing it in a hospital population. The study population in clinical studies should resemble the reference population with respect to severity and duration of illness, age, sex, other sociodemographic characteristics, accompanying illnesses and medications, and any other factors that might influence the result of the study.[1]

Practical questions may arise. Is the proposed study population one about which it will be possible to obtain the required information? Is it an 'accessible' population to which the investigator already has an *entrée*? Is it likely to cooperate in the study so that a low nonparticipation rate can be expected, or will it be a resistant one, possibly as a result of having been overresearched in the past? If patients with a specific disease are to be studied, will it be possible to identify enough cases to yield useful conclusions? If a long-term follow-up study is planned, is the population so mobile that it may be difficult to maintain contact with the subjects? A preliminary exploratory survey may sometimes be required in order to answer such questions.

The study population or populations should be clearly and explicitly defined in terms of place, time and any other relevant criteria.[2]

In a longitudinal study, the study population may be a *closed* or *fixed cohort*, which individuals cannot enter after the onset of follow-up. It can be regarded as closed even in cohort studies and trials where individuals enter, and their follow-up starts, at different calendar times, determined by the occurrence of some event (e.g. swimming in polluted water, or myocardial infarction). Alternatively, the study population may be a *dynamic* one (such as the population of a city) that individuals can enter or leave at any time. A dynamic population may or may not be stable, in the sense that its size and characteristics may or may not remain unchanged during the period of the study.

Denominator data, i.e. facts about the size and relevant characteristics (age, sex, etc.) of the study population, are essential for the computation of rates[3] and other meaningful measures of group health. As an illustration, a survey based on obituary columns in the *British Medical Journal* revealed that doctors of Indian origin tended to die young – at an average age of 61.8 years, compared with 75.2 years for doctors born in the United Kingdom (a difference very unlikely to be due to chance; $P < 0.001$). This finding, it was suggested, might be due to a higher risk of coronary heart disease. But no denominator data were presented, without which the likeliest explanation is simply that doctors of Indian origin in Britain during the period covered by the study were younger than other doctors. This was pointed out in letters to the editor.[4] When numbers of cases are presented instead of rates, they are sometimes referred to as *floating numerators*.

In studies where individuals remain in the study population for different periods it is important to obtain information on times of entry and exit, as a basis for the computation of a person-time denominator expressed in person-years[3] or other person-time units. This is the sum total of the periods during which individual members are in the study population.

Obtaining denominator data may present no special difficulty, e.g. in a morbidity survey where information is obtained about all subjects, irrespective of whether they have the disease under study. Sometimes, however, it may not be easy. The denominator data required for the above study of doctors' deaths, e.g. the age distribution of living doctors of different origins, were not readily available. In some studies, numerator and denominator data come from different sources – e.g. in a study of correlates of infant mortality, from death and birth certificates respectively – and it becomes necessary to check whether the sources provide the required data and whether they use comparable definitions. These problems should be explored and tackled while the study is still on the drawing board.

Especially in studies requiring the cooperation of the subjects, nonrespondents or nonparticipants may bias the findings, since respondents and nonrespondents may differ with respect to whatever is being studied, and it may be difficult to apply the findings even to the study population, let alone a wider reference population. In a study of cardiovascular diseases in California, nonrespondents were especially likely to be smokers and were much less likely to have a family history of heart disease.[5] In Sweden, over half the nonparticipants in a health survey said their reason was that they were ill or in regular contact with a doctor. Social insurance records revealed that nonparticipants in another Swedish study had over five times as many days of sickness, on average, as did participants.[6] In Switzerland, people who refused to participate in a health survey had particularly high health-care expenditures.[7] In most of 27 populations in which cardiovascular risk factors were monitored in community-based samples, nonrespondents were especially likely to be single and less well educated, and to have poorer lifestyles and health profiles.[8]

Exploration of the possibility of this kind of bias generally starts with a comparison of the demographic characteristics of the respondents with those of the nonrespondents (or those of the study population as a whole). From a practical point of view, the study plan should, therefore, include efforts to collect limited easy-to-get information concerning the nonrespondents, or a representative sample of them.

What Does the Study Population Represent?

If a study population is believed to be typical of a broader population to which the findings may be generalized, then the latter population may be termed the *reference population* or *external population*.[9] As an example, the study population may comprise the elderly people in a given neighbourhood, all or a sample of whom may be studied; the investigators may decide they can apply the findings to elderly people in the whole city or nation or world. There may be several possible reference populations – people with a given disease attending a given clinic during a given week may be studied with the intention of applying the findings to patients attending the clinic at other times, or to patients attending other clinics, or to all patients with the disease.

Consideration should be given to specific features of the study population that may affect the validity of generalizations of the findings to broader populations. For example:

1. *Volunteer populations.* People who volunteer to enter a study or submit to a procedure may differ in many respects from those who do not – even in their chances of living or dying.[10] Therefore, the findings in a volunteer population do not necessarily apply to the population at large. In some circumstances, people who are anxious about their health may be those most likely to volunteer; in others, they may be the most reluctant. Therefore, it is, for example, wrong to evaluate an immunization procedure by immunizing volunteers and then comparing them with persons who have not been immunized. Studies of volunteers have their place: the finding, in a 17-year cohort study of 11,000 'vegetarians and other health conscious people' recruited through health-food shops, vegetarian societies, and magazines, that daily consumption of fresh fruit was associated with a significantly reduced mortality might or might not be applicable to the general population (whose total mortality was double that of the cohort), but it was certainly of interest to vegetarians and other health-conscious people.[11]

2. *Hospital or clinic populations.* People receiving medical care are obviously not representative of the general population or, necessarily, of all ill persons. People with rheumatoid arthritis who are treated in hospital may differ from those receiving ambulant care, and both groups may differ from patients with this disease who do not receive medical care for it. Expectant mothers who receive care from physicians may have different characteristics from those who do not – they may have higher incomes and include fewer teenagers,[12] or they may differ in other ways. Furthermore, the chance of entering a clinic population may vary for different diseases (or other characteristics) and for various combinations of characteristics, and this may produce spurious associations. For example, if people who have two specific diseases at the same time have an especially high chance of hospitalization, then a study of hospital patients may reveal an association between the two diseases even if there is no such association in the population as a whole. If the two diseases carry different chances of hospitalization, a third characteristic (another disease, or a suspected aetiological factor) might, for this reason, turn out to be more frequently associated with one of the two diseases than with the other. This problem of the

interplay of admission rates, which is referred to as *Berkson's bias*[13] (*admission rate bias*) may arise in any population (not only hospital or clinic populations) in which individuals with different characteristics have different chances of inclusion. The use of hospital or clinic patients in case-control studies is discussed on p. 96.

3. *Populations with good medical records.* It is often tempting to carry out studies in specific practices or clinics in which practitioners maintain good clinical records or are prepared to keep especially detailed records for the purposes of the study. This may be an essential condition for some studies, e.g. surveys of the work of general practitioners. But the doctors who are selected in this way may be singular in other respects also, and their practices may be atypical.

4. *People living at home.* A study population comprising people living at home necessarily excludes those who are in hospitals, old folks' homes, and other institutions; there may, thus, be a selective exclusion of persons with diseases and other conditions of interest to the investigator. Young adults who are unfit for army service may be overrepresented in community samples in a country where such service is compulsory.

5. *Patients notified as having a disease.* Even if notification is compulsory, it is unlikely that all cases are notified, and the notified cases may not be representative. Socially unacceptable diseases, such as sexually transmitted ones, may be more fully notified by public agencies than by private physicians. A study in the United States showed underreporting (particularly by private physicians) of hepatitis B patients who were homosexual.[14]

6. *Autopsy populations.* Persons submitted to autopsy are obviously not necessarily representative of all decedents. Also, Berkson's bias may occur. It played a role in a well-known epidemiological blunder, the discovery in 1929 of an apparent 'antagonism' between tuberculosis and cancer, which led to the institution of a 'programme for treating cancer patients with tuberculin'.[15]

7. *Groups characterized by their behaviour or occupation* (smokers, joggers, migrants, bus drivers, etc.). It is often worth considering the selective factors that may have led to membership in these groups or exclusion from them, especially if health status may have played a role. This has been called *membership bias*.[16] Persistent cigarette smokers may be healthier than ex-smokers, not because smoking is salubrious, but because people stop smoking because of illness. The mental health status of immigrants may be a reflection of the characteristics that led to migration, rather than of the stresses or rewards of migration. Since ill health interferes with work, workers are *ipso facto* healthier, on average, than nonworkers (this is termed the *healthy worker effect*).[16] Since having children may keep women away from work, working women may be relatively infertile (*the infertile worker effect*).[17] Patients who take their medications regularly may be more likely to engage in a variety of health-promoting behaviours, whose influence might be confused with the influence of the medication (the *healthy user effect*).[18] If there are many cases where ill health has led to the adoption of a sedentary occupation, or retirement from work, or weaning from the breast, relationships that are subsequently detected between health and sedentary work, retirement or breast feeding may be misinterpreted. Membership

bias may crop up in unexpected places: a follow-up study in Finland showed that poor health at the age of 14 was predictive of a heavier coffee consumption at the age of 18, suggesting a *'sick drinker effect'*.[19]

8. *Populations in which the same individuals appear more than once*. If the same individuals appear more than once in a study population, then the findings in these individuals may have an undue effect on the results.[20] This might arise in a study of the correlates of gastroenteritis, based on an investigation of all cases of this disease treated in hospital, including repeated hospitalizations of the same patients. A list of women who received antenatal care may include repeated pregnancies of the same women. Similarly, patients who consult their doctor frequently will be overrepresented in a study based on records of medical visits; unless the study is focused on episodes of disease or medical visits, it may be decided to limit each person to a single appearance, e.g. by using the first visit or a randomly selected one.

9. *Internet users*. Employment of the Internet for conducting a study offers several potential advantages (see Chapter 35). But the study population is obviously a selected one; Internet users are computer literate, and they currently tend to be young, male and educationally and socio-economically advantaged. Nor will the study sample necessarily represent Internet users in general, since inclusion generally depends on coming across an invitation to participate and volunteering to do so. In a study of patients with ulcerative colitis, those who had been treated surgically and responded to an Internet invitation to fill in SF-36 and bowel disease questionnaires turned out to be younger, well off, well educated, and in worse health than post-surgery patients drawn from a surgical clinic.[21]

Notes and References

1. Bornhoft G, Maxion-Bergemann S, Wolf U, Kienle G S, Michalsen A, Vollmar HC, Gilbertson S, Mathiessen PF. Checklist for the qualitative evaluation of clinical studies with particular focus on external validity and model validity. BMC Medical Research Methodology 2006; 6: 56.

2. A written record should be kept of the criteria for inclusion in the study population. These should be stated explicitly; e.g. if residents of a stated neighbourhood are to be studied, what is a 'resident'? (6 months' stay is often used as a criterion). If unforeseen problems of definition arise subsequently (e.g. students who live at home at weekends only), the new decisions should also be recorded so that they can be applied uniformly.

3. See notes 3 and 4, Chapter 10.

4. Wright DJM, Roberts AP. Which doctors die first? Analysis of BMJ obituary columns. British Medical Journal 1996; 313: 1581. Khaw K-T. Letters: Lower mean age at death in doctors of Indian origin may reflect different age structures. British Medical Journal 1997; 314: 1132. McManus C. Letters: Recording the doctors' sex might have led authors to suspect their conclusions. British Medical Journal 1997; 314: 1132.

5. Criqui MH, Barrett-Connor E, Austin M. Differences between respondents and non-respondents in a population-based cardiovascular disease study. American Journal of Epidemiology 1978; 108: 367.

6. Janzon L, Hanson B S, Isacsson S-O, Lindell S-E, Steen B. Factors influencing participation in health surveys: results from prospective population study 'Men born in 1914' in Malmo, Sweden. Journal of Epidemiology and Community Health 1986; 40: 174. Bergstrand R, Vedin A, Wilhelmsson C, Wilhelmsen L. Bias due to non-participation and heterogeneous sub-groups in population surveys. Journal of Chronic Diseases 1983; 36: 725.

7. Etter J-F, Perneger TV. Analysis of non-response bias in a mailed health survey. Journal of Clinical Epidemiology 1997; 50: 1123.

8. Tolonen H, Dobson A, Kulathinal S. Effect on trend estimates of the difference between survey respondents and non-respondents: results from 27 populations in the WHO MONICA Project. European Journal of Epidemiology 2005; 20: 887.

9. Other terms for the *reference population* are *target population* and *theoretical population*. The term 'target population' is best avoided in this context, since it is sometimes used for the sampled population and sometimes for the reference population. In the context of health care, it refers of course to the population at which a programme is directed. 'Target population' has also been used to refer to the population that the investigator wished to study or sample, before the loss of members through nonresponse or other reasons, leaving a study population not necessarily representative of the target population.

10. In Pennsylvania, respondents to an advertisement inviting people aged 65 or more to participate in an epidemiological study had a significantly lower mortality, over the next 6–8 years, than randomly selected subjects of the same age (Ganguli M, Lutle ME, Reynolds MD, Dodge HH. Random versus volunteer selection for a community-based study. Journals of Gerontology, Series A, Biological Sciences and Medical Sciences 1998; 53: M39).

11. Key TJA, Thorogood M, Appleby PN, Burr ML. Dietary habits and mortality in 11000 vegetarians and health conscious people: results of a 17 year follow up. British Medical Journal 1996; 313: 775.

12. Peoples-Sheps MD, Kalsbeek WD, Siegel E. Why we know so little about prenatal care worldwide: an assessment of required methodology. Health Services Research 1988; 23: 361.

13. Real-life examples of Berkson's bias, from surveys in Ontario, include the detection of a strong association between diseases of the respiratory and locomotor systems in hospital data but not in the general population, and the finding that fatigue was positively associated with allergic and metabolic disease in the general population, but negatively in hospital data (Roberts RS, Spitzer WO, Delmore T, Sackett DL. An empiric demonstration of Berkson's bias. Journal of Chronic Diseases 1978; 31: 119).

    In a clinic, the rate of neurological disorders in boys was found to be double that in girls; this unusual finding was attributed to the fact that the ratio of boys to girls was 4:1 in this clinic (Brown GW. Berkson fallacy revisited: spurious conclusions from patient surveys. American Journal of Diseases of Children 1976; 130: 56).

    In a hospital, a problem arose in a study of a malignant disease because cancer was apparently regarded as a sufficient reason for hospitalization of patients, whereas noncancer patients with whom they might be compared tended to be admitted only if they had multiple diseases (Robertson SJ, Grufferman S, Cohen HJ. Hospital versus random digit dialing controls in the elderly: observations from two case-control studies. Journal of the American Geriatric Society 1988; 36: 119).

    Algebraic explanations of Berkson's fallacy are given by Fleiss JL, Levin B, Paik MC (Statistical methods for rates and proportions, 3rd edn. New York, NY: Wiley; 2003. pp. 9–13).

14. Alter MJ, Mares A, Hadler SC *et al*. The effect of underreporting on the apparent incidence and epidemiology of acute viral hepatitis. American Journal of Epidemiology 1987; 125: 133.

15. Lilienfeld AM, Lilienfeld DE. Foundations of epidemiology, 2nd edn. New York, NY: Oxford University Press; 1980. pp. 203–204. Mainland D. Elementary medical statistics, 2nd edn. Philadelphia, PA: WB Saunders; 1963. pp. 121–122.

16. As an example of the healthy worker effect, a longitudinal study of a cohort of workers exposed to granite dust revealed that those who were still at work after 5 years had significantly less deterioration in their lung function than 'drop-outs' (Eisen EA, Wegman DH, Louis TA, Smith TJ, Peters JM. Healthy worker effect in a longitudinal study of one-second forced expiratory volume (FEV1) and chronic exposure to granite dust. International Journal of Epidemiology 1995; 24: 1154).

17. Joffe M. Biases in research in reproduction and women's work. International Journal of Epidemiology 1985; 14: 118.

18. Brookhart MA, Patrick AR, Dormuth C, Avorn J, Shrank W, Cadarette SM, Solomon DH. Adherence to lipid-lowering therapy and the use of preventive health services: an investigation of the healthy user effect. American Journal of Epidemiology 2007; 166: 348.

19. Hemminki E, Rahkonen O, Rimpela M. Selection to coffee drinking by health – who becomes an adolescent coffee drinker? American Journal of Epidemiology 1988; 127: 1088.

20. Bias due to the overrepresentation of frequent attenders in a study that is based on records of medical visits can be controlled by a weighting procedure. This is described by Shepard DS, Neutra R (American Journal of Public Health 1977; 67: 743), who show how estimates of the numbers and characteristics of hypertensive patients attending a medical clinic can be derived from a study of visits.

21. Soetikno RM, Mrad R, Pao V, Lenert LA. Quality-of-life research on the Internet: feasibility and potential biases in patients with ulcerative colitis. Journal of the American Medical Inforatics Association 1997; 4: 426.

7

Control Groups

Controls are never needed in studies in which hypotheses are not tested, and are sometimes superfluous in studies that do test hypotheses. In Bradford Hill's words, 'If we survey the deaths of infants in the first month of life and find that so many are caused by dropping the baby on its head on the kitchen floor I am not myself convinced that we need controls to convince us that it is a bad habit. If, on the other hand, so many of the deaths are found to be of infants whose mothers had influenza during pregnancy then I should shriek for controls before I was satisfied that the two events were related'.[1] The fact that 79% of patients receiving lithotripsy treatment for kidney stones in Wyoming chose country-western music when asked what they would like to hear during the procedure[2] does not convincingly indicate that country-western music is associated with kidney stones, in the absence of a comparison with Wyomingites without kidney stones.

The term 'control' is used with various connotations in epidemiologic studies.[3] In the present context, it refers to a group (or its members) with which study subjects are compared. The controls generally differ from the study subjects in their exposure to a postulated aetiological factor (in a cohort study), in their disease experience (in a case-control study), or in their exposure to an experimental treatment or programme (in a trial).

Controls should be selected from the same study population as the study subjects with whom they are compared, or (failing this) from a similar study population. In any type of controlled study, and however the controls are selected, the analysis should include a comparison of all the possibly relevant characteristics of the study and control groups to see whether there are differences that may explain the findings of the study.

Use is sometimes made of *matched controls*; that is, controls chosen in such a way that with regard to selected characteristics they are the same as, or similar to, the study subjects or groups with whom they are compared.

This chapter will deal with matching and then with the selection of controls for cohort studies and trials. The use of controls in trials will be discussed more fully in Chapters 32 (clinical trials) and 33 (programme trials). The selection of controls in case-control studies will be considered in Chapter 9. Cross-sectional and cohort studies of total populations have built-in controls.

Research Methods in Community Medicine: Surveys, Epidemiological Research, Programme Evaluation, Clinical Trials   J. H. Abramson and Z. H. Abramson   Copyright © 2008, John Wiley & Sons Ltd

Matching

If there are differences between the characteristics of study and control groups, they may sometimes obscure or distort ('confound') the associations being studied. For example, one of the reasons for the 12-year delay in ending the iatrogenic epidemic of retrolental dysplasia, a blinding disease of premature infants caused by high-dose oxygen therapy, was that cases were compared with controls who were mainly full-term. Because of the difference in maturity status there were more congenital, placental and prenatal disorders in the cases than in the controls, leading to the conclusion that retrolental dysplasia was the result of anoxia during intrauterine development.[4]

One way of avoiding or reducing such differences, so as to ensure similarity with respect to possible confounding factors that may distort the findings, is to match the control group with the study group.

Matching reduces the confounding effect (less well in case-control than in follow-up studies; see p. 97) and (under certain conditions) adds to the precision with which the association under study is estimated.[5]

Matching can be done in two ways:

1. Each control may be selected so as to be similar to a specific member of the study group (*individual matching* or, if a single control is chosen per case, *pair matching*). This may be done by formulating matching criteria and then seeking suitable controls for each subject. A large pool of potential controls may be needed if there are more than two or three matching criteria and a very close match is demanded on each of them. Individual matching may also be achieved by selecting a spouse, sibling, friend, neighbour[6] or fellow worker, a child born on the same day in the same hospital, a patient in the same hospital ward, etc.
2. The controls may be so selected that, as a group, they are in specified respects (e.g. age and sex) similar to the study group (*group matching*). For *frequency matching*, the potential controls are divided into strata (say age–sex groups) and an appropriate number of individuals is then selected from each stratum, so that the frequency distributions are similar in the study and control groups. *Mean matching* ('balancing') tries to produce groups with similar mean values.

The control and study groups need not be equal in size; if individual matching is used, then two or more controls can be selected for each subject. There may be good reasons for having unequal groups. If there is a constraint on the number of subjects, then having more than one control per subject compensates for the small number of subjects. This may be especially important in a clinical trial where treatment is inconvenient, costly or potentially hazardous. The additional benefit is small if the ratio is increased beyond three or four; but a higher ratio may be indicated on economic grounds if the treatment is very expensive.

Whatever method is used, clear-cut rules[7] should be laid down, in order to ensure objectivity when deciding whether a match is sufficiently close and when choosing between two or more candidates who meet the matching criteria. It may be required, for example, that the value of the matching variable must be the same as in the case, or that the control must be in the same category as the case (e.g. the same 5-year age group: 30–34, 35–39, etc.; this is sometimes called *category*, *within-class* or *stratified matching*), or must have a defined degree of similarity (e.g. an age within 2 years of the case's; this is *caliper matching*).

Matching may be made easier (and less exact) by reducing the number of matching criteria or relaxing the requirements. For example, an age disparity of up to 10 years may be regarded as acceptable. Alternatively, it may be decided that a close match will be sought, but a less close match (using a less strict criterion) will be accepted if necessary. A method sometimes used is *'nearest available' matching*, i.e. selecting the potential control who is nearest (say, in age) to the case. This method has the advantage that matches can always be found, but it is less effective than other methods in the control of confounding.

The rules must clearly state the matching procedures and priorities. If one potential control is closely matched in age and less closely in educational level, and another is closely matched in education and less closely in age, which will be chosen? Standard procedures should also be laid down to cover instances where there are two or more potential controls who satisfy the criteria equally. It may be decided to select the one who is closest to the case in respect of a given matching variable (age) or the one who best meets one or more additional matching criteria, which are applied only in such instances. A random choice (e.g. by using random numbers) may also be made, to ensure objectivity.

Matching should not be undertaken when it is unnecessary, since it has disadvantages:

1. It complicates the selection of controls and may be costly. The study may suffer delay if large numbers of potential controls have to be screened, or if a pool of potential controls is not immediately available (e.g. if the controls are patients suffering from a specific condition and it is necessary to wait for the appearance of a suitable candidate).
2. It may lead to the exclusion of subjects for whom suitable controls cannot be found. If there are numerous matching variables, then many subjects may be 'wasted' in this way and the study group may become less representative of the reference population.
3. A confounding variable that has been controlled by matching can no longer be studied as an independent variable. If cases and controls are matched for age, then it becomes impossible to study the relationship of the disease to age: a comparison of the ages of the cases and controls will provide information only on the effectiveness of the matching procedure. Also, it becomes difficult to reach useful conclusions on associations with variables that are closely linked with age. Note, however, that the effect of age as a modifier (see p. 271) of other relationships can still be examined, i.e. it is possible to see whether an association – between, say, drinking and coronary heart disease – is consistent in different age groups.
4. The groups may inadvertently be made so similar that the difference that the investigation was designed to seek may be falsely reduced or masked ('matched out') in the crude data; this is sometimes called *overmatching*.
5. Unnecessary matching (i.e. in the absence of a strong confounding effect) may impair the precision with which the association can be measured.[5] This, too, is sometimes called *overmatching*.

Matching is useful if three conditions are met (the first two are prerequisites for a strong confounding effect):

1. There is likely to be a marked disparity between the groups with respect to some characteristic if the characteristic is not 'held constant' by matching.
2. The characteristic is believed to be strongly associated with whatever is being compared in the groups (e.g. disease incidence in a prospective study, or exposure to a causal factor in a case-control study).
3. The groups are so small (e.g. because of the cost of studying large groups), or there are so many potential confounders (see p. 274), or the confounders have so many categories, that the handling of confounding effects by statistical means during the analysis may be unfeasible or inefficient.

Controls in Cohort Studies

In a cohort study of the association between a suspected causal factor and a disease, the ideal control group for the cohort exposed to the factor is a group that would have the same disease rate as the exposed group, if the factor was unassociated with the disease. The closest approximation to this ideal is achieved in a cohort study of a total population (or a representative sample of a total population), since inclusion in the study is not influenced by exposure to the factor. Such a study has built-in controls (an *internal comparison group*). A well-known example is the cohort study of British physicians by Doll and Hill, which provided one of the first clear demonstrations of the effect of smoking on lung cancer mortality.[8] In cohort studies of total populations, the amount or duration of exposure (number of cigarettes per day, duration of smoking, etc.) can often be taken into account, instead of simplistically using two groups, 'exposed' and 'nonexposed'; this permits examination of the dose–response relationship (see p. 283).

If the study is not of a total population or a representative sample, then a control group of unexposed people should, if possible, be selected from the same population as the exposed group. If the exposed people are members of a special population (e.g. workers in a factory), then the controls should be drawn from the same special population. Failing this, the comparison population should be an external one that is as similar as possible to the population of which the exposed persons are members, with respect to factors (other than the exposure) that may influence the risk of incurring the disease.

Since it is not always possible to find a completely satisfactory control group, it is frequently decided to use two or more control groups drawn from different sources, and subsequently see whether the various comparisons yield similar conclusions. In a study of workers exposed to a specific occupational hazard, for example, one comparison might be with disease incidence in the general population – a comparison that may be biased by the 'healthy worker effect' (see p. 65). Another might be with workers in some other industry. Sometimes both internal and external comparison groups are used.

The choice of control groups is sometimes constrained by the need to ensure that the same methods of investigation, especially for case detection, are applied as in the exposed group or groups. It is advisable to gather information – for both exposed and nonexposed subjects – about all factors that may affect the risk of the disease, so that their influence can be taken into account when the findings are analysed and interpreted.

The need to define 'nonexposure' may sometimes lead the investigator to give closer thought to the meaning of 'exposure' and to formulate the research hypothesis more precisely. What control group is required in a cohort study of the effect of smoking? This depends on the definition of smoking. Are 'nonsmokers' people who have never smoked at all, or those who have never smoked regularly, or those who do not smoke at present, or those who have not smoked for a given number of years, or those who have not smoked (say) at least 20 cigarettes a day for a continuous period of at least 10 years?

Controls in Experiments

'I was a 90 lb. weakling, and look at me now!' is not convincing evidence of the effectiveness of a course of treatment, as the change may well have been due to processes of adolescence or other factors quite unrelated to the treatment. To be reasonably convincing, 'before–after' studies of this sort (without external controls) must be replicated, or extended in time so as to see what happens when the treatment is withdrawn.

In most experiments, separate control groups are used. The findings in the experimental group are compared with those in a control group not exposed to the experimental procedure. Infant mortality dropped after the introduction of a programme, but what happened in other (similar) regions? This approach is often the best available method of evaluating a programme or procedure. In the absence of an external control group we run the risk that we may think that a change is a specific effect of the intervention that we are testing, when actually it is not.[9] The main circumstances that may confuse the issue are:

1. *Changes that are due to other causes.* People may recover from illnesses for reasons quite unconnected with the care they receive. Changes happen because people age, they mature, they adapt to disability, they become integrated into new social settings, and external events and changes exert their influence on them. Food prices may alter, foodstuffs low in calories or saturated fats may become readily available, there may be a publicity campaign about cigarette smoking, a new medical service may be started, a war may break out or come to an end, etc.

2. *Nonspecific effects caused by the intervention or the experiment.* The administration of a treatment may produce a *placebo effect* or a *nocebo effect*[10] (from the Latin for 'to please' and 'to injure' respectively) that expresses the subject's belief or expectancy concerning its consequences. The placebo effect of a drug or procedure is cognate to a nonspecific *caring effect*[11] resulting from the subjects' belief that they are receiving care. If the subjects know that they are participating in an experiment, this awareness may in itself produce changes (the *guinea-pig effect*). This is part of the possible influence of the experimental situation as a whole – the examinations and other procedures,

the feedback of investigation findings, the special relations with investigators, etc. – that is sometimes called the *Hawthorne effect*. This name comes from a study of industrial efficiency at the Hawthorne Plant in Chicago in the 1920s,[12] which showed that work output increased when experimental changes were made to working conditions, even when these were worsened. Production rose both when illumination was improved and when it was reduced to the brightness of a moonlit night. In a study of smoking by schoolchildren, the Hawthorne effect was considered as a reason for the relatively low rates observed in schools that had been surveyed repeatedly.[13] A Hawthorne effect has been demonstrated in a randomized controlled clinical trial.[14]

3. *Artefacts*. The change may not be real, but only an expression of a change in methods of measurement – in diagnostic criteria or techniques, in the completeness of recording or notification, in laboratory procedures, etc.

4. *Regression towards the mean*.[15] Even if the methods have not altered, an artefact may arise if measurements are very unreliable or if the characteristics they measure are very unstable. If such measurements are repeated in the same subjects, the second value will tend to be lower than the first if the initial value was high, and vice versa. A study sample selected on the grounds of initially high values of blood pressure will tend to have lower blood pressures when examined a second time, and this may be misinterpreted as an effect of treatment. There are various ways of overcoming this problem, one of the simplest being to use a suitable control group that is selected in the same way as the intervention group.

Depending on circumstances and the detailed objectives of the study, a control group may be exposed to an alternative treatment or programme, to no intervention whatever, or to placebo treatment. In therapeutic trials the controls are commonly given the usual standard treatment for their disease.

The groups that are compared should be similar, apart from their exposure to the experimental treatment. A story is told of a sea captain who tested a seasickness remedy during a voyage and was very enthusiastic about the results: 'Practically every one of the controls was ill, and not one of the subjects had any trouble. Really wonderful stuff'. A sceptic asked how he had chosen the controls and subjects. 'Oh, I gave the stuff to my seamen and used the passengers as controls'.[16] Similarly, trials in which a vaccine was administered to volunteers (who may be a very select group) and in which the subsequent incidence of the disease was compared with that in a general population have led to erroneous conclusions. Experiments of this sort are similar to surveys in which different populations are compared, in that all the possibly relevant characteristics of the groups should be studied and a careful search made for differences that may explain the findings of the study.

Various experimental and quasi-experimental designs, and methods of allocating subjects to experimental and control groups, will be discussed in Chapters 32 and 33.

Notes and References

1. Hill AB. Statistical methods in clinical and preventive medicine. Edinburgh: Livingstone; 1962. p. 365.

2. Childs SJ. Editorial: New etiology of urinary calculi. Infections in Urology 1997; 10(3): 69.
3. Last JM. A dictionary of epidemiology, 4th edn. New York, NY: Oxford University Press; 2001.
4. Jacobson RM, Feinstein AR. Oxygen as a cause of blindness in premature infants: 'autopsy' of a decade of errors in clinical epidemiologic research. Journal of Clinical Epidemiology 1992; 45: 1265.
5. For references and more detailed discussions of the *effects of matching*, see Rothman KJ, Greenland S (Modern epidemiology, 2nd edn. Philadelphia, PA: Lippincott-Raven; 1998. pp. 147–161) or Costanza MC (Matching. Preventive Medicine 1995; 24: 425).
6. As an example of the use of *neighbourhood controls*, in a study in Toronto, 'five age-matched controls were obtained for each case. They were also matched by neighbourhood and by type of dwelling (house or apartment) in the expectation that this would lead to reasonably close socioeconomic matching. Controls were obtained by door-to-door calls, which started at the fourth door to the right of the case and proceeded systematically round the residential block or through the apartment building'. No one was found at home in two-thirds of the dwellings visited. To get an idea of whether this produced bias in the selection of controls and, hence, influenced the findings, a separate analysis was subsequently done in which cases were compared with only 'those controls who were enrolled immediately after the case (or another control) had been interviewed – i.e. controls obtained without an intervening failure'. (Clarke EA, Anderson TW. Does screening by 'Pap' smears help prevent cervical cancer? A case-control study. Lancet 1979; ii: 1).

    In urban areas of North Carolina, a door-to-door search for neighbourhood controls matched by sex, age and race and with no history of heart attack or angina pectoris, in which the interviewer proceeded in ever-widening circles around the home of the index case, required an average of 98 minutes (94 km of travel) for each successfully matched case (Ryu JE, Thompson CJ, Crouse JR. Selection of neighborhood controls for a study of coronary heart disease. American Journal of Epidemiology 1989; 129: 407).
7. For a detailed discussion of *matching methods*, see Anderson S, Auquier A, Hauck WW *et al.* (Statistical methods for comparative studies: techniques for bias reduction. New York, NY: Wiley; 1980. Chapter 6).
8. Doll R, Hill AB. Lung cancer and other causes of death in relation to smoking; a second report on the mortality of British doctors. British Medical Journal 1956; 2: 1071. Doll R, Peto R. Mortality in relation to smoking: 20 years' observations on male British doctors. British Medical Journal 1976; 2: 1525.
9. Illustrations of misleading conclusions yielded by uncontrolled trials are cited by Ederer F (American Journal of Ophthalmology 1975; 79: 758), who cites Professor Hugo Muench of Harvard University's second law: 'Results can always be improved by omitting controls'.
10. *Placebo effects* are expressions of the patient's belief or expectancy that the treatment is beneficial; they may reflect the belief or expectancy of the healer, and the relationship between healer and patient may be a crucial factor.

    Since the term 'placebo effect' implies an action of the placebo, whereas what happens is a reaction that is erroneously attributed to the placebo, it has been suggested that a better term would be 'post-placebo response' (Feinstein AR. Post-therapeutic response and therapeutic 'style': re-formulating the 'placebo effect'. Journal of Clinical Epidemiology 2002; 55: 427).

    A poser. Which was the placebo group in a trial in which preoperative patients were divided into two groups: Group A (experimental) – visited for 5 minutes by the anaesthetist, who carefully explained what pain might be expected and tried to establish a warm and sympathetic relationship; B (control) – cursorily visited by the anaesthetist? The patients in group A subsequently needed far less pain medication, and their hospital stay was 2.6 days shorter (Egbert LD, Battit GE, Welch CE, Bartlett MI. Reduction of postoperative pain by encouragement and instruction of patients. New England Journal of Medicine 1964; 270: 825).

    Another poser. Which is the placebo group in a randomized trial that compares patients who receive a homoeopathic remedy, the preparation of which involves repeated dilution in a solvent (to the extent that a dose may contain an infinitesimal amount of the agent, or maybe none) with patients who receive only the solvent? For the results of such trials, see Linde K, Clausius N, Ramirez G, Melchart D, Eitel F, Hedges LV, Jonas WB (Are the clinical effects of homoeopathy placebo effects? A meta-analysis of placebo-controlled trials. Lancet 1997; 350: 834). According to Vandenbroucke JP (Homoeopathy trials: going nowhere. Lancet 1997; 350: 824), 'a randomized trial of "solvent only" versus "infinite dilutions" is a game of chance between two placebos'.

Nocebo effects are occasioned by anxiety, fear, mistrust or doubt, and expectations of sickness. They may find expression in the reporting of side-effects of treatments. In clinical trials they are unlikely to reach the extreme of voodoo death. See Kaada B (Nocebo – the antipode to placebo. Nordisk Medecin 1989; 104: 192), Benson H (The nocebo effect: history and physiology. Preventive Medicine 1997; 26: 612) and Hahn RA (The nocebo phenomenon: concept, evidence, and implications for public health. Preventive Medicine 1997; 26: 607).

11. *Caring effects* are described by Hart JT, Dieppe P (Caring effects. Lancet 1996; 347: 1606), who cite a randomized control trial in which patients with chronic arthritis who were phoned twice a week showed significant improvements in pain and physical and psychological disability, although they did not use more drugs or other therapies than controls; Weinberger M, Tierney WM, Booher P, Katz P (Can the provision of information to patients with osteoarthritis improve functional status? A randomized controlled trial. Arthritis and Rheumatism 1989; 36: 243); Weinberger M, Tierney WM, Cowper EA, Katz BP, Booher PA (Cost effectiveness of increased telephone contact for patients with osteoarthritis: a randomized controlled trial. Arthritis and Rheumatism 1993; 36: 243).

12. Roethlisberger FJ, Dickson WJ. Management and the worker. Cambridge, MA: Harvard University Press; 1939.

13. Murray M, Swan AV, Kiryluk S, Clarke GC. The Hawthorne effect in the measurement of adolescent smoking. Journal of Epidemiology and Community Health 1988; 42: 304.

14. A Hawthorne effect was demonstrated in a placebo-controlled clinical trial in London in which randomly allocated participants who were followed up more intensively (i.e. three assessments during 6 months of medication instead of a single assessment after 6 months) had a significantly better outcome. This was a trial of the effect of an extract of *Ginkgo biloba* leaves on the cognitive functioning of mild and moderately demented patients living in the community, in which the treatment was not found to confer any benefit (McCarney R, Warner J, Iliffe S, van Haselen R, Griffin M, Fisher P. The Hawthorne effect: a randomised, controlled trial. BMC Medical Research Methodology 2007; 7: 30).

15. The term *regression toward the mean* comes from a 19th-century finding that although tall parents tended to have tall children, the children tended to be less tall than their parents; the children of short parents tended to be taller than their parents. The principle is that 'if all the flies in a closed room are on the ceiling at eight o'clock in the morning, more flies will be below the ceiling than above the ceiling at some time during the next 24-hr period' (Schor S. The mystic statistic: the floor-and-ceiling effect. Journal of the American Medical Association 1969; 207: 120).

Ways of preventing spurious conclusions, say in a study of the effect of treatment on people with high cholesterol levels, include: (1) comparing the changes in treated and control groups that were selected in exactly the same way; (2) using two or more initial measurements (e.g. one when deciding whether the level is high enough to warrant inclusion in the trial, and another for use as the baseline for measuring change; or basing the decision on a mean of two or more measurements); and (3) statistical solutions.

The effect of regression to the mean can be estimated or avoided in the analysis. For software, see Appendix C.

See Barnett AG, van der Pols JC, Dobson AJ (Regression to the mean: what it is and how to deal with it. International Journal of Epidemiology 2005; 34: 215).

16. Wilson EB Jr. An introduction to scientific research. New York, NY: McGraw-Hill; 1952. p. 42.

8

Sampling

It is often decided to study only a part, or sample, of the study population (the 'sampled' or 'parent' population). Samples may be chosen, for example, of residents of a neighbourhood, of people with (or without) a given disease, or of people exposed (or not exposed) to a suspected causal factor. The decision to sample may be forced on the investigator by a lack of resources. The procedure may make for better use of available resources – because of the restricted number of individuals to be studied, it is possible to investigate each of them more fully than might otherwise have been possible, and to make greater efforts to ensure that information is in fact obtained from each individual. Frequently, it is decided to have the best of both worlds, by obtaining easily acquired types of information about the total study population, but limiting certain parts of the study, which require more intensive investigations, to one or more samples.

Provided that certain conditions are met, there is no difficulty in applying the results yielded by a sample to the parent population from which it has been selected, with a degree of precision that meets the investigator's requirements. Statistical techniques are available that make it possible to state with what precision and confidence such inferences may be made. The conditions to be met are:

1. The sample must be *well chosen*, so as to be representative of the parent population.
2. The sample must be *sufficiently large*. If a number of representative samples drawn from the same parent population are investigated, it can be expected that, by chance, there will be differences between the findings in each sample; this problem of *sampling variation* is reduced if the sample is large.
3. There must be *adequate coverage* of the sample. Unless information is in fact obtained about all or almost all members of the sample, the individuals studied may not be representative of the study population.

Mere size is not enough. A sample that is badly chosen or inadequately covered remains a biased one, however big it may be. This was strikingly shown by the notorious poll conducted by the Literary Digest in 1936, which, although based on 2,000,000 ballots, dismally failed to predict Roosevelt's landslide victory in the presidential election. These ballots constituted 20% of the 10,000,000 that had been sent out to an unrepresentative sample comprising Literary Digest and telephone subscribers.

Research Methods in Community Medicine: Surveys, Epidemiological Research, Programme Evaluation, Clinical Trials J. H. Abramson and Z. H. Abramson Copyright © 2008, John Wiley & Sons Ltd

How can a survey finding that 22% of sword swallowers have a history of perforation be relied upon, if responses were received from less than half of the sample?[1]

This chapter deals with sampling methods and sample size, followed by remarks on substitutions and random numbers.

Sampling Methods

A sample chosen in a haphazard fashion, or because it is 'handy', is unlikely to be a representative one. Such samples have been termed 'chunks' or 'accidental' or 'incidental' samples, or *samples of convenience*. Their use has no place in community medicine research, except possibly in exploratory and other surveys where the investigator is doing no more than obtaining a 'feel' of the situation, and in some qualitative studies (see pp. 147–149 and 318).

The recommended method is *probability sampling*, the distinctive feature of which is that each individual unit in the total population (each *sampling unit*) has a known probability of being selected. Generalizations can then be made to the 'parent' population with a measurable precision and confidence (see p. 260).

First, however, a word on the nonprobability sampling methods that are sometimes used: quota, purposive and snowball sampling. In *quota sampling*, the general composition of the sample, e.g. in terms of age, sex and social class, is decided in advance; quotas, or required numbers, are determined for, say, men and women of different ages and social classes, and the only requirement is that the right number of people be somehow found to fill these quotas. The disadvantage of this method is that the persons chosen may not be representative of the total population in each category, and generalizations made from the findings may be incorrect. *Purposive samples* are those selected because the investigator presumes that they are typical of the study population. In a study of general practices, for example, what is believed to be a representative cross-section of practices may be selected; subsequent generalizations from the findings may or may not be valid. In some qualitative studies (see p. 147) subjects are purposively selected not in order to represent the study population, but in such a way that they will express a wide range of the beliefs, practices or experiences under study. In *snowball sampling*[2] (*chain referral sampling*), people who meet the criteria for inclusion in the study are asked to name others who meet these criteria. This may be a useful way of identifying hard-to-find individuals, e.g. those with deviant or illegal behaviour, or homeless people. But the sample, say of drug abusers, will not necessarily be representative of all drug abusers.

We will discuss four types of *probability sampling* (random, systematic, cluster and stratified) – with special mention of random digit dialling – and two-stage and multistage sampling.

It is important to set up the sampling rules in advance and to avoid any possibility that selection may be influenced by whim or convenience. The interviewers in a household survey, for example, should be told in advance which homes to visit. If inclusion in the sample depends on information that is collected during the visit, then the interviewer should be given precise instructions for making the choice.[3]

Random sampling

Random sampling (or *simple random sampling*) is a technique whereby each sampling unit has the same probability of being selected: the laws of chance alone decide which of the individual units in the parent (or 'target') population will be selected. To avoid confusion with the colloquial meaning of the word 'random', i.e. 'haphazard' or 'without a conscious bias', the term *strict random sampling* is sometimes preferred.

The basic procedure is:

1. Prepare a *sampling frame*. This is usually a list showing all the units from which the sample is to be selected, arranged in any order. For example, it might be a list of the registered patients in a particular practice. The preparation of a sampling frame may sometimes require considerable effort; it is seldom easy, for example, to obtain an up-to-date list of the elderly people living in a neighbourhood. If a population registry is maintained in a country or city, this may constitute the sampling frame; but such registers are often out of date, especially with regard to addresses; moreover, with the increase in concern for the individual's right to privacy, registers of this kind are becoming less accessible to investigators. Voters' lists, telephone directories, or lists of people with driving licences may be used, but these may tend to leave out some categories of people.[4] If the frame is an incomplete and biased representation of the study population, the sample will inevitably be biased too, however strictly the rules of random sampling are applied.
2. Decide on the size of the sample (see pp. 83–85).
3. Select the required number of units at random, by drawing lots or using random numbers. The use of random numbers is explained on pp. 86–87. When one matched control has to be chosen randomly from a small group of suitable candidates, it is often simplest to draw lots or (if there are up to six candidates) to throw a die.

The ratio 'number of units in sample/number of units in sampling frame' is referred to as the *sampling ratio* or *sampling fraction*. It is usually expressed either in the form '1 in n' (e.g. '1 in 3', '1 in 4', etc.) or as a percentage or proportion.

Random sampling does not ensure that the characteristics of the sample and the population will coincide exactly; chance differences will exist, but by the use of appropriate statistical methods[5] it is possible to calculate the probability that these divergences lie within given limits (see p. 260).

Random sampling may be applied not only to the selection of subjects from a population, but to the selection of times or locations. In the latter instance, geographic areas or the coordinates of points are used as the sampling units; the sampling frame may be a map rather than a list.

Random digit dialling

In a region where nearly everyone has a telephone at home, such as the United States, where under 5% of households were without a landline telephone in 2004, *random digit dialling* – i.e. phoning numbers selected at random – is a convenient way of selecting a random sample, either for telephone interviews or for subsequent home interviews or other investigations. Phone numbers are kept in the sample only if they turn out to be for residential addresses. If there is no reply, the call is repeated a number of times, at different times and on different weekdays. A two-stage procedure may be used, whereby a sample of households is first selected by random digit dialling and information is then obtained about the members of the household, the subsequent selection of subjects being determined by age, sex, or other eligibility criteria, or by using a random or systematic selection rule, such as the choice of the member with the latest birthdate in the year. The detailed procedure[6] is designed in a way that reduces the proportion of wasted calls; unlisted numbers are not excluded. Random digit dialling is generally regarded as preferable to sampling from telephone directories, which exclude unlisted numbers.

High success rates have been reported. In some studies in the United States, information on household composition was obtained for over 90% of the residential numbers phoned, and over 80% of the eligible subjects were subsequently interviewed. Samples selected by random digit dialling have been reported to be reasonably representative of the general population; but the possible selective exclusion of underprivileged population groups and overrepresentation of households with more than one phone line may be important in some studies.

The utility of random digit dialling has, however, been impaired by new technologies,[7] such as cell phones, answering machines, voicemail, and caller identification, and by the public's resentment of telemarketing and opinion polls, which have led to a drop in response rates. Response rates for the University of Michigan's Survey of Consumer Attitudes, for example, declined from 72% in 1979 to 48% in 2003. A comparison of 17 North American studies using random digit dialling to find controls for childhood cancer cases revealed a decrease in the response rate from over 80% in the 1980s to 50–67% after the mid-1990s, mainly due to a drop in the percentage of households in which the phone was answered.

Of particular importance is the exponential growth in the use of cell phones (at the end of 2005, 62% of households in the United States had more than one cell phone). In many countries, this has been accompanied by an increase in the proportion of households without landline phones. Random digit dialling surveys in the United States – where people who have only a cell phone tend to be either young and relatively well off, or poor members of minority groups – do not include cell phones in their sampling frame. The reasons include difficulties in finding sampling frames, the fact that cell phones are personal and not linked to households (making the selection of a random sample difficult), the receipt of calls while driving and in other awkward situations, and the subscriber's obligation (in many cell phone plans) to pay for incoming calls. The inclusion of cell phones in random digit dialling surveys is less problematic in countries where cell phone users do not have to pay for incoming calls, such as Brazil and Finland. Telephone survey researchers have been urged to see the cell phone problem as an opportunity rather than a roadblock, and to find solutions – basically, the use of mixed-mode and multiple-frame approaches – to maximize coverage.[7] In studies of groups with a high usage of cell phones, text (SMS, short message service) messaging may be a useful way of stimulating and obtaining survey responses.[7]

Systematic sampling

Instead of selecting randomly, a *predetermined system* may be used. The usual technique requires a list, not necessarily numbered, of all the sampling units. Having decided on the size of the required sample, the investigator divides the number in the list by this required size in order to calculate the sampling ratio, expressed as '1 in *n*', rounds *n* off to the nearest whole number, and uses this figure *k* as a *sampling interval*. Every *k*th item in the list is then selected, starting with an item (from the first to the *k*th) selected at random. This technique is often easier than simple random sampling.

Such a sample can be considered as essentially equivalent to a random sample, provided that the list is not arranged according to some system or cyclical pattern. If a 1-in-30 systematic sample is selected from a list of persons arranged according to decreasing age, there may be an appreciable age difference between a sample where the first member selected was the first on the list and one where the first person selected was the 30th. If the list is one of dwelling units, listed in such a way that ground-floor and upper-floor dwellings alternate, then a 1-in-2 systematic sample (or any systematic sample using an even number as the sampling interval) will contain either ground-floor dwellings only or upper-floor dwellings only.

Other methods of systematic sampling may be used that do not require prior listing of the sampling units. For example, it may be decided to select every third patient admitted to a hospital, or every patient whose personal identity number, social security number, hospital registration number, or birthdate (day of month) ends with a predetermined and randomly selected digit or digits. These methods are usually chosen because of their convenience.

Cluster sampling

In cluster sampling, a simple random sample is selected not of individual subjects, but of groups or clusters of individuals. That is, the sampling units are clusters and the sampling frame is a list of these clusters. The clusters may be villages, apartment buildings, classes of schoolchildren, schools, general practices, housing units, households or families (note that these latter terms are not synonymous),[8] etc.

This is often a convenient method, especially when at the outset there is no sampling frame showing all the individual subjects. It is, of course, also more convenient to investigate people living in a relatively small number of households or villages, rather than the same number of persons who have been selected randomly and whose places of residence are, therefore, more scattered.

The technique has the disadvantage, however, that if there is a degree of similarity between the people in each cluster, (*homogeneity, high intraclass correlation*), it becomes difficult, without special methods of analysis,[9] to estimate the precision with which generalizations may be made to the parent population.

Other things being equal, a large number of small clusters is preferable to a small number of large clusters.

Stratified sampling

To use this method, the population (the sampling frame) is first divided into subgroups or *strata* according to one or more characteristics, e.g. sex and age-group, and random or systematic sampling is then performed independently in each stratum (*stratified random sampling, stratified systematic sampling*).

This procedure has the advantage that there is less sampling variation than with simple random or systematic sampling. It eliminates sampling variation with respect to the properties used in stratifying; and if the strata are more uniform than the total population with respect to other attributes, it also reduces sampling variation with respect to other properties. The greater the differences between the strata and the less the differences within the strata, the greater is the gain due to stratification.

The same sampling ratio may be used in all strata. This is called *proportional allocation*, since the number of individuals chosen in each stratum is proportional to the size of the stratum. Alternatively, different sampling ratios may be used in different strata (*disproportionate stratified sampling*). This permits heavier sampling in subgroups with few members, so as to provide acceptable estimates, not only for the population as a whole, but also for each of its subgroups. In a clinical trial, for example, this can ensure that the sample will contain enough elderly subjects for separate study – the effectiveness and safety of a treatment often differs in younger and older people.

Estimates for the total population are prepared by combining the data for the various strata. If varying sampling fractions are used, then an appropriate weighting procedure is required.[9] If a uniform sampling fraction is used, then the sample is *self-weighting* and can, for some purposes, be treated as if it were a simple random or systematic sample. The use of varying sampling ratios greatly adds to the complexity of the analysis and should not be decided upon lightly. There is, of course, no objection to the use of different sampling ratios if the strata are to be kept separate throughout the analysis, e.g. if people of different religions are to be studied as separate groups.

Two-stage and multistage sampling

In *two-stage sampling*, the population is divided into a set of first-stage sampling units (*primary sampling units*), and a sample of these units is selected by simple random, stratified or systematic sampling. Individuals are then chosen from each of these primary units, using any method of sampling. The sample may be biased if very few first-stage units are selected.

The first-stage units may be census tracts, villages, classes of schoolchildren, households, or other aggregations. They may be time periods, e.g. if the samples are the patients who attend a clinic on randomly chosen days. This method has the same advantages as cluster sampling: less travel by interviewers, fewer school teachers to negotiate with, no need for a sampling frame showing all individuals in the population, etc. Two-stage cluster sampling (the selection of clusters within the chosen first-stage sampling units) will be discussed in Chapter 31.

The analysis is simplified if *self-weighting* procedures are used. These ensure that each individual has an equal chance of entering the sample (the *equal probability of selection method*, or '*epsem*' sampling). One method is to select primary units with a probability proportional to their size (*PPS* sampling), and then choose an equal number of individuals from each primary unit; for an example, see pp. 314–315). Another is to choose the primary units by simple random or systematic sampling and then choose samples proportional to the sizes of the primary units by applying the same sampling fraction in each primary unit.[10]

Multistage sampling is used in large-scale surveys. A sample of first-stage sampling units is chosen, each of the selected units is divided into second-stage units, samples of second-stage units are selected, and so on. Different methods (simple random, stratified, systematic or cluster sampling) may be used at any stage.

Substitutions

It usually happens that, after a sample has been selected, it is found that some of the selected subjects cannot be investigated. People may have died or moved away, may refuse, or may be unavailable for a variety of other reasons. It is tempting to replace such subjects with other randomly selected subjects. This is an acceptable procedure (although an unnecessary one if expected losses were taken into account when deciding on the required sample size) provided that it is remembered that if the omissions produce a sample bias then substitutions will not remove this bias. The outcome will merely be a large biased sample instead of a small biased sample. What is important, if there are more than a few omissions, is to examine the possible bias by determining the reasons for omission and, if possible, studying the demographic and other characteristics of the subjects omitted; the relevance of this bias to the study findings can then be appraised.

Sample Size

If numbers are too small it may be impossible to make sufficiently precise and confident generalizations about the situation in the parent population, or to obtain statistical significance (see p. 273) when associations are tested. It may thus be impossible to achieve the study's objectives. On the other hand, it is wasteful to study more subjects than these objectives require. Moreover, if numbers are large enough, then any difference, however small, will be statistically significant and there may, hence, be a tendency to ascribe false importance to trivial differences. ('Samples which are too small can prove nothing; samples which are too large can prove anything.')[11]

'How big should my sample be?' has been likened to the question 'How much money should I take when I go on vacation?'[12] (How long a vacation? Doing what? Where? With whom?) Calculations of sample size require both decisions and surmises.

For example, suppose a simple random sample is to be used to provide a confidence interval of a given width for the prevalence of a disease, i.e. to indicate the range within which it is probable (with a given degree of confidence, usually 95%) that the true prevalence lies. To calculate the size of the sample needed for this purpose, the following must be plugged into the formula or the computer program:

1. A reasonably close estimate of the actual prevalence (if in complete doubt, 50% can be used; this maximizes the sample size and, hence, errs on the safe side).
2. The maximum acceptable difference between the estimated prevalence (based on the sample) and the actual prevalence; this 'acceptable margin of error' is half the confidence interval.
3. The required confidence level (usually 95%).
4. Also, optionally, the size of the population; this is relatively unimportant – its effect on the calculated sample size (the *finite population correction*)[13] is small, unless the population is very small.

To calculate the sizes of the random samples required for a comparison of two groups, e.g. to test whether there is a significant difference between the rates of some outcome in two groups in a trial or analytic survey, the requirements are:

1. Whether a two-sided or one-sided testing procedure will be used. In a trial comparing two treatments, A and B, a two-sided test examines the study hypothesis, i.e. the alternative to the null hypothesis (see note 10, Chapter 27), that A and B have different effects, whereas the study hypothesis for a one-sided test is either that A is better than B, or that B is better than A.
2. A reasonably close estimate of the actual rate in one group.
3. The magnitude of the difference (or odds, rate or risk ratio) to be detected.
4. The relative size of the two samples.
5. The required significance level (e.g. 0.05).
6. The required power (e.g. 90%), of the test (its ability to detect the difference) or the required precision (the width required for the confidence interval).

When calculating the sample sizes for a comparison of two groups, a two-sided testing procedure is usually stipulated. But the sample sizes required for a one-sided test are somewhat smaller, and, especially in a trial, smaller samples are to be preferred for both ethical and practical reasons. Therefore, it has been suggested that sample sizes should be calculated for a one-sided test whenever this is appropriate.[14] Specifically, this would apply to a trial comparing treatment A with treatment B (or a placebo), where the research question is whether A is clearly better than B with respect to a defined clinical end-point and where there is no interest whatever in knowing whether B is better than A, because such a finding would have no practical implications. Although this seems a reasonable suggestion, some authors object to it, on such grounds as that a one-sided test might not detect harmful effects of treatment A.[15]

Computation of sample sizes can be done by using computer programs[9] or by manual calculation or the use of tables or nomograms.[16] The computed size should be increased to allow for the loss of members of the sample; a larger sample will be needed if separate analyses of subgroups are intended.

Consideration must be given to practical constraints. A large sample may be difficult or impossible to find, or there may be an insufficiency of resources or time. A balance may have to be struck between the cost and the usefulness of the sample. The larger the sample, the less the sampling variation, i.e. the less the likelihood there is that the sample will be a misleading one. As a very rough guide, the usefulness of a sample is proportional not to its absolute size but to the square root of its size. To double the usefulness of a sample, its size must be increased fourfold; above a sample size of about 200, the absolute size of the sample must be augmented considerably to make an appreciable difference to its usefulness. This means that it may be necessary to balance increased cost (largely determined by the size of the sample) against increased usefulness (largely determined by the square root of its size). A *sensitivity analysis* may be helpful, i.e. a series of calculations of sample size based on different assumptions and requirements.

Samples that are to be compared with one another, e.g. in case-control studies and clinical trials, are usually kept approximately equal in size, since (for a given total sample size) this provides the most precise results (i.e. a measure of association that has a narrow confidence interval). But equal groups are by no means essential, and there may be good reasons for having unequal ones.[17] The relative size of the groups must be taken into account when calculating sample size.

In some therapeutic and prophylactic trials in which the subjects enter the investigation serially, as they become available, no initial decision is made about the sample size. Instead, rules are set up in advance whereby at any stage it can be decided, on the basis of the findings to date, whether enough subjects have been studied to give a sufficiently definite answer so that the trial can be stopped. This procedure is termed *sequential analysis.*[18]

A basic difficulty in calculations of sample size, whether they are done in advance or by the sequential method, is that the result depends on the attribute that is to be measured or compared. Samples of very different sizes are needed to study differences between two groups in their blood lipid levels, in their incidence of coronary heart disease, or in their mortality rates. It is seldom that a study is conducted to investigate only a single characteristic, and the real question often becomes not 'How many subjects do I need?' but 'With such-and-such a sample size (determined by practical considerations), about what variables and about what associations can I expect to get useful findings? – and in these circumstances, is the study worth doing?'

Cluster samples present a special case.[19] The required sample size is generally larger than for a simple random sample in the same study population, for the same maximum acceptable difference and confidence level.

The *power* of a test (i.e. its ability to demonstrate a difference if it exists) for given sample sizes can be appraised by the same basic formulae as for calculating sample size, but used in reverse, i.e. sample sizes are entered instead of power, and power is calculated instead of sample sizes. This can be very useful information when a study is being planned. But calculating power *after* the study has been done has been called an abuse of power – it is generally inappropriate, and may be misleading.[20]

Random Numbers

Tables of random numbers (digits arranged in a random order) are to be found in most statistics textbooks, or can be provided by a computer.[21] A short specimen (provided as an illustration, and not for use) is shown here (Table 8.1), and a table for actual use is provided in Appendix B.

Readers who intend to use computer programs to select samples can safely skip this section.

To use a table of random numbers for selecting a sample, a number must first be allocated to each sampling unit (e.g. from one to the total number of sampling units). Successive random numbers are then read from the table, and the sampling units whose numbers coincide with these random numbers are chosen. This is continued until enough units have been selected. Numbers not appearing in the list of sampling units are ignored, and numbers that reappear after they have already been selected are generally also ignored. The starting point is chosen at random, e.g. by shutting one's eyes and using a pin.

As an example, if five units are to be chosen out of nine, numbered from 1 to 9, one could start at (say) the '8' in row 4 of Table 8.1 and read off numbers 8, 9, 3, 1 and 6 (moving horizontally). Or one could move vertically and select the units numbered 8, 6, 7, 9 and 5; the two zeros would be ignored, as there are no subjects numbered '0'. To choose a sample from 86 units, we would use pairs of digits. Moving horizontally from the same starting-point, we would select the units numbered 89 (ignored), 31, 62, etc. To choose a sample from between 100 and 999 sampling units, we would use

Table 8.1   Random numbers

Row	Columns		
	1–4	5–8	9–12
1	96 22	74 70	80 46
2	82 14	73 36	41 54
3	21 47	59 93	48 40
4	89 31	62 79	45 73
5	63 29	90 61	86 39
6	71 68	93 94	08 72
7	05 06	96 63	58 24
8	06 32	57 11	81 59
9	91 15	38 54	73 30
10	54 60	28 35	32 94

sets of three digits (893, 162, 794, 573, 632, and so on). With between 1000 and 9999 sampling units, we would use sets of four digits (8931, 6279, etc.).

Sometimes, many numbers have to be discarded and the process may become very tedious. For example, with 195 units to choose from, if we started from the same '8' in row 4 and moved horizontally we would find only two helpful numbers among the first 16 we looked at: 162 in row 4 and 050 (or 50) in row 7. In such instances, short-cut methods may be used.[22]

Notes and References

1. A postal survey of 110 sword swallowers (members or contacts of the Sword Swallowers' Association International) revealed a history of definite or probable perforation in 22% of the respondents (10 of 46) (Witcombe B, Meyer D. Sword swallowing and its side effects. British Medical Journal 2006; 333: 1285). The percentage with perforations in the total sample might conceivably be as high as 67% (74 of 110) if all the nonrespondents were perforated, or as low as 9% (10 of 110) if all the nonrespondents were unperforated.

   Note that the sample could not include mortally wounded sword swallowers – an example of *prevalence-incidence bias* (see p. 92). Moreover, it is unlikely that all sword swallowers are members or contacts of the Sword Swallowers' Association International (which can be joined by sending a photograph of oneself swallowing a sword and completing a membership application at the association's website). Furthermore, we do not know how valid the reports of perforation and nonperforation were (see *sensitivity* and *specificity*, p. 167). Add to this is the uncertainty related to the small size (46) of the effective sample – the 95% confidence intervals (see p. 260) of the above extreme estimates are 58–76% and 4–16% respectively – and we can conclude with certainty that we can only guess exactly how dangerous this pastime is. But some sensitive souls may feel that a risk even as low as 4% is enough to put them off trying.

2. Faugier J, Sargeant M. Sampling hard to reach populations. Journal of Advanced Nursing 1997; 26: 790.

   It is claimed that there are statistical manoeuvres that can derive valid population estimates from snowball samples of hidden populations, e.g. of injection drug users or (surprise!) jazz musicians (Heckathorn DD. Respondent-driven sampling II. Deriving valid population estimates from chain-referral samples of hidden populations. Social Problems 2002; 49: 11. Salganick MJ, Heckathorn DD. Sampling and estimation in hidden populations using respondent-driven sampling. Sociological Methodology 2004; 34: 193).

3. Specimen instructions for interviewers: 'Ask if any children aged under 15 years live in the home. If 'yes', carry on with the interview if there is an "A" in the sealed envelope'; this requires a prior allocation of the required proportion of As, in accordance with the sampling fraction; the envelopes should be well shuffled.

4. See Smith W, Mitchell P, Attebo K, Leeder S (Selection bias from sampling frames: telephone directory and electoral roll compared with door-to-door population census: results from the Blue Mountains Eye Study. Australian and New Zealand Journal of Public Health 1997; 21: 127).

   A New York study that used driver's licence files as a sampling frame for the selection of controls found differences (e.g. in age, income and alcohol consumption) between cases of breast cancer with and without licences (Bowlin SJ, Leske MC, Varma A, Nasca P, Wienstein JA, Caplan L. Breast cancer risk and alcohol consumption: results from a large case-control study. International Journal of Epidemiology 1997; 26: 915).

5. For a detailed exposition of the statistical aspects of sampling and the handling of sample data, see Cochran WG (Sampling techniques, 3rd edn. New York, NY: Wiley; 1977).

6. *Random digit dialling* is usually done by the procedure described by Waksberg J (Sampling methods for random digit dialing. Journal of the American Statistical Association 1978; 73: 40).

   In a study in Washington requiring blood tests, potential subjects were chosen by random digit dialling. The response rate was 83% in this phase, 81% in the next phase (a telephone interview) and 67% in the third phase (blood-taking). The overall rate was thus 83% × 81% × 67%, or only 45%, illustrating the effect of offering repeated opportunities for nonresponse (Brown IM, Tollerud DJ, Pottern LM, Clark JW, Kase R, Blattner WA, Hoover RN. Biochemical epidemiology in community-based studies: practical lessons from a study of T-cell subsets. Journal of Clinical Epidemiology 1989; 42: 561).

7. Kempf AM, Remington PL. New challenges for telephone survey research in the twenty-first century. Annual Review of Public Health 2007; 28: 113. Nathan G. Telesurvey methodologies for household surveys – a review and some thoughts for the future. Survey Methodology 2001; 27: 31. Bunin GR, Spector LG, Olshan AF, Robison LL, Roesler M, Grufferman S, Shu X, Ross JA. Secular trends in response rates for controls selected by random digit dialing in childhood cancer studies: a report from the Children's Oncology Group. American Journal of Epidemiology 2007; 166: 109.

   A national study in the USA found that, in comparison with adults in households with landline telephones, adults who only had cell phones were more likely to smoke and have drinking binges, and less likely to receive influenza vaccine and to have medical insurance (Blumberg SJ, Luke JV, Cynamon MC. Telephone coverage and health survey estimates: evaluating the need for concern about wireless substitution. American Journal of Public Health 2006; 96: 926).

   Daily text messaging was found to be a useful procedure in a survey that found that the frequency of mild hypoglycaemia in young diabetics was three times higher than previously recognized (Tasker APB, Gibson L, Franklin V, Gregor P, Greene S. Pediatric Diabetes 2007; 8: 15).

8. One research institute used the following operational definitions:

   'A *household unit* is a room or group of rooms occupied or vacant and intended for occupancy as separate living quarters. In practice, living quarters are considered separate and therefore a housing unit when the occupants live and eat apart from any other group in the building, and there is either direct access from the outside or through a common hall, or complete kitchen facilities for the exclusive use of the occupants, regardless of whether or not they are used'. (The definition then goes on to explain what is meant by 'living apart', 'eating apart', 'direct access', etc.) A household is everyone who resides in a housing unit at the time the interviewer speaks to a household member and learns who lives there, including those who have places of residence both there and elsewhere. The household also includes people absent at the time of contact, if a place of residence is held for them in the housing unit and 'no place of residence is held for them elsewhere'.

   'A *family unit* consists of household members who are related to each other by blood, marriage, or adoption. A person unrelated to other occupants in the housing unit – or living alone – constitutes a family unit with only one member'. If there is more than one family unit in the household, the 'primary family unit' is the one that owns or rents the home. 'If families share ownership or rent equally, the one whose head is closest to age 45 is usually considered to be the primary family'. (Survey Research Center, Institute for Social Research. Interviewer's manual. Ann Arbor, MI: University of Michigan; 1976. pp. 39, 91, 94).

9. For software, see Appendix C.

10. If there are many primary units (e.g. households) it is easier to divide them into strata according to their size, and use a different sampling fraction for each stratum, the sampling fractions being proportional to the size of the units. If a single member of each selected household is required, use may be made of a simple method described by Cochran WG (1977, pp. 364–365; see note 5).

11. Sackett DL. Bias in analytic research. Journal of Chronic Diseases 1979; 32: 51.
12. Moses LE. Statistical concepts fundamental to investigations. New England Journal of Medicine 1985; 14: 890.
13. The *finite population correction*, the factor introduced into the calculation to allow for the effect of the size of the parent population, is one minus the sampling fraction. If the sampling fraction is low then this factor is close to unity, and the correction has a negligible influence and may be omitted (Armitage P, Berry G, Matthews JNS. Statistical methods in medical research, 4th edn. Blackwell Science; 2002. pp. 95–96).
14. Knottnerus JA, Bouter LM. The ethics of sample size: two-sided testing and one-sided thinking. Journal of Clinical Epidemiology 2001; 54: 109. Knottnerus JA, Bouter LM. The ethics of sample size: the whole picture should be considered. Journal of Clinical Epidemiology 200; 56: 207.
15. Moyé LA, Tita TN. Hypothesis testing complexity in the name of ethics: response to commentary. Journal of Clinical Epidemiology 2002; 55: 209. Schouten HJA. The ethics of sample size: reaction to commentary. Journal of Clinical Epidemiology 2003; 56: 206.
16. *Calculations of sample size.* To estimate a proportion from a simple random sample, the required sample size is

$$z^2 p (1 - p)/d^2$$

where $z = 1.96$ for 95% confidence, 1.645 for 90% confidence, p is the estimated proportion in the study population, and d is the acceptable margin of error.

If the finite population correction is used, the required sample size is

$$Nz^2 p(1 - p)/[d^2(N - 1) + z^2 p(1 - p)]$$

where N is the size of the study population.

For other sample size formulae, refer to a statistics text (see note 2, Chapter 26).

Formulae for use with a wide variety of statistical tests are given by Lachin JM (Introduction to sample size determination and power analysis for clinical trials. Controlled Clinical Trials 1981; 2: 93).

For *tables* showing sample sizes for a comparison of two proportions, see Fleiss JL, Levin B, Paik MC (Statistical methods for rates and proportions, 3rd edn. Wiley; 2003. Table A.4) or Schlesselman JJ (Case-control studies: design, conduct, analysis. New York, NY: Oxford University Press; 1982. Appendix A). For a *nomogram*, see Altman DG (Practical statistics for medical research. London: Chapman & Hall; 1991. p. 486).

For computer programs, see Appendix C.

Compensating for losses. Allowance can be made for an expected loss of $R\%$ of the study sample (due to nonresponse, dropouts, etc.) – but of course without compensating for possible selection bias – by multiplying the computed sample size by $(100 - R)^2/10,000$ (Lachin JM (1981; see above)).

17. See p. 70.
18. Armitage P. Sequential medical trials, 2nd edn. Oxford: Blackwell; 1975.
19. The required size of a *cluster sample* (for software, see Appendix C) depends not only on the factors influencing the required size of a simple random sample, but also on the cluster size and the evenness or unevenness of the distribution of the disease or characteristic (does it occur more in some clusters than in others?).

When a cluster sample has been used in a study, it is customary to compute and report the *design effect*, which is the ratio of the required sizes for cluster and random samples. Design effects of 2 or more are not uncommon. The simplest way to estimate sample size for a cluster-sample survey is to calculate the required size of a simple random sample and then multiply this by the design effect reported in a previous cluster-sample survey of the same disease in a similar population, using a similar cluster size, or in a previous round of the same survey. If different studies yielded different design effects, it is prudent to use the highest value.

The larger the cluster size, the larger the design effect. If a design effect $D\,1$ is based on a cluster size $b\,1$ and you wish to estimate the sample size required for a cluster size $b\,2$, the required design effect $D\,2$ is approximately

$$D_2 = 1 + (D_1 - 1)(b_2 - 1)/(b_1 - 1)$$

Methods of estimating the design effect are described by Bennett S, Woods T, Liyanage WM, Smith DL. (A simplified general method for cluster-sample surveys of health in developing countries. World Health Statistics Quarterly 1991; 44: 98) and Katz J, Zeger SL (Estimation of design effects in cluster surveys. Annals of Epidemiology 1994; 4: 295).

For *comparisons of cluster samples*, see Kerry SM, Bland JM (Sample size in cluster randomization. British Medical Journal 1998; 316: 549).

For *stratified cluster randomization*, see Donner A (Sample size requirements for stratified cluster randomization designs. Statistics in Medicine 1992; 11: 743).

20. *Post hoc* calculations of power are often performed to explain nonsignificant test results; but this procedure is logically flawed, and reliance should rather be placed on an appraisal of confidence intervals (Hoenig JM, Heisey DM. The abuse of power: the pervasive fallacy of power calculations for data analysis. The American Statistician 2001; 55: 19). 'We should adopt confidence intervals for effect sizes more widely, to encourage us to think more about the range of effect sizes that are supported by the data and those that are not and think less about *p* values' (Colegrave N, Ruxton GD. Confidence intervals are a more useful complement to nonsignificant tests than are power calculations. Behavioral Ecology 2003; 14: 446).

21. Computer programs that generate random numbers (see Appendix C) actually produce *pseudorandom numbers*, generally using algorithms whose capacity to produce sequences of numbers that are to all intents and purposes random have been thoroughly tested.

22. *Shortcuts* can be taken when using a table of random numbers to choose a sample. For example, if there are between 101 and 200 sampling units to choose from, read the successive three-digit numbers, and subtract the largest possible multiple of 200 from every number above 200 (also, read 000 as 200). Using the example in the text (p. 86), the sampling units selected would then be 93 (893 − 800), 162, 194 (794 − 600), 173 (573 − 400), 32, 190, 18, 39, etc. If there are between 201 and 300 sampling units, subtract a multiple of 300 from numbers above 300, discarding numbers above 900. If there are between 301 and 400 sampling units, subtract 400 from numbers above 400, discarding numbers above 800. And if there are between 401 and 500, subtract 500 from numbers above 500 (take 000 as 500).

9

Selecting Cases and Controls for Case-control Studies

Selecting cases and controls for case-control studies[1] is not always as easy as it may seem. Inappropriate selection of subjects is an important reason for the conflicting results that these studies often produce, and for doubts about the applicability of their findings.

The usual procedure is to identify cases and then select controls. Exceptionally, an investigator may start with a data set that can be used as the control data and then seek suitable cases for comparison ('control-initiated' studies).[2]

Selecting Cases for a Case-control Study

Five interrelated decisions are required:

1. What is the definition of a case?
2. Which cases will be eligible for inclusion in the study?
3. From what source will they be drawn?
4. How will they be chosen from this source?
5. How many cases are required?

What is the definition of a case?

A case-control study is generally performed in order to reach conclusions that are applicable not only to the specific individuals studied or the specific study population from which they are drawn, but also to a reference population. The cases must, therefore, be suitable representatives of this reference population, and this must be kept in mind when making the above decisions.

A *clear operational definition* (see Chapter 11) of the disease (or other characteristic) under consideration is essential. The cases may be new ones developing during a defined period (incident cases) or existing (prevalent) cases. If possible, incident cases should be used. The time lapse since exposure to the suspected causal factors is then

Research Methods in Community Medicine: Surveys, Epidemiological Research, Programme Evaluation, Clinical Trials   J. H. Abramson and Z. H. Abramson   Copyright © 2008, John Wiley & Sons Ltd

shorter, so that it may be easier to obtain correct information about this exposure and its duration and time relationship to the onset of the disease. Also, the use of new cases avoids *prevalence-incidence bias* (*Neyman bias*): if prevalent cases are used, patients who recover rapidly are likely to be underrepresented, and those who die soon after onset (e.g. sudden deaths from coronary heart disease) will not be represented at all; hence, if a difference is detected between cases and controls in their exposure to some factor, it may be difficult to infer that the factor is a cause of the disease rather than a determinant of recovery or survival. Prevalent cases are sometimes the only choice, e.g. in studies of chronic conditions with ill-defined onset times, congenital anomalies diagnosed at or after birth, and underuse or overuse of health services. If a condition is rare, incident cases may be too few to permit a useful comparison.

Which cases will be eligible for inclusion?

Eligibility criteria (inclusion and exclusion criteria) are determined mainly by the investigator's concept of the reference population, e.g. a wish to apply the findings to elderly people, fertile women, or truck drivers. Subjects are sometimes excluded on the grounds that they could not have been exposed to the 'causal' factor under study; for example, postmenopausal women and those who were sterilized many years previously might be excluded from a case-control study of the short-term effects of 'the pill' – and men certainly would be. Such exclusions will reduce the cost of the study, unless it is difficult to identify ineligible subjects, but other advantages have been questioned.[3] Among other reasons for limiting eligibility, it may be decided to restrict the study to a certain category of case in order to avoid effects that might be confused with the effects of the factor under study; for example, a study might be restricted to nonsmokers to avoid effects connected with smoking (see confounding, p. 274).

Eligibility criteria should preferably be decided in advance, even if they can be applied only after the collection of data. Care must obviously be taken not to exclude cases because of characteristics or behaviour that may be consequences of the exposure under study.

From what source will they be drawn?

Two alternative strategies can be used for case identification, with respect to the source of the cases. First, the cases can be sought in a defined population, e.g. the residents of a defined neighbourhood or region, the registered patients of a general practice, members of a prepaid health-care plan, the children in a school, a group of factory workers or, for a nested case-control study, the people included in a cohort study. The aim would be to identify all, or a representative sample of, the eligible cases in this *population base* (*source population, study base*). A preselected source population of this kind may be termed a *primary study base*. In a study in which individuals move into or out of the source population, and this is taken into account by using person-time measures (e.g. person-years), the study base is a *population-time base* rather than a population base.

The other strategy is to use any convenient source of eligible cases, such as a hospital or general practice, and then try to define the population base from which the cases are drawn (a *secondary study base*). Sometimes this is easy; if the cases in a food-poisoning outbreak turn out to have attended a wedding party, for example, it is obvious that the partygoers as a whole constitute the population base for a case-control study to identify the offending foods. Usually, it is more difficult than this, and only a vague definition of the population base is feasible. In a study of hospital patients, for example, the population base may be visualized as comprising those people who, if they had the disease being studied, would be admitted to the hospital or hospitals under consideration. A tertiary-care referral hospital that also provides general care for surrounding neighbourhoods may have patients who come from different population bases with different referral patterns, and it might be decided that a case-control study should be limited to patients from close by.[4] It is important to define the population base, however vaguely, both because the controls should be drawn from the same base and because the characteristics of the base will determine to whom the results can be generalized.

How will they be chosen from this source?

The identification of cases in the population base is sometimes complete or reasonably complete, e.g. if use is made of a case-finding survey, a cancer register, or information accumulated by a community health service that provides ongoing care for a defined population, or if the disease is one that always, or almost always, leads to hospitalization.

If case identification is incomplete, the investigator should try to know what the major selective factors are. Disease cases drawn from clinical sources, for example, may not be representative of all people with the disease, since there may be underrepresentation of those with mild symptoms and of people with a low availability or use of medical services. Cases drawn from a hospital or consultative clinic may not be typical of all cases under clinical care, and cases drawn from a teaching hospital may not be representative of all hospital cases (*referral filter bias*); also, the study may be affected by Berksonian bias (see p. 65). If the cases are drawn from other 'special populations' (see p. 64), then this too will, of course, affect the ability to generalize.

Cases may be identified by case-finding procedures using examinations, interviews or questionnaires, or from documentary sources such as clinical records, special registers, and death certificates. Whatever method is used, the cases should be chosen in an unbiased way (see selection bias, p. 261), e.g. by taking all consecutive eligible cases diagnosed in a given period or by selecting a random sample (see Chapter 8) representing all eligible cases identified.

Practical problems (the availability of cases, the accessibility of disease registers and other records, etc.) often influence the selection of cases. These and other constraints may necessitate reservations when the findings are interpreted.

How many cases are needed?

The *required number of cases* can be determined by the methods described in Chapter 8 (see p. 84). If cases are difficult to find, this can, to an extent, be compensated for by increasing the number of controls (see below).

Selecting Controls for a Case-control Study

The main decisions to be made are:

1. Who can be a control?
2. How will controls be found?
3. How many controls are needed?
4. Should the controls be matched?

Who can be a control?

A case-control study typically compares the prior exposure of cases and controls to a factor suspected of being a cause of a disease (or other outcome). The purpose of the controls is to provide an estimate of what the exposure status of the cases would be if the factor was not associated with the disease. They should represent people who, if they had the disease in question, could have become cases in the study. The main requirements are that, at the time of selection, the controls should be free of the disease (confirmation of which may require special procedures) and that they should (ideally) come from the same study base as the cases. The controls should be representative of disease-free people in the study base (rather than of 'all disease-free people').

Any eligibility criteria that are applied to the cases (apart from the presence and characteristics of the disease) should be applied to the controls also. Exposure to the suspected cause must, of course, play no part in the selection of controls. A person who develops the disease after being selected as a control and is then selected as a case should be included in the study both as a control and as a case.[5]

How will controls be found?

If the study base is well defined and the study includes all or a representative sample of the cases in this base, it should be easy to find suitable controls by taking a representative sample of (or all) the individuals without the disease in the study base. If the study has a population-time base, in which people are members (and are hence prospective controls) for different periods, it may be decided to use a sampling procedure that takes account of duration of membership in the base[6] (this does not apply to a *case-cohort study*, whose controls represent all members of the cohort at the start of follow-up, irrespective of their duration of membership).[5] Interest is confined to the control's exposure status at or before the time of selection. Control selection may be difficult if the population-time base is very dynamic; in a case-control study of risk factors for injury while driving tractors, for example, it may be difficult to obtain information about the time spent on tractors by prospective controls.[7]

It may be hard to find suitable controls if the study base is vaguely defined or difficult to sample. Use is then usually made of population controls, friends or neighbours etc., or hospital or clinic controls. Each of these methods presents its own problems. Some studies are based on no more than a hope, well founded or poorly founded, that the controls resemble members of the study base. 'If only we lived in an epidemiologist's utopia …', laments an epidemiologist, 'Alas, we do not live in such a place but must instead struggle on in a world of imperfect information and limited resources … The literature on myriad threats to the validity of case-control studies conducted under real-world circumstances will no doubt continue to grow.'[8]

The choice of a source can obviously affect the study findings, sometimes in unexpected ways. In a case-control study of hospitalized children with acute lymphoblastic leukaemia in Montreal, a comparison with population controls, matched for age, sex, and region of residence, showed a significant negative association with breast feeding, but a comparison with age- and sex-matched children with other severe illnesses treated in the same services showed no such relationship, although the two control groups were very similar to each other and to the cases in their socioeconomic characteristics.[9] The use of inappropriate controls has been suggested as a reason for the surprisingly low preventive effect of condoms against sexually transmitted diseases (STDs) reported in some case-control studies, where the cases are drawn from STD clinics and the controls are a sample of people tested in these clinics and found not to have an STD. Since the cases can be assumed to have infected partners, the controls should be restricted to those with infected partners, e.g. noninfected people who were examined because of contact with a person diagnosed with an STD.[10] Many case-control studies use more than one control group, to see whether they yield consistent findings.

Population controls (*community controls*) may be selected by any sampling method (see Chapter 8), including random digit dialling. The obvious advantages of population controls must be weighed against the disadvantages, which include cost, inconvenience and the probability of a high nonresponse rate. Moreover, if the cases are drawn from a hospital, then a representative population sample may not reflect the true study base, because not everyone would land up in this hospital if they had the disease. Also, it may be difficult to ensure that the controls will be investigated in the same way as the hospital cases, and the controls may differ from hospital patients in their motivation to recall and report past events.

Use may also be made of controls identified through their relationship with the cases, e.g. friends, neighbours, spouses, siblings, fellow workers or classmates. Such controls may tend to resemble the cases in their circumstances, lifestyles or (for blood relatives) genetic characteristics. This similarity may be an advantage, since the reduction of irrelevant differences between cases and controls may make it easier to test the study hypothesis. But it may also blur the very difference sought by the study; friends may, for example, tend to have similar smoking habits. The use of friends as controls presents particular difficulties; not only may there be reluctance to name friends, but particularly sociable or prestigious people are most likely to be named, which may cause bias if these characteristics are related to the variables under study. Selecting the control at random from a list of friends may reduce this bias, but cannot remove it. People living nearby may be useful controls for hospital cases, even if they would not go to the same hospital if they had the disease; but there may be important bias if the factors influencing hospitalization are strongly associated with the variables under study.

The use of *hospital or clinic controls* (patients with other diseases) for comparison with hospital or clinic cases is convenient, and it may be possible to assume that they are drawn from the same catchment population and are subject to the same selective factors as the cases. It should be remembered, however, that the probability of reaching a specific institution may vary for different diseases, depending on the reputation of its specialists, the availability of other services, etc. To minimize this problem, diseases that are similar are sometimes used, e.g. cancer controls for cancer cases. The problem is avoided if cases and controls have the same clinical picture, e.g. in a study of women referred for breast biopsies of suspicious nodules, in which those found to have breast cancer (cases) are compared with those not found to have cancer or precancerous conditions (controls).[11]

The main disadvantages of controls who have other diseases is that they are obviously a selected group, not necessarily representative of people without the disease under study. If the analysis reveals (or fails to reveal) interesting differences between the cases and controls, this may have more to do with the epidemiology of the diseases of the control patients than with the disease under study. This problem is reduced if patients with diseases known or suspected to be associated with the postulated causal factor are not used as controls – patients with lung cancer would not be good controls in a study of smoking and cervical cancer. Also, it may be wise to use a variety of diseases rather than a single disease. Patients admitted because of traffic accidents or for elective surgery are sometimes used as controls, in the probably unjustified hope that they represent the population base. Other controls sometimes used because of their easy accessibility include blood donors and hospital visitors.[12]

To avoid bias in the choice of hospital controls, systematic methods are sometimes used, e.g. the first eligible patient admitted after the study case, or the eligible patient closest in age in the same hospital ward. The best hope for avoiding Berkson's bias is to use controls who have a disease that has the same probability of hospitalization as the disease under study; the direction of the bias depends on whether the probability of hospitalization is higher for the disease under study or for the comparison condition. It is usually found that drawing controls from all hospital patients who are free of the disease under study underestimates the association between the disease and the causal factor, and use of population controls overestimates it.[13]

When deciding on a control group, attention must of course be paid to the feasibility of obtaining information comparable to that collected about the study group. An issue sometimes raised in studies where information about dead cases is obtained from proxy informants (relatives or friends) is whether dead controls (who died of other causes) should be sought, so as to ensure comparability. This procedure may, however, introduce its own biases, and it is usually preferable to use live controls and obtain the information about them from proxy informants.[14]

It is seldom easy to find a source of controls that is both convenient and free of possible bias. Each instance must be considered on its merits, and a careful choice made of the lesser of the alternative evils. It is often best to use two or more control groups (of different kinds), and to see whether different comparisons yield the same conclusion; discrepancies may throw light on the study's biases.

How many controls are needed?

The number of controls per case is based on statistical requirements (see p. 84) and practical considerations. For a given total sample size, equal numbers of cases and controls yield the most precise results. If there are few cases, then the study's power and precision can be boosted by using more controls (after four controls per case, there is generally little extra benefit). If controls are individually matched, then analytic methods can cope with any number (or a variable number) of controls per case.

Should the controls be matched?

Matching (see Chapter 7) *per se* does *not* prevent confounding in a case-control study; on the contrary, it introduces a bias by diminishing the difference between the total groups of cases and controls in their exposure to the postulated causal factor. However, the payoff is that if an appropriate technique to control confounding is used in the analysis (e.g. stratification, see p. 277) this bias is removed and the results are then generally more precise than they would be if the controls were not matched.[15] If a variable is matched, then it becomes impossible to examine its association with the disease, but it remains possible to see whether it modifies the association between the exposure and the disease. Matching may be counterproductive if the controls are matched for variables that do not affect risk.

Notes and References

1. The *selection of subjects for case-control studies* is considered in more detail by Lasky T, Stolley PD (Selection of cases and controls. Epidemiologic Reviews 1994; 16: 6), Wacholder S *et al.* (in a series of three papers on 'Selection of controls in case-control studies' in the American Journal of Epidemiology 1992; 135: 1019, 1029, 1042) and Rothman KJ, Greenland S (Modern epidemiology, 2nd edn. Lippincott-Raven; 1998. pp. 93–114).
2. Greenland S. Control-initiated case-control studies. International Journal of Epidemiology 1985; 14: 130.
3. For a debate on the *exclusion of subjects with no opportunity for exposure*, see Poole C (Exposure opportunity in case-control studies. American Journal of Epidemiology 1986;

123: 352), Schlesselman JJ, Stadel BV (Exposure opportunity in epidemiologic studies. American Journal of Epidemiology 1987; 125: 174), and Poole C (Critical appraisal of the exposure-potential restriction rule. American Journal of Epidemiology 1987; 125: 179).

4. A study of patients treated for lymphoma in a Jerusalem teaching hospital showed differences between Jerusalem residents and patients referred from other regions, with respect to age, country of birth, religion, histologic type, and form of treatment (Paltiel O, Ronen I, Polliack A, Epstein L. Two-way referral bias: evidence from a clinical audit of lymphoma in a teaching hospital. Journal of Clinical Epidemiology 1998; 51: 93).

   The possible bias caused by the inclusion of referred patients in a case-control study in such a hospital is explained diagrammatically by Morabia A (Case-control studies in clinical research. Preventive Medicine 1997; 26: 674).

5. Rothman KJ, Greenland S (1998, pp. 97–98, 108–110; see note 1).

6. A simple way of allowing for variable duration of membership in the study base (*density sampling*) might be by stratified random sampling (using a uniform sampling fraction) after stratifying the prospective controls by their duration of membership in the base.

   A more elaborate method is *risk-set* sampling: each case's controls are selected from the risk set of people in the source population who are at risk of becoming a case at the time the case is diagnosed; see Rothman KJ, Greenland S (1998, pp. 97–98; see note 1).

7. Mittelman MA, Maldonado G, Gerberich SG, Smith GS, Sorock GS. Alternative approaches to analytical designs in occupational injury epidemiology. American Journal of Industrial Medicine 1997; 32: 129.

8. Thompson WD Nonrandom yet unbiased. Epidemiology 1990; 1: 262.

9. Infante-Rivard C. Hospital or population controls for case-control studies of severe childhood diseases? American Journal of Epidemiology 2003; 167: 176.

10. Kleinbaum DG. Epidemiologic methods: the 'art' in the state of the art. Journal of Clinical Epidemiology 2002; 55: 1196.

11. For an example, see Cade J, Thomas E, Vail A (Case-control study of breast cancer in south east England: nutritional factors. Journal of Epidemiology and Community Health 1998; 52: 105).

12. *Hospital visitors* have been used as convenient substitutes for community controls in a number of studies: see Rathbone B, Martin D, Stephens J, Thompson JR, Samani NJ (*Helicobacter pylori* seropositivity in subjects with acute myocardial infarction. Heart 1996; 76: 308), Perez-Padilla R, Regalado J, Vedal S, Pare P, Chapela R, Sansores R, Selman M (Exposure to biomass smoke and chronic airway disease in Mexican women. A case-control study. American Journal of Respiratory and Critical Care Medicine 1996; 154: 701); Sankaranarayanan R, Varghese C, Duffy SW, Padmakumary G, Day NE, Nair MK (A case-control study of diet and lung cancer in Kerala, south India. International Journal of Cancer 1994; 58: 644), Narendranathan M, Cheriyan A (Lack of association between cassava consumption and tropical pancreatitis syndrome. Journal of Gastroenterology and Hepatology 1994; 9: 282), and Armenian HK, Lakkis NG, Sibai AM, Halabi SS (Hospital visitors as controls. American Journal of Epidemiology 1988; 127: 404).

   A study in the Philippines found that hospital visitors and neighbourhood controls were similar with respect to numerous social and behavioural characteristics; visitors of the cases studied were not chosen (Ngelangel CA. Hospital visitor-companions as a source of controls for case-control studies in the Philippines. International Journal of Epidemiology 1989; 18: S50).

13. These conclusions about *Berkson's bias* are based on algebraic analyses by Feinstein AR, Walter SD, Horwitz RI (An analysis of Berkson's bias in case-control studies. Journal of Chronic Diseases 1986; 39: 495) and Peritz E (Berkson's bias revisited. Journal of Chronic Diseases 1984; 37: 909).

14. There does not seem to be strong justification for using dead controls for dead cases (Gordis L. American Journal of Epidemiology 1982; 115: 1).

The study base consists of living subjects, and people who die represent a special sample from that base (Wacholder S, McLaughlin JK, Silverman DT, Mandel JS. 1992; see note 1). In a study that used both living and dead controls, more smoking, drinking and diseases were reported if the control was dead – 'it appears that exposures associated with premature death are overrepresented in dead controls'; this difference appeared to be real, and not attributable to the obtaining of information from next of kin (McLaughlin JK, Blot WJ, Mehl ES, Mandel JS. American Journal of Epidemiology 1985; 121: 131; 1985; 122: 485).

15. For a more detailed discussion of the pros and cons of matching in case-control studies, see Rothman KJ, Greenland S (1998, pp. 150–160; see note 1).

10

The Variables

The characteristics that are measured are referred to as *variables*, whether they are measured numerically, e.g. age or height, or in terms of categories, e.g. sex (or, for the squeamish, gender)[1] or the presence or absence of a disease.

When an association between variables is studied, the variables may be referred to as *dependent* and *independent*. The variable we try to 'hang on' to another variable (i.e. the variable whose presence or amount we wish to study) is the *dependent variable*. For example, in a study of the prevalence of a disease in different age and sex groups, the presence of the disease is the dependent variable and age and sex are independent variables. On the other hand, if we study the frequency of a given symptom among persons with different diseases, then the type of disease is the independent variable. If we want to know whether transcendental meditation affects the blood pressure, blood pressure is the dependent variable. Whenever we consider a causal association, the outcome (the postulated effect) is the dependent variable. In a therapeutic trial, the treatment is the independent variable and the measure of outcome is the dependent variable. (But be warned that statisticians may use the terms 'dependent' and 'independent' differently.)[2]

A variable based on two or more other variables may be termed a *composite variable*. Adiposity, for example, may be measured in terms of a body mass index (Quetelet's index) calculated by dividing the person's weight (in kilograms) by the square of their height (in metres). Dental caries may be measured by a DMF index, calculated by adding the number of permanent teeth that are decayed (D), the number that are missing (M), and the number that have been filled (F).

Incidence and prevalence rates, sex ratios, and all other rates[3] and ratios are composite variables, since they are based on separate numerator and denominator information.

During the planning of the study it is necessary to select and clarify the variables that will be measured.

Selection of Variables

The variables to be studied are selected on the basis of their relevance to the objectives of the investigation. If the study objectives have been formulated in writing, as previously recommended (see p. 43), the key variables (dependent and independent) will have been specifically mentioned in the objectives. The more specific the formulation of objectives, the greater the number of variables that will have been mentioned.

There may also be variables that have not been mentioned but which require to be measured if the study is to attain its aims. In selecting these additional variables, it is helpful to start with a list of all the characteristics (other than the independent variables that have already been specified) that are known or suspected to affect or cause the characteristics (dependent variables) that the investigator wants to study. Each of these variables can then be considered in turn to decide whether it should be included in the study on any of the following five grounds:

1. Whether it is important enough to warrant study as an *independent variable* in its own right. Its omission was an oversight.
2. Whether it is a *possible confounding factor*, i.e. it may obscure the relationship between some other independent variable and the dependent variable, or have other deceptive effects on that relationship, producing an association that has little meaning in itself (see p. 274 for a fuller explanation of confounding). To confound the picture, a variable must be associated both with the dependent variable and with the other independent variable. In a study of the relationship between work accidents and age, for example, we may decide to take the type of work into account, since older workers may have fewer accidents merely because they are in safer jobs – the possible confounder (type of work) may influence the dependent variable (accidents) and may also be associated with the independent variable (age). Although various procedures may be used to eliminate or reduce the effect of possible confounders (see p. 277), this does not obviate the need to measure them; in fact, most of these procedures are possible only if the possible confounders have been measured. The effect of possible confounders can be neutralized by matching (see p. 69) or, in a trial, by random allocation of the subjects to experimental and control groups (see p. 328), but they should still be measured, so that the effectiveness of matching or randomization can be checked.
3. Whether it may be a *modifier variable* (see p. 271), i.e. it may modify the relationship between some other independent variable and the dependent variable (or, in a trial, it may modify the effect of the treatment). It specifies the conditions for the relationship. Are older workers especially prone to accidents only in their first year of employment? Or does their special proneness (or immunity) vary in different departments of the factory? Or is the relationship between age and accidents different in the two sexes? If we want to answer these questions, we must add length of employment, department, and sex to the list of variables.
4. Whether it may be an *intervening cause* (see p. 276) that will explain a causal mechanism. Can a difference in the use of protective equipment explain the relationship between age and accidents?
5. Whether it has a strong enough *influence* on the dependent variable to warrant its inclusion, without necessarily meeting the above criteria. If variables that strongly affect the dependent variable are included in the statistical analysis of associations (even for this reason only), then this may (under certain conditions) appreciably increase the precision with which the effects of other independent variables (i.e.

those of interest to the investigator) can be estimated, and increase the statistical significance of these effects. In a study of the effects of smoking or a disease on pulmonary function, for example, it would probably be decided to include sex, age, height, and the presence of a cold or cough, all of which may affect the test results.

Apart from variables with an obvious relevance to the study objectives, consideration should be given to the following four types of variables:

1. *Universal variables.* These are variables that are so often of relevance in health-related studies that their inclusion should always be considered. They should not be automatically included, but should be automatically considered for inclusion. A suggested basic list of these variables is:
   - sex;
   - age;
   - parity;
   - ethnic group;
   - religion;
   - marital status;
   - social class, and attributes that may be used as indicators of social class or as variables in their own right, e.g. occupation, education, income, and household crowding index;
   - place of residence (e.g. region, or urban/rural);
   - geographical mobility (e.g. nativity, date of immigration).

   This list may, of course, require modification to suit the investigator's specific interests and the reality of the population studied. In certain communities it may be necessary to replace social class, for example, by some other measure of social stratification, or to add 'race' (which refers primarily to a group's relative homogeneity with respect to biological inheritance, whereas 'ethnic group' refers primarily to its shared history, social and cultural tradition, and way of life), or to replace 'marital status' by 'type of union' in communities where other types of stable union are prevalent.

2. Measures of *time*. Apart from obviously relevant measurements (such as the date of onset in any study of disease incidence), it may be necessary in a follow-up survey or clinical trial to record the dates on which the subject entered and left the study. This is essential information for both of the analytic techniques commonly employed in studies with varying observation periods: the use of person-time, e.g. person-years of observation,[4] as a denominator for the calculation of rates, and the life table method.[5] In some studies, *time to event*, or what statisticians may call the *failure time*, i.e. the time lapse between the beginning of the observation period and the occurrence of the event under study (e.g. death, onset of a disease, a relapse, a complication, return to work, conception, etc.), is the dependent variable; this applies to studies of survival[5] and to studies using Cox proportional hazards regression (see p. 254).

3. *Ecologic* (*contextual*) measures. In a study based on individuals, consider the inclusion of relevant variables concerning the context (see *multilevel surveys*, p. 22). These may be environmental measures (e.g. the air pollution level), aggregate

measures (e.g. the prevalence of tuberculosis in the place of residence), or other (global) measures, such as the level of poverty or crime, or the availability of specific health-care facilities.
4. Variables that delineate the *study population* (see p. 62) or populations. The characteristics of the study population may indicate the extent to which generalizations may be made from the findings. If groups are to be compared, then their demographic and other similarities and dissimilarities should be known; if a sample is to be used, then its characteristics should be compared with those of the parent population; if there are many nonrespondents, then they (or a sample of them) should be compared with respondents. Measures of the attributes of the study population or populations should be included for these purposes. These may be attributes with a bearing on the study topic, or may be quite unrelated ones, introduced solely as checks on the adequacy of the matching, sampling or allocation procedures.

Number of Variables

How many variables should be studied? The only answer, and not a very helpful one, is 'as many as necessary and as few as possible'. Unnecessary variables increase costs, impair participation, and complicate the analysis. One thing is clear: the initial list is usually too long and will have to be pruned to facilitate the collection and processing of the data. Bradford Hill tells of a plan submitted to him for a proposed inquiry into the causes of prematurity:

> It ran to a trifle of 180 questions, which covered a catholic range. For instance, it seemed that the author was confident that some person or persons – undefined in the draft I saw – could accurately inform her for each of the woman's previous confinements of the time interval between birth of the child and the placenta; the incidence of congenital malformations in her blood relations; whether she wore high- or low-heeled shoes; how often she took a hot bath; the state of health of the father at the time of conception; and the frequency of sexual intercourse, which was engagingly included under the sub-heading 'social amenities'. This, in my view, is not the scientific method; it is mere wishful thinking, mere hoping that some rabbit may come out if only the hat be made big enough.[6]

Clarifying the Variables

Once the variables have been selected, each of them should be clarified. There are two aspects to be considered. First, an *operational definition* must be formulated, clearly defining the variable in terms of objectively measurable facts, and stating, if necessary, how these facts are to be obtained (see Chapters 11 and 12). Second, the *scale of measurement* to be used in data collection should be specified (Chapters 13 and 14).

An example is given showing part of the list of variables to be measured in a survey of illnesses among hospitalized infants (Table 10.1). Whether the record should take this or another format is a matter of taste, but the information it contains should certainly be recorded somewhere. It will be noted that the list contains two variables, i.e. age and social class, on which no direct data are obtained. In this study, age is a composite variable based on the date of birth and date of admission, and social class is inferred from the father's occupation. The construction of the list in this way serves as a reminder of the basic data that must be collected.

Table 10.1 Selected variables in a survey of illnesses among infants

Variable	Definition	Scale
Date of birth	Infant's date of birth, as recorded in hospital records	Full date (day, month, year)
Date of admission	Date of infant's admission to hospital, according to hospital records	Full date (day, month, year)
Age	Infant's age at admission to hospital, calculated from date of birth and date of admission	Completed months (0 to 11) (99 if unknown)
Mother's age	Age at birth of infant, as stated by mother	1. Under 20 years 2. 20–24 years 3. 25–29 years 4. 30–34 years 5. 35–39 years 6. 40 years or more 9. No information
Father's occupation	Father's usual occupation, as stated by mother	Detailed occupation
Socio-economic class	Based on father's occupation, using National Statistics Socio-economic Classification [five classes]	1. Class 1 2. Class 2 3. Class 3 4. Class 4 5. Class 5 7. Never worked and long-term unemployed 8. Unclassifiable 9. No information
Reason for admission to hospital	Final diagnosis, according to hospital records. If two or more, the one stated by hospital physician to have been the principal reason for admission	Detailed categories of International Classification of Diseases (tenth revision)
Haemoglobin	In capillary blood, measured by [specified] method within 24 hours of admission	Grams per 100 ml, rounded off downwards to nearest gram
Mother's satisfaction with hospital	Response to specific question put to mother within 1 week after infant's discharge or death	1. Very satisfied 2. Satisfied on the whole 3. Somewhat dissatisfied 4. Very dissatisfied 8. Don't know 9. No answer

If the investigation is concerned with more than one study population, then more than one list of variables may be needed; but the full details about each variable need not be obsessively inserted in each list.

Complex Variables

Some variables are too complex to be easily measured as single entities and are best broken up into component aspects that can be regarded as separate variables and measured separately.

If we wish to investigate the attitude to abortions, for example, we would be well advised to obtain separate measures of the attitudes to abortions performed for medical, economic and psychological reasons, to those carried out by medical practitioners and by unqualified persons, to those performed on married and unmarried women, etc. It may be possible afterwards to combine these separate measures into a single integrated measure (now a composite variable).

Similarly, if we wish to study electrocardiogram (ECG) findings we may, instead of making a global and probably subjective appraisal of the ECG pattern, give separate consideration to a series of different measurable aspects, Q and QS patterns, S–T junction and segment depression, etc. This approach is the basis of the Minnesota code for the classification of ECG findings, which is widely used in epidemiological studies.[7] Different combinations of ECG findings may be used afterwards to provide electrocardiographic diagnoses of myocardial infarction and other disorders (composite variables). In longitudinal studies in which ECG examinations are repeated, electrocardiographic diagnoses may be based on the combined findings of serial Minnesota codes.

Notes and References

1. In the same way as, in Victorian times in England, it was deemed improper to say 'leg' in mixed company, rather than the euphemism 'limb' (and although this is probably a myth, even piano legs were scandalous and were draped with tiny pantalettes), so the grammatical term 'gender' has come into use as a politically correct euphemism for 'sex'. The Dictionary of Epidemiology points out that this genteelism 'is bewildering to readers whose first language has nouns that may carry any of three genders that are not necessarily related to the sex of the individual' (Last JM (ed.). A dictionary of epidemiology. Oxford University Press; 2001).
2. By the definition used in the text, chronic bronchitis is the dependent variable in a study of the effect of smoking on the occurrence of chronic bronchitis, even in a case-control study that examines this effect by comparing the smoking habits of people with and without chronic bronchitis. In this case-control study, a statistician might regard smoking habits as the dependent variable in the statistical analysis, the presence of the chronic bronchitis being the independent variable. If a regression analysis is used, then the variable predicted by the regression equation is called the dependent variable.
3. A *rate* expresses the frequency of an event or characteristic. It is generally calculated by dividing the number of events (e.g. deaths or disease onsets) by the total of the periods during which individual members are in the study population (expressed in person-years or other person-time

units – see note 4) or by dividing the number of persons with a characteristic (e.g. a disease) by the 'population at risk' (the total number of persons in the group or population), and then multiplying by 100, 1000, or another convenient figure. There is an increasing tendency to use the term 'rate' only for 'true' rates whose denominators are person-time units, and to use other terms (e.g. 'proportion' or 'risk') for other measures.

The importance of *denominator data* cannot be overstressed (see p. 62). It has been said that in the same way as a clinician keeps a stethoscope handy, an epidemiologist should always carry a denominator or two. If the numerator is confined to a specific category, e.g. males, the denominator should be similarly restricted (sex-specific rates, age-specific rates, etc.).

Prevalence tells what proportion of individuals have a disease or other attribute at a given time. It is a measure of what *exists*.

Incidence refers to what *happens* (e.g. disease onsets or deaths) during a specified period. Incidence may be expressed as a *cumulative incidence*, or *risk* – the proportion of initially disease-free individuals who develop the disease during a stated period – or as a person-time incidence rate (*incidence density*, *mortality density*). For clarification, see any recent epidemiology textbook.

Standardized and other adjusted rates are estimates of what the rate would be under specified conditions, e.g. if the age or sex composition of the study population conformed with a specified standard, or if the groups under comparison were similar with respect to defined independent variables. They are *counterfactual* ('pertaining to, or expressing, what has not in fact happened, but might, could, or would in different conditions' – Oxford English Dictionary).

The magnitude of directly age-standardized rates depends on the choice of a standard population, and comparisons of age-standardized rates may lead to different conclusions, depending on whether a young or an old population is used as the standard. In New Zealand, Maoris and non-Maoris have the same standardized mortality rate from diseases of the nervous system when the WHO-recommended world standard population is used, but the Maori rate is higher by 23% when the (young) Maori population is used as a standard (Robson B, Purdue G, Cram F, Simmonds S. Age standardisation – an indigenous standard? Emerging Themes in Epidemiology 2007; 4: 3). An alternative simple standardization method, which gives each year of age the same weight instead of using a standard population, has certain advantages (Abramson JH. Age-standardization in epidemiological data. International Journal of Epidemiology 1995; 24: 238. Hill C, Benhamou E. Age-standardization in epidemiological data. International Journal of Epidemiology 1995; 24: 241). For software, see Appendix C.

Crude rates are rates that have not been adjusted.

A *specific rate* (*age-specific rate*, *sex-specific rate*) is a rate in a specific group. Both the numerator and the denominator refer to this group.

4. To calculate *person-years* (or person-months, etc.) of observation, it is necessary to know the length of each subject's period of observation, from the start of follow-up until its end (i.e. until occurrence of the 'endpoint' event under study – death, loss of contact, conclusion of the study, or withdrawal from follow-up for some other reason). The sum total of these periods can be used as a person-time denominator for calculating a rate. It has been called *candidate time* (Miettinen OS. Theoretical epidemiology: principles of occurrence research in medicine. New York, NY: Wiley; 1985. p. 319).

    A member of an Internet discussion group on epidemiological methods thanked other members for explaining how to compute the rates he wanted, and then added: 'P.S. It was cows, not persons!'

5. The analysis of *survival* (nonoccurrence of a defined endpoint event, such as the onset of a disease or complication, or death) is discussed by (among others) Selvin S (Statistical analysis of epidemiologic data, 3rd edn. New York, NY: Oxford University Press, 2004. Chapters 11–13). For software, see Appendix C.

6. Hill AB. Statistical methods in clinical and preventive medicine. Edinburgh: Livingstone; 1962. p. 360.
7. Prineas RJ, Crow RC, Blackburn H. The Minnesota code manual of electrocardiographic findings: standards and procedures for measurement and classification. Boston, MA: John Wright PSG; 1982.
    The use of serial readings is described by (among others) Crow RS, Prineas RJ, Hannan PJ, Grandits G, Blackburn H (Prognostic associations of Minnesota Code serial electrocardiographic change classification with coronary heart disease mortality in the Multiple Risk Factor Intervention Trial. American Journal of Cardiology 1997; 80: 13).

11

Defining the Variables

Each of the variables measured in a study should be clearly and explicitly defined. Unless this is done, there can be no assurance that similar findings would be obtained if the study were performed by a different investigator, or repeated by the same investigator.

The same term may have more than one meaning, even in day-to-day usage; there are no hard and fast, universally accepted, 'correct' definitions. The investigator must choose a definition that will be useful for the purposes of the study. Like Humpty Dumpty, the investigator can say, 'when I use a word, it means just what I choose it to mean – neither more nor less'.

There are two kinds of definition: conceptual and operational.

The *conceptual definition* defines the variable as we conceive it. This definition is often akin to a dictionary definition. For example, 'obesity' might be variously defined as: 'excessive fatness' or 'overweight' or 'a bodily condition that is socially regarded as constituting excessive fatness'. In effect, it is a definition of the characteristic we would like to measure.

In contrast, the *operational definition* (or *working definition*) defines the characteristic we will actually measure. It is phrased in terms of objectively observable facts and it is clear and explicit enough to avoid ambiguity. Where necessary, it states how the facts are obtained. 'Obesity', for example, might be operationally defined in different surveys as one of the following:

- A weight, based on weighing in underclothes and without shoes, which exceeds, by 10% or more, the mean weight (in a specified population at a specified time) of persons of the subject's sex, age and height.
- A skinfold thickness of 25 mm or more, measured with a Harpenden skinfold caliper at the back of the right upper arm, midway between the tip of the acromial process and the tip of the olecranon process (this level being located with the forearm flexed at 90°), with the arm hanging freely and the skinfold being lifted parallel to the long axis of the arm.
- A positive response to the question 'Are you definitely overweight?'
- A positive response to the question 'Does your husband/wife think you are too fat?'

It is often helpful, but it is not always essential, to formulate a conceptual definition. But it is always necessary to formulate an operational definition.

Research Methods in Community Medicine: Surveys, Epidemiological Research, Programme Evaluation, Clinical Trials   J. H. Abramson and Z. H. Abramson   Copyright © 2008, John Wiley & Sons Ltd

In doing this, the investigator is heavily influenced not only by the need to come as close as possible to the conceptual definition, but also by considerations of practicability. In most research on blood pressure, the characteristic in which the investigator is interested is the pressure within the arteries; as intra-arterial measurements are usually not feasible, blood pressure is usually defined in terms of measurements made externally with a sphygmomanometer. This operationally defined blood pressure may be markedly different from the intra-arterial pressure, particularly in fat subjects.

Similarly, social class may be operationally defined in terms of a classification of occupations. The British Registrar-General's classification was widely used for this purpose for many years.[1] It had five classes, which were generally regarded as comprising an ordinal scale. Since 2001 this classification has been supplanted in the UK by the UK National Statistics socioeconomic classification (NS-SEC),[2] whose eight-group and five-group versions are summarized in Table 11.1. The categories should be regarded as nominal rather than ordinal. In the case of children, the classification is often based on the father's occupation, and on the husband's occupation in the case of married women. Social class, defined in this way, does not necessarily correspond with the researcher's conception of social class, which may have to do with prestige or wealth or power or social connections or knowledge or living conditions or lifestyle.[3] But, in a particular investigation, this definition (or some other simple one, such as educational level) may be a practical one to use, while the information the researcher really wants may be difficult or impossible to obtain.

In other words, the investigator is playing what has been called a 'substitution game'. What they *can* measure – a *proxy variable* – is substituted for what they *would like* to measure. Discrepancies may be unavoidable, but the investigator should at least be aware of them. If they are perforce large, it may be necessary to reconsider whether it

Table 11.1   The UK National Statistics socio-economic classification (NS-SEC) classes

Eight classes	Five classes
1 Higher managerial and professional occupations	1 Managerial and professional occupations
1.1 Large employers and higher managerial occupations	
1.2 Higher professional occupations	
2 Lower managerial and professional occupations	
3 Intermediate occupations	2 Intermediate occupations
4 Small employers and own-account workers	3 Small employers and own-account workers
5 Lower supervisory and technical occupations	4 Lower supervisory and technical occupations
6 Semi-routine occupations	5 Semi-routine and routine occupations
7 Routine occupations	+ Never worked and long-term unemployed
8 Never worked and long-term unemployed	[can be kept as a separate group]

is worthwhile measuring the variable at all, and even whether the whole investigation is worthwhile.

As an example, suppose we wish to perform a survey to test the hypothesis that drivers whose emotional health is disturbed have a higher risk of being involved in road accidents. Clearly, 'emotional health' will be difficult to define in operational terms. The defining of 'accidents', on the other hand, seems an easier nut to crack; after all, everyone knows what an accident is. In actual fact, the task is not so easy. Do we want to include all mishaps occurring on the road, including 'near misses', or only those that result in damage? If the latter, are we to include any damage, whether to vehicles, lampposts, cats, dogs, hedgehogs, etc., or only injury to human beings? If we confine the study to accidents causing injuries to humans, will we include mild and transient injuries, such as temporary emotional shock, or only more severe ones? And if the latter, what precisely do we mean by 'more severe'? Whatever definition of 'accident' we are considering, is it a practical one? Will we be able to get the required information? Maybe we will have to fall back on accidents reported to the police or insurance companies (which are not necessarily representative samples of accidents), or even confine ourselves to fatal accidents. In the latter instance, our ascertainment may be fairly complete, but we will be investigating only the tip of the iceberg and ignoring the main bulk of accidents. Maybe accidents defined in different ways have different associations with emotional health.[3] Can we find a definition that meets our need, or should we give the whole thing up as a bad job?

It is thus clearly impossible to suggest a list of 'recommended' definitions. Instead, we will draw attention to a number of questions that may arise when definitions are sought for certain frequently used variables.

1. *Occupation*. Present or usual occupation? Occupation for which the subject was trained (profession or trade), or work actually performed? If retired or unemployed, will the previous occupation be used?
2. *Education*. Number of years of education, or last grade attained, or type of educational institution last attended, or age at completion of full-time education? What kinds of education are included: evening classes and other part-time studies, religious seminaries?
3. *Income*. Personal income, family income, or average family income per member? Income from all sources, or only from gainful employment? Total (gross) earnings, or net earnings, after subtraction of income tax and social security payments and other 'deductions at source'? Is income 'in kind', e.g. free lodgings or self-grown vegetables or crops, included?
4. *Crowding index* (mean number of persons per room in housing unit). What rooms are excluded (bathrooms, showers, toilets, kitchens, storerooms, rooms used for business purposes, entrance halls)? Are children taken as wholes or halves in the computation?
5. *Social class*.[4] Based on occupation, education, crowding index, income, neighbourhood of residence, home amenities, or subject's self-perception? Based on one of these, or a combination? If based on occupation, will women be graded by their own or their husbands' occupations? If the latter, how will unmarried women,

widows and divorcees be graded? Will all members of the household be graded according to the occupation of one of its members? And if so, how should that member be selected?[5] What occupational classification is suitable for use in the specific community under study?

6. *Ethnic group.*[6] In terms of 'race' (see p. 103), skin colour, country of birth, father's country of birth, mother's country of birth, tribe, religion, or subject's self-perception?

7. *Marital status.* In terms of legal status (single, married, widowed, divorced; and, in some communities, 'common-law marriages',' separated', and same-sex unions) or in terms of stability of union (e.g. stable union, casual union)? Present status or total marital experience ('second marriage', etc.?).

8. *Parity.* Total number of previous pregnancies, or only those terminating in still or live births, or number of children delivered?

9. *Date of onset of disease.* Date when first symptoms were noticed, or date when first diagnosed, or date of notification?

10. *Presence of chronic disease.*[7] Based on duration since onset? If so, what duration makes it chronic: 3 months, 6 months, a year? Based on presence of certain diseases that are defined as chronic whatever their duration? If so, what diseases? Do they include dental caries, myopia, obesity? Are chronic symptoms enough (cough, constipation)? What about conditions that come and go, e.g. frequently recurrent sore throats?

11. *Disability.* Capacity to function, or actual performance? Difficulty in performance, or need for assistance?[8] Appraised by self, by family, or by examiner? What functions are considered: ability to get around alone, or perform physical activities,[9] or carry out major activity (work, housework, schoolwork – but what is a pensioner's 'major activity'?), or see, hear, carry out activities of daily living? Emphasis on impairments (physical and mental abnormalities) or on disability (reduced capacity to function) or on handicap (reduced capacity to fulfil a social role)? Long-term disability only, or temporary disability also (days of work loss or school absence, days in bed, days with restricted activity on account of illness or injury)? Measured as percentage disability, using rating scales established for entitlement to benefits (workmen's compensation, etc.)? Emphasis on effect on quality of life, for use in computation of quality-adjusted life-years?[10]

12. *Overall or general health.* Appraised by physician, nurse, or self?[11] And if by self, appraisal in comparison with others of same age and sex? Physical, mental, social, or comprehensive health? Based only on presence or absence of specific diseases? Subjective wellbeing? Functional capacity? Positive aspects of health?

13. *Quality of life.*[12] 'Health-related quality of life' (personal experience more specifically related to health or health care)? Or (more generally) overall life satisfaction, living standards, goal achievement, social utility? Related to a specific health problem and its care, or 'generic'? The same definition for all subjects, or different definitions for specific groups (e.g. elderly, children)?[13] A global appraisal, or measures of different dimensions (physical, emotional and social function, role performance, pain, etc.)? Assessed by whom?[14] Subjective wellbeing as well as functional status?

14. *Physician visit.* Including telephone consultations? What if the service was pro-
    vided by a nurse or other person acting on the doctor's instructions? If a patient
    comes for a certificate or to collect a letter, is this a visit? Can a visit be paid *in
    absentia* – if a mother comes to consult a doctor about her child, is the visit ascribed
    to the mother or the child? If she consults the doctor about herself, and the doctor
    uses the opportunity to discuss her son's health, or to prescribe treatment for him,
    is the visit ascribed to the son also?
15. *Hospitalization.* Is hospitalization for childbirth included? Is the hospital stay of a
    healthy newborn baby included? Is overnight stay essential? Is overnight stay in a
    casualty ward included? What institutions qualify as hospitals?
16. *Breastfeeding.* Is a single breastfeeding enough to label an infant as 'breastfed'? When
    is a child 'exclusively breastfed' and when 'partially breastfed': does *any* bottle-feeding,
    even with small quantities of liquid, make the child 'partially' breastfed? Is a child who
    receives minimal supplementary ('token') breastfeeding to be regarded as breastfed?[15]
    Is a child who is fed with breast milk in a bottle considered breastfed?

If it is hoped to obtain information that can be directly compared with the findings
of previous studies, care must be taken to use the operational definitions used in the
other studies. For a few variables, such as 'underlying cause of death'[16] and 'neonatal
death', internationally recommended and generally accepted definitions are available.
If it is hoped or expected that the study will be repeated by others, then it is particularly important that the operational definitions should be very explicit and that their
application elsewhere should be feasible. If application of the study findings in clinical
care is anticipated, then it may be advisable to choose operational definitions that are
practicable and acceptable in clinical situations.

Finally, it must be noted that there are some variables for which, paradoxically, detailed
operational definitions can be formulated only after the findings have been analysed.
These are composite variables based on combinations of a number of separate items,
using rules that are determined only after the actual interrelationship between the items
has been examined (see pp. 134–136).

Notes and References

1. The *British Registrar-General's classification* had five classes (I, Professional occupations;
    II, Intermediate; III, Skilled occupations (divided into IIINM, skilled nonmanual; and IIIM,
    skilled manual); IV, Partly skilled occupations; V, Unskilled occupations). The classification
    was originally based on the social prestige of occupations, and later on occupational skill
    (Brewer RI. A note on the changing status of the Registrar-General's classification of occu-
    pations. British Journal of Sociology 1986; 37: 131). See Susser MW, Hopper K, Watson W
    (Sociology in medicine, 3rd edn. New York, NY: Oxford University Press; 1985. Chapter 5).
2. Details of the *NE-SEC classification* are available on the Internet at http://www.statistics.
    gov.uk/methods_quality/ns_sec/default.asp. As well as giving detailed coding instructions,
    the website provides a self-administered questionnaire that leads to grouping into five classes
    (1. Managerial and professional occupations; 2. Intermediate occupations; 3. Small employers

and own account workers; 4 Lower supervisory and technical occupations; 5. Semi-routine and routine occupations), on the basis of information about occupation (self-classified into eight categories), employment status (employer, self-employed, or employee), size of organization, and supervisory status. Although there is only 75% agreement with interviewer-coded groups, the self-coded and interviewer-coded five-class NS-SECs display similar patterns and strength in their relationships with other variables (e.g. with smoking).

3. In a national study in Britain, the definition of 'childhood accident' was found to be a crucial factor in determining results. Accidents 'resulting in an injury for which the child was admitted to hospital' were associated with large family size, whereas accidents 'resulting in an injury which warranted medical attention' were not (Stewart–Brown S, Peters T J, Golding J, Bijur P 1986 Case definition in childhood accident studies: a vital factor in determining results. International Journal of Epidemiology 15: 352).

4. *Measures of social class or socioeconomic position or status* are reviewed at length by Golobardes B, Show M, Lawlor A, Lynch JW, Smith GD (Indicators of socioeconomic position [parts 1 and 2]. Journal of Epidemiology and Community Health 2004; 60: 7, 95), Krieger N, Williams DR, Moss NE (Measuring social class in US public health research: concepts, methodologies and guidelines. Annual Review of Public Health 1997; 18: 401) and Berkman LF, Macintyre S (The measurement of social class in health studies: old measures and new formulations. IARC Scientific Publications 1997; 138: 51). For a briefer discussion, see Susser M, Warren W, Hopper K (1985, see note 1). Also, see Abramson JH, Gofin R, Habib J, Pridan H, Gofin J (Indicators of social class: a comparative appraisal of measures for use in epidemiological studies. Social Science and Medicine 1982; 16: 1739).

Also, see a set of papers on 'Measuring social inequalities in health', introduced by Krieger N, Moss N (Accounting for the public's health: an introduction to selected papers from a U.S. conference on 'measuring social inequalities in health'. International Journal of Health Services 1996; 26: 383).

In many populations, *neighbourhood of residence* is a useful rough-and-ready measure of social class, one advantage being that it is as easily applicable to women as to men. In Scotland, for example, coronary heart disease in both sexes bears similar relationships to occupation-based social class and to a 'deprivation index' based on features of the area (postal-code sector) of residence, namely the prevalence of unemployment, household crowding, semiskilled or unskilled labour, and nonownership of a car (Woodward M. Small area statistics as markers for personal social status in the Scottish heart health study. Journal of Epidemiology and Community Health 1996; 50: 570). See Carstairs V (Deprivation indices: their interpretation and use in relation to health. Journal of Epidemiology and Community Health 1995; 49(suppl. 2): S3).

A *combination of criteria* may be more useful than a single criterion. A cohort study in Britain, for example, showed wider mortality differentials when house and car ownership were taken in conjunction with occupation-based social class than when the latter was used alone (Wannamethee SG, Shaper AG. Socioeconomic status within social class and mortality: a prospective study in middle-aged British men. International Journal of Epidemiology 1997; 26: 53).

Status inconsistency, e.g. a disparity between education and occupational status, may be an important variable in its own right. For example, raised rates of emotional ill-health have been found in better-educated people with a low occupational status and in poorly educated people with a high occupational status, and there is evidence that disparities between education and occupational status or income affect the risk of ischaemic heart disease. See Abramson JH (Emotional disorder, status inconsistency and migration. Milbank Memorial Fund Quarterly 1966; 44: 23) and Peter R, Gassler H, Geyer S (Socioeonomic status, status inconsistency and risk of ischaemic heart disease: a prospective study among members of a statutory health insurance company. Journal of Epidemiology and Community Health 2007; 61: 605).

5. In the past, the household's social class was determined by that of the *head of the household* – generally the eldest householder, with males taking precedence over females in the case of couples or nonrelated joint householders. If in doubt, members of the household or family could be asked whom they regarded as the head. Sometimes, detailed operational definitions were devised.

   Because of the overt sexism involved in this definition, UK statistics now instead use the *household reference person* – the person responsible for owning or renting or who is otherwise responsible for the accommodation. In the case of joint householders, the person with the highest income takes precedence. Where incomes are equal, the older is taken as the household reference person.

6. Distinctive features of an *ethnic group* include shared origins and history, traditions, language and other components of culture, and a sense of identity and group membership. It may be best determined by self-assessment. See Bhopal R (Glossary of terms relating to ethnicity and race: for reflection and debate. Journal of Epidemiology and Community Health 2004; 58: 441).

   Ethnicity recorded in medical records may (for some groups) have a low correspondence with self-assessments (Gomez SL, Kelsey JL, Glaser SL, Lee MM, Sidney S. Annals of Epidemiology 2005; 15: 71).

7. In a well-known survey of *chronic disease* in the USA, the initial working definition was: 'Chronic disease comprises all impairments or deviations from normal which have one or more of the following characteristics: are permanent, leave residual disability; are caused by nonreversible pathological alteration; require special training of the patient for rehabilitation; may be expected to require a long period of supervision, observation or care'. This was found to be too vague and to include too many trivial disorders. In practice the examining physicians recorded all chronic conditions they detected, but conditions were disregarded if they were not 'medically disabling', i.e. if it was thought they did not affect the patient's wellbeing or interfere with their activities and were unlikely to do so. The report states: 'It is difficult to state concisely and specifically what conditions are included in these data on "chronic diseases". In the final analysis, the definition is the list of 47 diagnostic categories, plus two "all other" groups, for which data are presented'. These hold-all 'other diagnoses' groups included a quarter of all cases (Commission on Chronic Illness. Chronic illness in the United States, Vol III. Chronic illness in a rural area: the Hunterdon study. Cambridge, MA: Harvard University Press; 1959. pp. 149–151; and Commission on Chronic Illness. Chronic illness in the United States, Vol IV. Chronic illness in a large city: the Baltimore study. Cambridge, MA: Harvard University Press; 1957. pp. 49–50, 513–520).

   In the US Health Interview Survey, a condition was considered chronic if it was reported to have been first noticed more than 3 months previously, or if it was in a list of 34 conditions that were always considered chronic. These were phrased in lay terms, e.g. 'heart trouble' and 'repeated trouble with back or spine'. (National Center for Health Statistics. Health interview survey procedure 1957–1974. Vital and Health Statistics series 1, no 11. Washington, DC: Department of Health, Education, and Welfare; 1975. pp 127–128).

8. Some measures of *disability* in activities of daily living focus on difficulty in performance, others on the need for assistance by another person. Obviously, many people have difficulty without requiring assistance; in one study, 13% of elderly people reported trouble getting into or out of bed, but only 3% needed assistance. A focus on difficulty is appropriate in studies of the effects of illnesses, impairments, or care, whereas a need for assistance is especially relevant in studies concerned with planning or costing of services (Jette AM. How measurement techniques influence estimates of disability in older populations. Social Science and Medicine 1994; 38: 937).

9. Abramson JH, Ritter M, Gofin J, Kark JD. A simplified index of physical health for use in epidemiological studies. Journal of Clinical Epidemiology 1992; 45: 651.

10. See note 12, Chapter 5.

11. Numerous studies have shown that negative *self-appraisals of health* are predictive of subsequent mortality (Idler EL, Benyamini Y. Self-rated health and mortality: a review of twenty-seven community studies. Journal of Health and Social Behavior 1997; 28: 21).

12. Measures of *quality of life*, which have proliferated in recent years, are reviewed at length by Bowling A (Measuring health: a review of quality of life measurement scales. Buckingham: Open University Press; 1997) and briefly by Carr AJ, Thompson PW, Kirwan JR (Quality of life measures. British Journal of Rheumatology 1996; 35: 275). Core elements are summarized by Muldoon MF, Barger SD, Flory JD, Manuck SB (What are quality of life measurements measuring? British Medical Journal 1998; 316: 542). Also, see Guyatt GH, Feeny DH, Patrick DL (Measuring health–related quality of life. Annals of Internal Medicine 1993; 118: 622), Fitzpatrick R, Fletcher A, Gore S, Jones D, Spiegelhalter D, Cox D (Quality of life measures in health care I: Applications and issues in assessment. British Medical Journal 1992; 305: 1074), Fletcher A, Gore S, Jones D, Fitzpatrick R, Spiegelhalter D, Cox D (Quality of life measures in health care II: Design, analysis and interpretation. British Medical Journal 1992; 305: 1145), and Spiegelhalter D, Gore SM, Fitzpatrick R, Fletcher A, Jones DR, Cox DR (Quality of life measures in health care III: Resource allocation. British Medical Journal 1992; 305: 1205).

    Cultural factors should not be ignored. When asked about the effects of their symptoms on the quality of life, French patients considered all sexual aspects of life more important than English patients did (Calais DSF, Marquis P, Deschaseaux P, Gineste JL, Cauquil J, Patrick DL. Relative importance of sexuality and quality of life in patients with prostatic symptoms: results of an international study. European Urology 1997; 31: 272).

13. Quality of life in specific age groups: see Pal DK (Quality of life assessment in children: a review of conceptual and methodological issues in multidimensional health status measures. Journal of Epidemiology and Community Health 1996; 50: 391) and Kutner NG, Ory MG, Baker DI, Schechtman KB, Hornbrook MC, Mulrow CD (Measuring the quality of life of the elderly in health promotion intervention clinical trials. Public Health Reports 1992; 107: 530).

14. Doctors and patients may disagree about the quality of life (Janse AJ, Gemke RJBJ, Uiterwaal CSPM, van der Tweel I, Kimpen JLL, Sinnema G. Quality of life: patients and doctors don't always agree: a meta-analysis. Journal of Clinical Epidemiology 2004; 57: 653).

    Patients with multiple sclerosis, for example, are less concerned than their doctors about their physical disability; their ratings of physical disability do not correlate with their quality-of-life appraisals (Rothwell PM, McDowell Z, Wong CK, Dorman PJ. Doctors and patients don't agree: cross sectional study of patients' and doctors' perceptions and assessments of disability in multiple sclerosis. British Medical Journal 1997; 314: 1580).

    In a study in which cardiac outpatients, family members and medical staff were asked what they considered were important elements in the patients' quality of life, the patients, in contrast to family and staff, chose aspects that reflected the positive aspects of life (Woodend AK, Nair RC, Tang AS. Definition of life quality from a patient versus health care professional perspective. International Journal of Rehabilitation Research 1997; 20: 71).

    Yet subjects were asked to make their own ratings in only 13 of 75 quality-of-life studies reviewed by Gill TM, Feinstein AR (A critical appraisal of the quality of quality-of-life measurements. Journal of the American Medical Association 1994; 272: 619).

15. Labbok MH, Belsey M, Coffin CJ. A call for consistency in defining breast–feeding. American Journal of Public Health 1997; 87: 1060.

16. World Health Organization. International statistical classification of diseases and related health problems: tenth revision, vol 1. Geneva: World Health Organization, 1992. p. 1235.

12

Definitions of Diseases

It is as important to establish clear operational definitions for diseases as for other variables. This is a far from easy task. Clinicians tend to establish a diagnosis by making a clinical judgement of the extent to which the picture presented by the patient conforms with their *concept* of the disease in question. Use is seldom made of rigid diagnostic rules. That is, the diagnosis tends to be based on a conceptual rather than on an explicit operational definition. Inevitably, doctors often disagree.

The findings of a survey or trial will not be reproducible unless clear working definitions are used, nor will it be easy to apply the conclusions in clinical or other real-life situations. If we have formulated and used an operational definition of rheumatic fever, then we can report how many cases of rheumatic fever we have found, with the assurance that another investigator, using the same definition, would have obtained similar findings. This is the basis of good research. Our rigid rules may mean the inclusion of cases who some clinicians think do not have the disease, as well as the exclusion of patients who some clinicians think *do* have the disease, or who they believe should be given the benefit of the doubt and treated as if they *did* have the disease. Such discrepancies, although we should try to minimize them by choosing a satisfactory definition, are probably inevitable. The clinicians' decisions (or some of them) may be best for their patients, but when we report our findings concerning rheumatic fever, we must know and be able to explain exactly what we mean by the term. If application of the study findings in clinical care is anticipated, then it is advisable to choose working definitions whose use is practicable and acceptable in clinical situations.

Unfortunately, few diseases have satisfactory and widely accepted operational definitions. The definitions provided in medical textbooks (if they are given at all)[1] are usually conceptual ones. Here is one example:[2]

> A common cold is an acute, self-limited, infectious disorder characterized by nasal obstruction and/or discharge and frequently accompanied by sneezing, sore throat, and nonproductive cough.

It is obvious that this definition does not aim to provide rules for diagnosing a cold. No method is mentioned for determining the infectious nature of the disorder, and the phrase about sneezing, sore throat and cough is equivocal – are these manifestations essential for the diagnosis?

Research Methods in Community Medicine: Surveys, Epidemiological Research, Programme Evaluation, Clinical Trials   J. H. Abramson and Z. H. Abramson   Copyright © 2008, John Wiley & Sons Ltd

Operational Definitions

By contrast, operational definitions of diseases, like those of other variables, should be phrased in terms of objectively observable facts, and should be sufficiently clear and explicit to avoid ambiguity. Operational definitions of this sort are formulated in terms of *diagnostic criteria*; that is, the definition constitutes a set of rules for the diagnosis of the disease, based on the presence or absence of specified criteria.

These criteria may be *manifestations* or *causal experiences*.[3] Manifestational criteria include physical findings, symptoms, behaviour, the course of the illness, the response to specific therapy, etc. 'Causal' criteria are types of experience begun at a time preceding the illness, and often loosely called 'the cause' of the illness, e.g. difficult birth, an accident, exposure to lead, or contact with a case of measles. For a specific disease, manifestational criteria, experiential criteria, or both may be used.

The diagnostic criteria of a disease are chosen from those manifestations and experiences that are relatively frequent among people whom clinicians diagnose as suffering from the disease, by comparison with their frequency among well people and patients with other diseases. Certain of these manifestations and experiences are selected as diagnostic criteria, and rules are established for the diagnosis of the disease. For example, the disease may be diagnosed:

1. Only when all the criteria are present.
2. Or only when a sufficient number of them are present.
3. Or only when specific combinations of criteria are present.
4. Or only when certain specific criteria (or specific combinations) are present, and certain other additional conditions are met (e.g. a sufficient number of 'minor' criteria are present).
5. Or only when a score, obtained by adding defined weights allocated to each of the criteria, reaches a specified level. Such a weighting system makes it possible to attach more diagnostic importance to some criteria than to others.
6. Or only when one of the above conditions is met, and in addition the presence of certain defined other diseases can be excluded.

As an illustration, a diagnosis of an initial attack of rheumatic fever can be made (with 'a very high probability') in the presence of any two of the following major manifestations, or the presence of any one major manifestation and any two minor manifestations, provided (in all instances) that there is also supporting evidence of preceding group A streptococcal infection:[4]

Major manifestations

- Carditis
- Polyarthritis
- Chorea
- Erythema marginatum
- Subcutaneous nodules.

Minor manifestations

- Arthralgia
- Fever
- Elevated acute phase reactants
  - erythrocyte sedimentation rate
  - C-reactive protein
- Prolonged PR interval.

Evidence of antecedent group A streptococcal infection

- Positive throat culture or rapid streptococcal antigen test
- Elevated or rising streptococcal antibody titre.

As another example, seven diagnostic criteria are laid down for rheumatoid arthritis, and the disease is diagnosed if any four of them are present.[5]

Medical textbooks sometimes provide both conceptual and operational definitions. For example, for congestive cardiac failure[6] (conceptual):

> ... the condition in which an abnormality of cardiac structure or function is responsible for the inability of the heart to fill with or eject blood at a rate commensurate with the requirements of the metabolizing tissues

and (operational):

> at least one of eight major criteria (paroxysmal nocturnal dyspnoea, neck vein distension, etc.) plus at least two of eight minor criteria (extremity edema, night cough, etc.).

Rules of this sort have sometimes been validated by a comparison with diagnoses established by a 'better' set of criteria (a 'gold standard'), i.e. an operational definition that, *prima facie* or because it incorporates more sophisticated or accurate tests (but is too elaborate or expensive for general use), appears to approach closer to the conceptual definition of the disease. Usually, the decision on the usefulness of the rules is based solely on the degree to which the diagnoses they establish conform with those made on the basis of clinical judgements. Despite the obvious limitations of this method it is frequently the only practicable one.

Depending on the purpose of the study, a more or less specific definition should be used. If the aim is to identify people who almost certainly have the disease, a highly specific definition is required, using criteria that may fail to identify many people whom clinicians say have the disease. On the other hand, if the aim is to detect all persons who have the disease, even at the expense of falsely including many who do not have it, less stringent criteria are required.

The operational definition should not only distinguish the disease from other diseases, but should also serve to delimit it along its own biological gradient. If the disease is poliomyelitis, it may be wished to include only the relatively few persons with persistent paralysis, or the larger number with transient paralysis, or the considerably larger number who take ill but have no paralysis, or the even larger number who have subclinical infections.

The definitions may serve to delimit categories along a broad biological spectrum that extends into the 'normal' range. Using fasting plasma glucose concentrations, for example, the defined categories in an epidemiological study may be 'normal' (less than 100 mg/dl), 'impaired fasting glucose' (100 mg/dl or more, but under 126 mg/dl), and 'diabetes' (126 mg/dl or more). These cutting-points are based on the recommendations of the American Diabetes Association in 2007.[7] But cutting-points of this kind are somewhat arbitrary. They are determined mainly by current knowledge about the risk of complications and the effects of treatment, and they are often changed by expert committees as this knowledge accumulates. The above cutting-point of 100 mg/dl replaces the 110 mg/dl recommended by expert committees of the American Diabetes Association in 1997 and 2003.[8]

The choice of the criteria to be used is heavily influenced by the methods by which the data are to be collected. Very different criteria may be used in a study based solely on interviews, one in which clinical examinations are performed, and one utilizing biochemical, microbiological, radiological and other diagnostic tests. The definitive criterion of acute rheumatic fever is finding Aschoff bodies in a microscopic study of heart muscle,[9] and this is obviously of limited applicability, as is a definition of chronic bronchitis that specifies 'chronic inflammatory, fibrotic and atrophic changes in the bronchial structures'. At the other extreme, no medical training is required to diagnose chronic bronchitis if it is defined as 'the production of phlegm from the chest at least twice a day on most days for a least three months each year for two or more years',[10] the data being obtained by the use of a standard questionnaire.

The use of standard definitions is especially important in multicentre trials and other studies conducted in a number of cooperating general practices or other health services, in studies that compare the occurrence of diseases in different regions or countries, and in studies of time trends. A change in diagnostic criteria – insistence on demonstration of the malaria parasite in the blood – caused an 11-fold reduction in the annual number of cases of malaria in the United States between 1946 and 1949.[11]

We have said that few diseases have satisfactory and widely accepted working definitions. Paradoxically, difficulties frequently arise not because of a lack, but because of a surfeit of operational definitions. Different investigators use different definitions, and their findings are difficult to compare. A comparison of six different commonly used sets of diagnostic criteria for dementia showed that the prevalence of this disorder in the same large sample of elderly people in Canada varied from 3 to 29%, depending on which set of criteria was used – only 1% had dementia according to all six sets of criteria.[12] Similarly, the prevalence of benign prostatic hyperplasia in a community sample of men ranged, according to different definitions, from 4 to 19%.[13] A review of criteria independently developed by various authors for common musculoskeletal disorders of the upper limbs revealed that complete correspondence seldom occurred.[14]

The use of standardized criteria proposed for some diseases by committees or panels of experts facilitates comparisons. Even then there may be difficulties, since there may be differences in the way the criteria are understood or applied, and changes from time to time. A comparison of 'old' and 'new' World Health

Organization (WHO) criteria for definite myocardial infarction, for example, showed that only 82% of the cases who met the old criteria also met the new criteria; the new definition required Minnesota coding of the ECGs (see p. 106) rather than subjective appraisal.[15] The frequency of diabetes in Pima Indians in Arizona was 12.5% by the American Diabetes Association's 1997 criteria, and 15.3% by the WHO 1999 criteria.[16]

To come back to the common cold, one of the textbooks we have cited[2] provides two operational definitions:

> 1. *Suggestive.* A constellation of acute upper respiratory symptoms with a predominance of sneezing, nasal obstruction, and discharge suggests a diagnosis of a common cold.
> 2. *Definitive.* For decisions on clinical care, presence of the common cold syndrome and absence of a history of hay fever or exposure to noxious substances may be considered as providing a definitive diagnosis. Although not necessary for optimal care, isolation of one of the causative viruses from a person with the common cold syndrome would solidify the diagnosis.

The purpose of the first definition is unclear, since it does not apparently provide a sufficient basis for decisions on care. The second is more useful, but not completely unambiguous; the 'common cold syndrome' presumably refers to the constellation mentioned in the first definition. But what does 'a predominance of sneezing, nasal obstruction, and discharge' mean: must all three be present? Can a cold be diagnosed in the absence of sneezing or in the absence of nasal obstruction? Note that the isolation of a relevant virus is not an essential criterion.

In an investigation based on questions put weekly to a population sample, a common cold might be defined as 'a report of a stuffy or running nose'. The diagnosis may not be completely valid, as some cases of allergic rhinitis may be included, and some people with running noses may not report them, but the definition has the advantages that it is unequivocal and eminently practical. A different definition might, of course, be used if virological tests were warranted by the study's purpose and resources.

Side-stepping the Issue

In many (or even most) investigations, the need to formulate diagnostic criteria is side-stepped, and diseases are operationally defined in terms of reports of their presence. That is, the process of diagnosis is left to someone else (usually a doctor, sometimes the patient, a relative, teacher, etc.), and a report of the disease is taken as evidence of its presence. As an example, haemorrhoids might be operationally defined as:

- A recorded diagnosis of 'haemorrhoids' or 'piles' (in a specified clinical record).
- A positive response to the question 'Did a doctor ever tell you you had haemorrhoids or piles?'
- A positive response to the question 'Do you have piles?'

The use of second-hand diagnostic information of this sort, not based on defined criteria, has obvious limitations. But it is often the only practicable approach, and should by no means be rejected, particularly if the information is obtained from well-equipped clinical services with a high standard of medical practice. If this 'imperfect' method is the only practical method, then it should be used, provided that consideration is given to the effects the 'imperfection' may have on the findings, and that (if necessary) caution is used in interpreting the findings.

Self-reports and diagnoses based on experts' criteria may obviously not coincide. The prevalence of chronic constipation in a population sample was 14% or 19% using two sets of experts' criteria, and 29.5% according to self-reports.[17]

Notes and References

1. You will search in vain for an operational definition of the common cold in the 2745-page Harrison's principles of internal medicine (16th edn. Kasper DL, Braunwald E, Hauser S, Longo D, Jameson JL, Fauci AS (eds). McGraw-Hill; 2005).
2. Couch RB. In: Hurst JW (ed.), Medicine for the practicing physician, 4th edn. Stamford, CT: Appleton & Lange; 1996. pp. 479–481.
3. MacMahon B, Pugh TF. Epidemiology: principles and methods. Boston, MA: Little, Brown; 1970. pp. 47–54.
4. These are the Jones criteria (Special Writing Group of the Committee on Rheumatic Fever, Endocarditis, and Kawasaki Disease of the Council on Cardiovascular Disease in the Young of the American Heart Association. Guidelines for the diagnosis of rheumatic fever: Jones criteria, 1992 update. Journal of the American Medical Association 1992; 268: 2069). Cited in Harrison's principles of internal medicine (2005, p. 1977; see note 1).
5. Harrison's principles of internal medicine (2005, p. 1973; see note 1).
6. Harrison's principles of internal medicine (2005, pp. 1364, 1371; see note 1).
7. American Diabetes Association. Diagnosis and classification of diabetes mellitus. Diabetes Care 2007; 30(Suppl. 1): S42.
8. Expert Committee on the Diagnosis and Classification of Diabetes Mellitus. Report of the Expert Committee on the Diagnosis and Classification of Diabetes Mellitus. Diabetes Care 2003; 26(Suppl. 1): S55.
9. Schlant RC. In: Hurst JW (ed.) (1996, pp. 1255–1258; see note 2).
10. Fletcher CM. Some problems of diagnostic standardization using clinical methods, with special reference to chronic bronchitis. In: Pemberton J (ed.), Epidemiology: reports on research and teaching. Oxford: Oxford University Press; 1963. p. 253.
11. Mainland D. Elementary medical statistics, 2nd edn. Philadelphia, PA; WB Saunders; 1964. pp. 131–132.
12. The following six sets of diagnostic criteria were compared in this study: DSM-III (Diagnostic and statistical manual of mental disorders, 3rd edn); DSM-III-R (ditto, 3rd edn, revised); DSM-IV (ditto, 4th edn); CAMDEX (Cambridge Examination for Mental Disorders of the Elderly); ICD-9 (International classification of diseases, 9th edn); and ICD-10 (ditto, 10th edn). The respective results for the prevalence of dementia in the same 1879 men and women were 29.1%, 17.3%, 13.7%, 4.9%, 5.0% and 3.1%. The main reasons for the disparities were different requirements concerning long-term memory, abstract thinking and other executive functions, work and activities of daily living, and duration of symptoms (Erkinjuntti T, Ostbye T, Steenhuis R, Hachinski V. The effect of different

diagnostic criteria on the prevalence of dementia. New England Journal of Medicine 1997; 337: 1667).

13. Bosch JL, Hop WC, Kirkels WJ, Schroder FH. Natural history of benign prostatic hyperplasia: appropriate case definition and estimation of its prevalence in the community. Urology 1995; 46(3 suppl. A): 34.

14. Van Eerd D, Beaton D, Cole D, Lucas J, Hogg-Johnson S, Bombardier C. Classification systems for upper-limb musculoskeletal disorders in workers: a review of the literature. Journal of Clinical Epidemiology 2003; 56: 925.

15. Beaglehole R, Stewart AW, Butler M. Comparability of old and new World Health Organization criteria for definite myocardial infarction. International Journal of Epidemiology 1987; 16: 373.

16. Gabir MM, Hanson RL, Dabelea D, Imperatore G, Roumain J, Bennett PH, Knowler WC. The 1997 American Diabetes Association and 1999 World Health Organization criteria for hyperglycemia in the diagnosis and prediction of diabetes. Diabetes Care 2000; 23: 1108.

17. Garrigues V, Galvez C, Ortiz V, Ponce M, Nos P, Ponce J. Prevalence of constipation: agreement among several criteria and evaluation of the diagnostic accuracy of qualifying symptoms and self-reported definition in a population-based survey in Spain. American Journal of Epidemiology 2004; 159: 520.

13

Scales of Measurement

As part of the process of clarifying each of the variables to be studied, its scale of measurement should be specified. This chapter will discuss the types of scale and the criteria of a satisfactory scale, and will briefly describe the International Classification of Diseases and some other commonly used classifications.

Types of Scale

The scale of measurement may be *categorical* (consisting of separate categories) or *metric* (sometimes called *numerical*, although numbers can also be used to denote categories).

A *categorical scale* consists of two or more mutually exclusive categories (classes). If these do not fall into a natural order, the scale is *nominal*. Numbers may be used to identify the categories, but these are 'code numbers' with no quantitative significance. Examples are:

- Marital status – single, married, widowed, divorced.
- Religion – Christian, Jewish, Muslim, Hindu, Buddhist, freethinker, other.
- Type of anaemia – 1, iron-deficiency anaemia; 2, other deficiency anaemias; 3, hereditary haemolytic anaemias; 4, acquired haemolytic anaemias; 5, aplastic anaemia; 6, other anaemias.

If the categories fall into what is regarded as a natural order, the scale is *ordinal*. The scale shows ranks, or positions on a ladder; each class shows the same situational relationship to the class that follows it. If numbers are used, they indicate the positions of the categories in the series. Examples are:

- Social class, using the British Registrar-General's classification) – I, II, III, IV, V (see note 1, Chapter 11).
- Years of education – 0, 1–5, 6–9, 10–12, more than 12.
- Severity of a disease – mild, moderate, severe.
- Limitation of activity – 0, none; 1, limited activity, but not home-bound; 2, home-bound, but not bed-bound; 3, bed-bound.

Research Methods in Community Medicine: Surveys, Epidemiological Research, Programme Evaluation, Clinical Trials   J. H. Abramson and Z. H. Abramson   Copyright © 2008, John Wiley & Sons Ltd

A commonly used type of ordinal scale, usually employed to measure attitudes, is the *Likert-type scale*. This is typically a set of graded alternative responses to a question, with specified scores – for example, 'How strongly do you agree or disagree with the following statement?' with possible responses of '1, strongly agree'; '2, agree'; '3, undecided'; '4, disagree'; and '5, strongly disagree'. The intervals between successive alternatives are not necessarily equal, and statistical methods appropriate for ordinal data should be used when analysing the responses.

An ordinal scale is 'stronger' than a nominal one, in the sense that it provides more information. Where there is a choice, use of an ordinal scale is preferable.

If some categories are ranked and others are not, the scale is a nominal one. If a category of 'unclassifiable' is added to an ordinal scale, then the new scale is nominal – but it remains ordinal if the 'unclassifiable' class is ignored.[1] The NE-SEC scales shown in Table 11.1 (p. 110) are clearly nominal, not ordinal.

A scale with only two categories is a *dichotomy* (or *binary* or '*yes–no*' scale).[2] Many statistical procedures are applicable to dichotomies but not to scales with three or more categories. Numbers – generally 0 and 1 (indicating the absence or presence of an attribute), or 1 and 2 – may be used as code numbers. Examples are:

- Agreement with a statement – agree, disagree.
- Sex – 1, male; 2, female.
- Presence of a disease – 0, absent; 1, present.
- Occurrence of headaches – 0, no; 1, yes.

Metric (noncategorical) scales, which are also called *dimensional* or *numerical,* use numbers that indicate the quantity of what is being measured. They have two features. First, equal differences between any pairs of numbers in the scale mean equal differences in the attribute being measured, i.e. the difference between any two values reflects the magnitude of the difference in the attribute – the difference in temperature between 22 and 26 °C, for example, is the same as that between 30 and 34 °C; this makes the scale an *interval scale*. Second, in some of these scales, zero indicates absence of the attribute, as a result of which the ratio between any two values indicates the ratio between the amounts of the attribute – an income of \$1000 is twice as high as an income of \$500; this additional feature makes the scale a *ratio scale*. Most noncategorical scales have both these features; exceptional ones, like the Centigrade scale for temperature, are interval but not ratio scales: 0 °C does not mean 'absence of heat'; therefore, 30 °C is not 'twice as hot' as 15 °C. Examples of ratio scales are:

- Weight – measured in kilograms or pounds.
- Mortality rate – number of deaths per 1,000 persons at risk.
- Beauty – measured in milli-helens.[3]

An interval or ratio scale provides more information than an ordinal one, and is to be preferred when there is a choice.

Interval and ratio scales may be *continuous* or *discrete*. The scale is continuous if an infinite number of values is possible along a continuum, e.g. when measuring height or cholesterol concentration. It is discrete if only certain values along the scale are possible – a woman's parity, for example, cannot be 2.35. (But note that some authors use the term 'continuous' to denote *any* noncategorical data.)

An interval or ratio scale may be 'collapsed' or 'binned' into categories (or classes), each containing a range of values, e.g.

- Income (in monetary units): 0–49, 50–99, 100–149, etc.

If equal class intervals are used, as in this example, then the scale can sometimes still be treated as an interval one, taking the midpoints (25, 75, 125, etc.) as the values of the successive classes. Strictly speaking, however, it may now be an ordinal scale, since the individual values may not be uniformly spread within the classes, and the intervals between the average incomes of people in adjacent classes may hence not be equal. The scale is degraded to an ordinal scale if an 'open-ended' category is used (for instance, a top income group of '500 or more'). An accurate mean value cannot be calculated from such a scale. Similarly, the scale becomes an ordinal one if the class intervals vary, e.g. 0–49, 50–199, 200–399, etc.

The selection of a scale for measuring a variable is partly determined by the variable itself and the methods available for measuring it. Marital status, type of work, and type of anaemia cannot be measured by interval or ratio scales. For most variables, however, alternative methods of measurement are available.

Clearly, decisions concerning scales of measurement may influence the methods by which data will be collected. Different questions are required to measure the frequency of headaches (using an interval or ordinal scale), or merely to determine whether the subject suffers from headaches (using a 'yes–no' scale). When categories are used, they are usually specified in the questionnaires or examination schedules (see pp. 227–230).

Different statistical procedures are appropriate for different kinds of scale. A procedure appropriate for a dichotomy or categorical data can be applied to interval-scale or ordinal-scale data only if the data are grouped, and a procedure designed for ordinal data cannot ordinarily be applied to unordered data. Similarly, a procedure designed for numerical data cannot be applied to a nominal scale – we may know how many people have black, brown, blonde, carroty, blue, and grey hair (or none), but we cannot compute an average of these hair colours. But various options are usually available for the analysis, since the scale used when the data are collected is not necessarily the one that will be used throughout the analysis. Observations concerning a variable measured by one kind of scale may be analysed by a procedure suited to another kind of scale, in accordance with the research hypothesis and the purpose of the analysis. Age (measured by an interval scale) may be treated as an interval-scale variable – e.g. when calculating the mean age or examining a correlation between age and some other variable – but for some purposes it may be appropriate to use a nominal scale, merely dividing the subjects into different age groups, and not assuming a monotonic relationship between age and the other variable (i.e. a consistent increase or decrease in the other variable when people in younger and older categories are compared). Ethnic group is measured by a nominal scale; but it may be treated as an ordinal-scale variable by arranging the categories in a specific sequence, in an analysis designed to see whether its categories have an ordered relationship with some other variable.

During the planning phase, thought should be given to the scales that will be used when the data are analysed, as well as when they are collected. At this stage it is often helpful to construct *skeleton* or *dummy tables*, i.e. tables without figures or containing fictional figures respectively, incorporating the variables under consideration. If there are categories, then they should be specified in the column or row headings. At this stage it is not essential to decide precisely how the finer categories will be 'collapsed' into broader categories for the purposes of analysis. It is often desirable to defer such decisions, since they may be difficult to make without knowing the actual distribution of the values. If doubt exists about the way a variable will be treated in the analysis, then care should be taken to collect data in such a way as to leave the options open.

Criteria of a Satisfactory Scale

A satisfactory scale of measurement is one that meets the following seven requirements:

Requirements of a scale

1. Appropriate
2. Practicable
3. Sufficiently powerful
4. Clearly defined components
5. Sufficient categories
6. Comprehensive
7. Mutually exclusive

1. It is *appropriate* for use in the study, keeping in mind the conceptual definition of the variable and the objectives of the study. Occupations, for instance, may be classified in different ways, depending on whether the purpose is to use occupation as a measure of social class, of habitual physical activity, or of exposure to specific physical and chemical hazards. Similarly, different classifications may be used for the region of birth of immigrants, depending on whether the variable is to be used as an indicator of environmental conditions in childhood, of ethnic group, or of genetic attributes. In measuring birth weights, it may be decided to use categories extending evenly along the whole weight spectrum, or, if the specific subject of inquiry is the effect of low birth weight, to use narrow categories for babies of low birth weight and broad categories for heavier babies.
2. It is a *practicable* scale – one that is geared to the methods that will be used in collecting the information. For example, if the data are to be obtained from records that list marital status as 'single', 'married', 'widowed' and 'divorced', then there is no point in deciding upon a more elaborate scale of measurement, e.g. including 'married once', 'married more than once', etc. Account should be taken of the precision of the methods to be used in collecting the data. Can accurate ages be obtained

in terms of years and months, or only in terms of years? If people tend to 'round off' their ages ('I am 40 years old', '50 years old', etc.), a scale showing each year separately will have only spurious precision (see p. 164). Will it be possible to get detailed data on income or the number of cigarettes smoked per day, or is it only possible to use broad categories? Is the balance to be used for weighing sufficiently discriminatory to warrant measurements in tenths of kilograms, or should whole kilograms be used? Is there any point in recording liver enlargement in centimetres, if tests have shown a negligible correlation between measurements made by different physicians on the same patients?

3. The scale is *powerful* enough to satisfy the objectives of the study. If there is a choice, an ordinal scale should be used rather than a nominal one, and an interval or ratio scale rather than a categorical one. An analysis using the whole spectrum of haemoglobin levels is likely to be more informative than one using a dichotomy, such as 'below 12 g per 100 ml' and '12 g or more per 100 ml'. In measuring an attitude an ordinal scale should be used, based on the provision of graded alternative responses to a question or on a score derived from the responses to a series of questions, rather than a simple dichotomy such as 'agree–disagree' or 'important–unimportant'.

4. The components are *clearly defined*. Wherever necessary, operational definitions should be formulated not only for the variable, but for the categories. This applies especially to nominal and ordinal scales. If cases of a disease are to be classified as 'active' and 'healed', or patients with a malignant neoplasm according to the stage of the disorder, then these categories need careful definition. In the case of numerical measurements, decisions may be needed on the number of decimal places to be used and on whether and how values are to be rounded off – downwards or to the nearest number. It is usually preferable to round off downwards, so that the class '73 kg', for example, includes all weights between 73.0 and 73.9 kg; if this is done, then it must be remembered that the assumed average value of the weights in this category will be 73.5 kg.

5. The scale contains *sufficient categories*. While the number of categories should not be multiplied unnecessarily, the compression of data into too few categories may lead to a loss of useful information. For example, if immigrants from North Africa have a particularly high rate of mortality from cerebrovascular disease, then this fact may become less obvious or may be completely masked if they are included in a broader category of 'immigrants from Africa and Asia'. Often, 'articulated' scales are used – scales containing categories that 'branch', like the bones of the limbs – i.e. categories that are divided into subcategories and, if necessary, sub-subcategories. The use of such a scale leaves the options open for a later decision as to the use of broad or narrow categories. With numerical data, it is often similarly advisable to collect the information in a detailed form and to decide later whether to use the full scale or a 'collapsed' one (or both). With numerical data, the use of too few categories may prevent the calculation of an accurate mean.

6. The scale is *collectively exhaustive* (*comprehensive*). It provides a niche for the classification of every subject. This may necessitate the inclusion of one or more of the following categories:

- Other.
- Not applicable, e.g. information on the duration of marriage may be collected only from people who are at present married; in this case, the scale used may be 'under 5 years', '5–9.9 years', '10–19.9 years', '20–29.9 years', '30–39.9 years', '40 years and more', and 'not applicable'.
- Unknown (it may sometimes be desirable to subdivide this category, e.g. to distinguish between subjects who did not know the answer to a question and those with information lacking for other reasons: the question was not asked, the response was illegible, a page of the completed questionnaire was mislaid, etc.).

7. The categories are *mutually exclusive*. Each item of information should fit into only one place along the scale. For example, a scale including both '70 to 80' and '80 to 90' is generally unacceptable, as '80' could fit into either of these classes. Similarly, if a scale includes 'married' and 'remarried', a remarried person could fit into either category. If a scale for measuring the conditions producing disability includes the categories 'blindness' and 'deafness', then either a clear rule should be formulated whereby persons who are both blind and deaf are assigned to one of these categories, or the scale should include the categories 'blind, not deaf', 'deaf, not blind' and 'blind and deaf'. In the Minnesota code for ECG findings (see p. 106), where different codable items may coexist in the same scale of measurement (e.g. that for T wave items), only one is coded, the order of precedence being clearly stated.

International Classification of Diseases

The International Classification of Diseases (ICD), published by the WHO[4] and now in its tenth revision (ICD-10), is widely used as a nominal scale for the categorization of diseases. Each disease category is given a three-character code (a letter and two numerals), and almost all categories are divided into subcategories.

Since our principles of nosology are far from rational, the arrangement of the ICD is arbitrary. Some diseases are classified by their aetiology ('infectious and parasitic diseases'), some by their site ('diseases of the respiratory system'), some by a pathological feature ('neoplasms'), some by age at onset ('certain conditions originating in the perinatal period'), etc. Neoplasms are subclassified by their sites, but an optional supplementary morphological classification is provided. Injuries are classified in two ways: by their nature and by their external causes. Codes are provided for factors (other than illness) that may bring a person into contact with a health service or influence health status (e.g. immunization, contraceptive management, living alone, extreme poverty). Special short lists are provided for the tabulation of mortality and morbidity.

Some diseases have dual codes: a mandatory dagger code for classifying the underlying general disease and an optional asterisk code for classifying it according to its manifestation in a particular organ or site. If both codes are used, the categories of the classification are not mutually exclusive.

'Glossary descriptions' are provided for mental disorders and some other conditions. These descriptions fall far short of ideal operational definitions.

Coding is best left to experienced coders. One can do it oneself, but care must be taken. To code a disease, it is first looked up in the index, which is published as a separate volume. The index includes diagnostic terms that are not specifically stated in the classification itself. After using the index, reference should be made to the appropriate item in the classification, since this may contain a note leading to a modification of the code number. The conventions used in the classification must be clearly understood if the book is to be used effectively.[5] Before drawing inferences from tabulations based on the ICD it is wise to examine the details of the classification, so as to be sure of what is and what is not included in the various categories.

Adaptations of the ICD include a 'clinical modification' (ICD-10-CM),[6] which is more detailed than the ICD; it divides the ICD's categories into more specific subcategories.

Classifications for Use in Primary Care

The *International Classification of Health Problems in Primary Care (ICHPPC-2)* is a classification designed primarily to permit a general or family practitioner to code diagnoses or other problems at the time of the patient encounter.[7] It includes diseases (classified more simply than in the ICD), important signs and symptoms, social and family problems, forms of preventive care, and administrative procedures. *ICHPPC-2-Defined* is a version that contains definitions of most of the rubrics. These were designed as 'the briefest possible definitions which would reduce variability in coding', and stipulate criteria that must be fulfilled if miscoding is to be avoided. As examples, a diagnosis is coded as 'acute upper respiratory infection' (a category that includes colds, nasopharyngitis, pharyngitis and rhinitis) only if two criteria are met: (1) evidence of acute inflammation of the nasal or pharyngeal mucosa and (2) absence of criteria for more specifically defined acute respiratory infections listed in the classification. The authors stress that the definitions are not intended to serve as a guide to diagnosis, but can reduce chances of miscoding after a diagnosis has been made.

The *International Classification of Primary Care (ICPC)*[8] permits patients' encounters to be classified not only according to the physician's diagnosis or assessment of the health problem, but also according to the reason for the encounter as expressed by the patient, and the nature of the diagnostic and therapeutic interventions undertaken in the process of care. One or more of these axes may be used. The patient's reason for encounter (which may need clarification by the care provider) may be a symptom, a disease, getting a prescription or test result or certificate, etc. The 'process' components include various diagnostic, preventive, therapeutic and administrative procedures, and referrals. The ICPC is consistent with the use of problem-oriented clinical records, which use the SOAP acronym: S = subjective (the patient's reason for the encounter), O = objective signs, A = assessment (diagnosis) and P = plan (the process of care or intervention); but objective signs are not classified by the ICPC. The authors suggest use of the ICPC as a basis for an information system based on disease episodes (from onset to resolution) for which there may be more than one encounter.

The International Classification of Functioning, Disability and Health (ICF)[9] may be found useful in studies concerned with disability and rehabilitation. It replaces the International Classification of Impairments, Disabilities and Handicaps (ICIDH-2).

Notes and References

1. As an example, Katz's index of independence in activities in daily living has six ordered categories, A to F, and a seventh 'other' category. The categories are: Independent in: (A) continence, transferring (bed–chair), going to toilet, dressing, bathing; (B) all but one of these functions; (C) all but bathing and one additional function; (D) all but bathing, dressing and one additional function; (E) all but bathing, dressing, going to toilet, transferring, and one additional function; (F) dependent in all six functions; and (other) dependent in at least two functions, but not classifiable as C, D, E or F (Katz S, Ford AB, Moskowitz RW, Jackson BA, Jaffe MW. Studies of illness in the aged: the Index of ADL: a standardized measure of biological and psychosocial function. Journal of the American Medical Association 1963; 185: 914).

2. *Dichotomies* can be treated not only as nominal, but also as ordinal, interval, or (in some instances) ratio scales. Many statistical procedures are applicable to dichotomies but not to nominal scales that have three or more categories. Dichotomies and other nominal scales can usefully be regarded as different types of scale.

3. A milli-helen is 'the quantity of beauty required to launch exactly one ship' (Dickinson RE. The Observer, letter, 23 Feb. 1958). This useful unit of measurement of pulchritude is based on the well-known line, 'Was this the face that launched a thousand ships...?' (referring to Helen of Troy) in Christopher Marlowe's play The Tragical History of Doctor Faustus.

4. World Health Organization. The international statistical classification of diseases and related health problems: ICD-10, 2nd edn. Geneva: WHO; 2005. Available at http://www.who.int/classifications/apps/icd/_icd10online.

5. The ICD uses parentheses (...) to enclose words or phrases whose presence or absence does not matter. Square brackets [...] enclose alternative wordings or explanatory phrases. Terms preceding a colon are incomplete, and must be completed by one of the modifiers that follow the colon. 'NOS' stands for 'not otherwise specified' (i.e. without qualification). 'How to use the ICD' is explained in vol 2 of the classification (see note 4).

6. National Center for Health Statistics. The international classification of diseases, tenth revision, clinical modification (ICD-10-CM), July 2007 Release. Hyattsville, MD: National Center for Health Statistics, 2003. Available at http://www.cdc.gov/nchs/about/otheract/icd9/icd10cm.htm.

7. World Organization of National Colleges, Academies and Academic Associations of General Practitioners/Family Physicians (WONCA). Classification Committee 1983 ICHPPC-2-Defined, 3rd edn. Oxford: Oxford University Press.

8. WONCA. International classification of primary care: ICPC-2-R. Oxford University Press; 2005.

9. World Health Organization. The international classification of functional, disability and health – ICF. Geneva: WHO; 2001.

14

Composite Scales

Variables based on two or more other variables may be termed *composite variables*. Examples are: (1) caloric intake, which is calculated from the quantities of a variety of foodstuffs, (2) the presence or stage of a disease, which may be based on a set of symptoms and clinical signs, (3) an attitude, when measured by the responses to a series of separate questions, and (4) overall health, based on separate measures of physical and mental health. Scales that are used for measuring composite variables may be termed *composite scales*.

The manner in which the component data are brought together into a composite scale is usually decided upon in advance, using rules that enter into the operational definition of the composite variable. There are also techniques (e.g. Guttman scaling, factor analysis) that require the collection and analysis of the component data to see how they 'hang together', before deciding how to combine them.

The scale may be based on *combinations of categories*. For instance, hypertension may be defined as a systolic blood pressure of 140 mmHg or more and/or a diastolic pressure of 90 mmHg or more, and a normal blood pressure as a systolic pressure below 130 mmHg together with a diastolic pressure below 85 mmHg. If other combinations of systolic and diastolic pressures are placed in an intermediate or 'high normal' group, this provides a composite scale of the ordinal type. The scale might be elaborated by adding 'and/or receiving specific treatment for hypertension' to the definition of hypertension, and adding 'and not under treatment' to the definitions of the other categories. A composite scale of the nominal type is sometimes referred to as a *typology*.

Formulae are used for composite variables that express relationships between other variables. Examples are: the length of gestation, usually estimated from the date of onset of the last menstrual period and the date at which pregnancy ended; average family income per head; adiposity indices based on weight and height; and all rates.[1]

Use is often made of *combination scores* computed from the separate scores allotted to a set of component variables. Combining several variables in this way generally carries advantages over reliance on any single component variable (but if the components are heterogeneous, one or more of them may be more useful for some purposes than the combination score). The simplest technique is to add up the component scores, using the raw or weighted scores; appropriate weights are sometimes determined by rather complicated procedures.

This chapter will review Guttman scaling and combination scores in more detail, provide guidelines for the construction of a composite scale, and briefly consider scales that describe the community.

Research Methods in Community Medicine: Surveys, Epidemiological Research, Programme Evaluation, Clinical Trials   J. H. Abramson and Z. H. Abramson   Copyright © 2008, John Wiley & Sons Ltd

Guttman Scale

One way of combining component items into a composite scale is to see whether the results conform with a *Guttman scale (scalogram)*,[2] i.e. a 'hierarchy', and then use the Guttman scale type as a score. As a simple example, consider the following three 'yes–no' questions:

1. Do you weigh more than 50 kg?
2. Do you weigh more than 75 kg?
3. Do you weigh more than 100 kg?

The only four possible combinations of correct replies (to questions 1, 2 and 3 respectively) are 'no–no–no', 'yes–no–no', 'yes–yes–no', and 'yes–yes–yes'; these are four 'scale types' that constitute an ordinal scale. Question 2 cannot be answered 'yes' unless question 1 is also answered 'yes', and question 3 cannot be answered 'yes' unless both questions 1 and 2 are also answered 'yes'. All the responses should conform with the above scale types – there should be no deviant responses. The scale types might be numbered 0 to 3, i.e. (in this instance) according to the number of 'yes' responses, and they then provide an ordinal measure of weight. If analysis of the findings of a study reveals a set of variables that are acceptably *scalable* in this way, then each scale type expresses a position along the dimension that is measured. If a few responses do not fall into scale types they can be assigned to the closest scale type by the use of preset rules.

Guttman scales have been used for attitudes, dietary habits, clinical manifestations of a disease, the severity of low back pain, the ability to engage in self-care activities, the level of domestic violence, and other attributes. Among British students, it was found possible to construct a Guttman scale for 'meat avoidance' from questions about the eating of poultry, beef, lamb and pork – these questions apparently measured a single dimension; but (contrary to previous assumptions) the eating of fish did not fit into the scale.[3] In a study of schoolchildren, the scale types for 'risk behaviours' were: none; alcohol; alcohol and cigarettes; alcohol, cigarettes and sex; alcohol, cigarettes, sex and drugs.[4]

The number attached to a scale type not only constitutes a measure, it also provides qualitative information. For example, in a community survey, the reported ability to perform six activities constituted an excellent Guttman scale.[5] The activities were: 1, light work in the home (e.g. washing dishes); 2, walking in the vicinity of the house; 3, moderate work in the home (e.g. moving a chair or table); 4, walking uphill or upstairs; 5, running a short distance; and 6, active sports. The scale types were: 0, can do none of these activities; 1, can do activity 1 only; 2, can do activities 1 and 2 only; and so on. A scale type (score) of 3 not only tells us that the subject is less capable than one with a scale type of 4, it is also a shorthand way of telling us that they can do light or moderate work in the home and take a walk in the vicinity of the house, but no more vigorous activities.

The building blocks in developing the scale need not be separate items. They can also be combinations (connected by 'or', 'and/or', or 'and') of 'yes–no' items, combinations (connected by 'or') of possible responses to multiple-category items, etc. As a result, there may be different ways of constructing a hierarchy from the same variables. While the categories of Katz's index of independence in daily living[6] constitute a Guttman scale, an analysis of all the possible permutations revealed four hierarchies that were at least as good, and 103 that satisfied the minimum for scalability.[7]

The testing of a Guttman scale is best left to a computer program.[8]

When analysing the data, it should be remembered that a Guttman scale is an ordinal scale, not an interval scale.

Combination Scores

The simplest combination score is the number of positive responses to a set of 'yes–no' items (every 'yes' is taken as 1 and every 'no' as 0). This method is often used for scoring questionnaires like the Cornell Medical Index (CMI),[9] which comprises questions about the presence of symptoms, illnesses, etc. Similarly, the diagnosis of rheumatoid arthritis can be based on the number of diagnostic criteria that are fulfilled.[10] But note that 'number of symptoms' scores are not always acceptable, and they should not be used uncritically.[11]

If a set of items that deal with different aspects of a variable has a Likert-type scale (see p. 125), i.e. if they have graded alternative responses, with preset scores, then the scores for all the items can be added to provide a global measure. This combination is a *summative Likert scale*, and is often treated as a metric scale. A commonly used summative Likert scale is the Apgar score used to appraise the status of newborn infants. This is the sum of the points (0, 1 or 2) allotted for each of five items: heart rate, respiratory effort, muscle tone, response to stimulation by a catheter in the nostril, and skin colour. An internationally used Prostate Symptom Score is based on seven symptoms, each with a 0 to 5 score expressing its frequency.[12] Summative Likert scales are used in the SF-36 Health Survey questionnaire, which has achieved considerable popularity in recent years.[13]

Arbitrary weights are sometimes given to the items before their scores are added, based on the importance attributed to each item by the investigator or by a group of experts. For instance, in a study of the quality of medical care, scores were given for the quality of records, the quality of diagnostic management and the quality of treatment and follow-up. These three scores were then combined, using weights of 30%, 40% and 30% respectively.[14]

The component items may also be given scores based on or validated by a careful analysis of data collected in the current or a previous study. For example, a detailed study of patients in a metabolic laboratory was used to authenticate a 'clinical diagnostic index of thyrotoxicosis', with scores (based on 'diagnostic significance') for various clinical signs and symptoms (e.g. preference for cold, +5; palpable thyroid, +3; increase in weight, −13) and a recommendation that a total of 20 or more could be taken to indicate the presence of thyrotoxicosis.[15]

A variety of statistical methods (not necessarily simple) can be used to determine item scores. Among the more complicated procedures are *Rasch (item response theory) methods*[16] and *factor analysis*.[17] Rasch methods may be used to appraise whether the items form a hierarchy, whether they measure a single dimension, whether they are appropriately spaced along this dimension, and reproducibility. Factor analysis reports the fundamental dimensions that underlie the data collected for a group of variables (labelling them 'factor 1', 'factor 2', etc.), as well as stating what weights should be attached to the items in order to measure each dimension. The investigator then determines (some would say, divines) what characteristic is measured by each factor and gives it a name. This kind of analysis is most convincing if the findings are replicated in different samples. The measurement of *health locus-of-control* can be cited to demonstrate its use. Sets of questions were devised in order to grade people according to their belief that their health was under their own control (internal locus-of-control) or determined by external factors. But factor analysis revealed that there were also other dimensions, including beliefs in control by health providers and by others, and belief in the role of chance.[18]

A combination scale often used for attitudes is based on a set of 'agree–disagree' or 'true–false' questions concerning statements that represent different points along the dimension to be measured.[19] The statements may be selected in such a way that each respondent may be *a priori* expected to agree with only one or two of them and disagree with the others (*Thurstone-type differential scale*), or in such a way that agreement may be expected with all statements up to (or after) a particular point in the series (*cumulative scale*), as in the Guttman model. The selection and scoring of the questions are usually based on the judgements of a population sample or a panel of experts.

Various manipulations may be applied to the component scores or the combination score, however these are obtained. For example, scores may be converted to percentages or standardized according to the findings in a standard population.

Constructing a Composite Scale

Creating a satisfactory composite scale for general use can be a difficult and laborious process. But for an investigator who wants only to produce a combination score based on 'yes–no' or Likert-scored items, to serve the purposes of a specific study in a specific population, the task may not be overwhelming.

Here are simple guidelines.[20] When following these, take account of the purpose of the scale: is it 'discrimination' (i.e. to compare individuals or groups with different intensities of a characteristic), measurement of change, or prediction of a future event or status? If possible, the scale should be tested in a sample of the study population and then tried in another; if numbers permit, separate tests should be performed in subgroups (men and women, age groups, etc.).

1. Start with what seems to be an appropriate list of component items (questions, symptoms, etc.). The items should be relevant ones (see *face validity*, p. 164), and

should cover all important facets (see *content validity'*, p. 165). If the purpose of the scale is discrimination between individuals or groups, try to include items that express different intensities or quantities of the characteristic. If the purpose is to measure change, then the items should represent changeable characteristics and offer a sufficient number of graded response alternatives. If the aim is prediction, then all important predictors should be included. Decide on the scoring of the items: 1/0 ('yes–no') or a Likert scale.

2. Collect data, in a pretest or the study proper.
3. Examine the distribution of the combination scores. Is there enough variation to make the scale useful? If the aim is to detect change, is there a concentration at the worst possible score (a *floor effect*) or the best possible score (a *ceiling effect*), which might make it difficult to detect deterioration or improvement? The scale's *discriminatory power* can be measured with Ferguson's *delta* coefficient, which ranges from 0 if all subjects have the same score to 1 if subjects are equally divided among all possible scores.[21]
4. Examine the relationships between the items.[8] This may provide a basis for the deletion of items. This examination is relatively unimportant if the scale measures a heterogeneous attribute, such as the presence of a disease with diverse unrelated manifestations, or to predict a future event – good predictors do not necessarily have to be present at the same time.

   (a) Measure the correlations between items and between each item and the total score of the other items. Negatively correlated items have no place in the same scale.[22] On the other hand, if the aim is discrimination, very highly correlated items may not be helpful, since they may be measuring almost exactly the same thing; medium correlations suggest that the items reflect diversity with respect to the characteristic being measured.

   (b) Compute Cronbach's *alpha* coefficient,[23] which measures the scale's internal consistency; its value depends on the average correlation between items and on the number of items. A value of 0.7 or higher is often regarded as satisfactory, indicating that the items may be measures of much the same attribute; but a value in excess of 0.8 is preferable, and 0.9 or 0.95 is desirable. Alpha may be regarded as an indicator of reliability (see Chapter 16). According to a meta-analysis of studies using composite scales,[24] the deletion of items increased the mean alpha from 0.7 to 0.87.

   (c) If possible, determine whether the findings are consistent with the assumption that the scale measures a single attribute, e.g. by testing for Guttman scalability[2] (easily done for 'yes–no' items, but more difficult for multiple-response items). If so, this is probably the best scale to use, although there can be no guarantee that the attribute that the scale measures is indeed the attribute that the investigator wants to measure.

   (d) Make any required modifications to the scale and then retest. If the scale is internally consistent but contains an unwieldy number of items, then it may be worth dropping some; the items to be kept should be ones that examine different facets, rather than those that maximize internal consistency.

5. If possible, test the scale's reliability (see Chapter 16) and validity, with and without modifications. Validity tests should take account of the purpose of the scale (see Chapter 17). Any composite score based on decisions (possibly arbitrary) about the inclusion and weighting of items is open to criticism unless such tests are done– and yet only 25% of a series of clinical trials using quality of life as an outcome measure reported the reliability of the quality-of-life measure, and only 23% gave information on its validity![25]

6. When the scale is ready, test it in a different sample, so as not to be misled by chance 'quirks' in the initial sample.

The construction of a good composite scale is never easy. However, it is comforting that if the items measure a single dimension and have a clear-cut ranking of their categories, how they are brought together into a composite scale is not always of great consequence. This was shown in a survey of disability in London, where information was obtained about the capacity to perform various activities. Four separate composite scales were developed, including a Guttman scale and an additive scale in which each activity, and the degree of disability in performing it, was given an arbitrary score based on the criteria used by local social workers for defining handicap. The scores yielded by the different methods turned out to be highly correlated with one another.[26]

Scales that Describe the Community

Ecological and multi-level studies of the effects on health, health behaviour, and health care of the local community environment have usually relied on crude proxy measures derived from a census or other available databases. The need for more specific measures of possibly health-relevant features of the community context in which people live – such as safety, violence, the availability of healthy foods, 'walkability', and social cohesion – is currently leading to the development of simple composite scales.[27] This, it is hoped, may lead to a better understanding of the causal or modifying effects of these specific features of the context, and permit control of their confounding effects when examining associations found at the individual level.

The scales are usually based on questions put to residents. One 'safety' scale, for example, was based on Likert-type questions about agreement with three statements:[27]

1. I feel safe walking in my neighbourhood, day or night.
2. Violence is not a problem in my neighbourhood.
3. My neighbourhood is safe from crime.

A 'social cohesion' scale was based on four statements:

1. People around here are willing to help their neighbours.
2. People in my neighbourhood generally get along with each other.
3. People in my neighbourhood can be trusted.
4. People in my neighbourhood share the same values.

The residents to whom the questions are put should preferably not be the subjects of the epidemiological study in which the scales are to be used.

The scales may be based on observations as well as on questions. For example, a scale expressing the degree to which neighbourhoods were conducive to the integration of physical activity into daily routines was based on systematic observations (of convenience, safety, and the number of useful destinations in the neighbourhood).[28] A 'physical disorder' scale was based on sightings of various kinds of litter, graffiti, and abandoned cars, and a 'social disorder' scale on sightings of adults loitering or congregating, people drinking alcohol, adults fighting or hostilely arguing, prostitutes on the street, etc.[27]

The development of *ecometric scales*[29] of this sort requires appraisal not only of their internal consistency (e.g. using Cronbach's *alpha* coefficient) and test–retest reliability, but also of the extent to which residents rate their neighbourhood similarly, and the extent to which different neighbourhoods are rated differently.[27] Comparisons with other scales and variables can be used to assess the scale's convergent, discriminatory and construct validity (see p. 168).

Statistical processing, both in the development and in the use of these scales, is far from simple. 'Understanding if and how contexts … affect health is challenging and complex, but it is also enormously important … [It] means dealing with a messy, correlated, and confounded reality and doing the best we can to glean truth from our observations'.[30]

Notes and References

1. See note 3, Chapter 10.
2. The essence of a *Guttman scale* (scalogram) is a set of unambiguous and hierarchical questions. Contrast the questions about weight in the text with the following three, which would elicit 'helter-skelter' nonscalable replies: 1. 'Are you taller than a table?' 2. 'Are you taller than the head of a pony?' 3. 'Are you taller than a good-sized bookcase?' (Ford RN. A rapid scoring procedure for scaling attitude questions In: Riley MW, Riley JW Jr, Toby J (eds), Sociological studies in scale analysis. New Brunswick, NJ: Rutgers University Press; 1954. pp. 273–305).

    The main criteria of *scalability* are: (1) that the *coefficient of reproducibility* (the proportion of nonerroneous responses) must be at least 90%; (2) that the *coefficient of scalability* (which allows for the possibility of chance compliance with a Guttman scale) should be well above 60%. It has also been suggested that the frequency of no single deviant ('nonscale') type should exceed 5% of the number of respondents, that erroneous responses to any item should not exceed 15%, and that over half the positive responses and over half the negative responses to each item should be nonerroneous (Ford (1954, pp. 294–295)). For these purposes, an erroneous response to an item may be defined as one that differs from the response to be expected in the perfect scale type that has the same number of 'yes' responses; a more elaborate method of counting errors (for specific items) is suggested by Ford (1954, pp. 285–290).

    The coefficient of scalability may be defined as the difference between the coefficient of reproducibility and the *coefficient of reproducibility by chance* (CRC), expressed as a proportion of (1 – CRC). CRC is calculated by estimating the probability of each perfect scale type (by multiplying the appropriate marginal probabilities, based on the total numbers of 'yes' and 'no' responses to each item) and then summing the probabilities of all perfect scale types

(Riley MW. Sociological research, vol 1. New York, NY: Harcourt Brace and World; 1963. pp. 476–477).

If the scale is satisfactory, then respondents falling into nonscale types can be assigned to the closest scale type, i.e. the one requiring correction of the smallest number of erroneous responses. Ford (1954, pp. 290–291) provides rules for use if there are alternative 'closest scale types'. Assignment is sometimes made to the scale type with the same number of 'yes' responses.

The *Guttman scale* technique is described in detail by Gorden RL (Unidimensional scaling of social variables: concepts and procedures. New York, NY: Free Press; 1997) and Stouffer SA, Guttman L, Suchman EA, Lazarsfeld PF, Star SA, Clausen JA (Measurement and prediction. New York, NY: Wiley; 1966) and briefly by Goode WJ, Hatt PK (Methods of social research. New York, NY: McGraw-Hill; 1952. pp. 285–295) and Riley MW *et al.* (1963, vol 1, pp 470–488 and vol 2, pp 97–99; see above).

3. Santos ML, Booth DA. Influences on meat avoidance among British students. Appetite 1996; 27: 197.

4. Palti H, Halevy A, Epstein Y, Knishkowy B, Meir M, Adler B. Concerns and risk behaviors and the association between them among high-school students in Jerusalem. Journal of Adolescent Health 1995; 17: 51.

5. Abramson JH, Ritter M, Gofin J, Kark JD. A simplified index of physical health for use in epidemiological studies. Journal of Clinical Epidemiology 1992; 45: 651.

6. Katz's index: see note 1, Chapter 13.

7. Lazaridis EN, Rudberg MA, Furner SE, Cassel CK. Do activities of daily living have a hierarchical structure? An analysis using the Longitudinal Study of Aging. Journal of Gerontology 1994; 49: M47.

8. For software, see Appendix C.

9. Brodman K, Erdman AJ Jr, Wolff HG. Cornell Medical Index questionnaire (manual). New York, NY: Cornell University Medical College; 1956. Abramson JH. The Cornell Medical Index as an epidemiological tool. American Journal of Public Health 1966; 56: 287.

10. Arnett FC, Edworthy SM, Bloch DA *et al.* The American Rheumatism Association 1987 revised criteria for the classification of rheumatoid arthritis. Arthritis and Rheumatism 1988; 31: 315.

11. An analysis (using a Rasch model) of 20 common symptoms reported by a sample of elderly people provided strong evidence against the hypothesis that the number of symptoms measured a single dimension. Some of the symptoms were negatively correlated with one another (Dean K, Edwardson S. Additive scoring of reported symptoms: validity and item bias problems in morbidity scales. European Journal of Public Health 1996; 6: 275).

12. *Prostate Symptom Score*: to view the questionnaire (and test yourself), visit http://www.patient. co.uk/showdoc/40002437/.

13. *SF-36 Health Survey*: information and the questionnaire are available at www.sf36.com.

14. Morehead MA. The medical audit as an operational tool. American Journal of Public Health 1967; 57: 1643.

15. Crooks J, Murray IPC, Wayne EJ. Statistical methods applied to the clinical diagnosis of thyrotoxicosis. Quarterly Journal of Medicine 1959; 28: 211.

16. For examples of the use of Rasch methods, see note 11 and Haley SM, McHorney CA, Ware JE Jr (Evaluation of the MOS SF-36 Physical Functioning Scale (PF-10): 1. Unidimensionality and reproducibility of the Rasch item scale. Journal of Clinical Epidemiology 1994; 47: 671).

17. Darlington RB. Factor analysis; 2004. Available at http://www.albany.edu/~jz7088/documents/02-12-2004/Factor.nbsp.doc

18. Lau RR, Ware JE Jr. Refinements in the measurement of health-specific locus-of-control beliefs. Medical Care 1981; 19: 1147. Ware JE Jr. Methodological considerations in the selection of health status assessment procedures. In: Wenger NK, Mattson ME, Furberg CD, Elinson J

(eds), Assessment of quality of life in clinical trials of cardiovascular therapies. New York, NY: LeJacq Publishing; 1984. pp. 87–111.

19. For further details on Thurstone-type and cumulative scales, see Gorden RL (1997, pp. 35–38; see note 2) or Selltiz C, Wrightsman LS, Cook SW (eds) (Research methods in social relations, 3rd edn. New York, NY: Holt, Rinehart & Winston; 1976. pp. 413–417, 421–422).

   Thurstone's method of paired comparisons, one of the procedures for deriving scores from the judgements of respondents, is explained by McKenna SP, Hunt SM, McEwen J (Weighting the seriousness of perceived sleep problems using Thurstone's method of paired comparisons. International Journal of Epidemiology 1981; 10: 93). Unfortunately, these judgements, and hence the scores, may vary in different populations (Bucquet D, Condon S, Ritchie K. The French version of the Nottingham Health Profile: a comparison of item weights with those of the source version. Social Science and Medicine 1990; 30: 829. Prieto L, Alonso J, Viladrich MC, Anto JM. Scaling the Spanish version of the Nottingham Health Profile: evidence of limited value of item weights. Journal of Clinical Epidemiology 1996; 49: 31); and a different procedure, using the same judgements, may yield different scores (Kind P. A comparison of two models for scaling health indicators. International Journal of Epidemiology 1982; 11: 271).

   If the scale is based on the opinions of judges, then it may be possible to treat it as an interval scale (*Thurstone-type equal-appearing interval scale*).

20. Kirshner B, Guyatt G. A methodological framework for assessing health indices. Journal of Chronic Diseases 1985; 38: 27.

21. A scale may be considered discriminating if Ferguson's delta is above 0.9. Simple formulae are provided by Hankins M (Questionnaire discrimination: [re]-introducing coefficient delta. BMC Medical Research Methodology 2007; 7: 19). For software, see Appendix C.

22. If it is believed that negatively correlated items are alternative manifestations of a singular underlying characteristic – such as headache and diffuse aches in the study by Dean and Edwardson (1996; see note 11) – it may be worth combining them into a single 'and/or' component of the scale and then retesting.

23. Simple explanations of *Cronbach's alpha* are provided by Bland JM, Altman DG (Cronbach's alpha. British Medical Journal 1997; 314: 572), who point out that *alpha* is the expected correlation between two random samples of all the possible items that could be used to make up the scale, and Guilford JP, Fruchter B (Fundamental statistics in psychology and education, 6th edn. Auckland: McGraw-Hill; 1986. pp. 427–428).

   See Cronbach LJ (Coefficient alpha and the internal structure of tests. Psychometrika 1951; 16: 297) and Cronbach LJ (My current thoughts on coefficient alpha and successor procedures. Educational and Psychological Measurement 2004; 64: 391).

24. Peterson RA. A meta-analysis of Cronhach's coefficient alpha. Journal of Consumer Research 1994; 21: 381.

25. Kong SX, Gandhi SK. Methodologic assessments of quality of life measures in clinical trials. Annals of Pharmacotherapy 1997; 31: 830.

26. Bebbington AC. Scaling indices of disablement. British Journal of Preventive and Social Medicine 1977; 31: 122.

27. Mujahid MS, Roux AVD, Morenoff JD, Raghunathan T. Assessing the measurement properties of neighbourhood scales: from psychometrics to ecometrics. American Journal of Epidemiology 2007; 165: 858.

28. Gauvin L, Richard L, Craig CL, Spivock M, Riva M, Forster M, Laforest S, Laberge S, Fournel M-C, Gagnon H, Gagne S, Potvin L. From walkability to active living potential: an 'ecometric' validation study. American Journal of Preventive Medicine 2005; 28: 126.

29. The term *ecometrics*, referring to the quantitative assessment of ecological settings, such as neighbourhoods and schools, was apparently coined by Raudenbush SW, Sampson R (Ecometrics: toward a science of assessing ecological settings, with application to the systematic social

observation of neighbourhoods. Sociologic Methodology 1999; 29: 1), who describe observation-based as well as question-based scales.

For discussions of concepts, methods, pitfalls and potentialities, also see Roux AVD (Investigating neighborhood and area effects on health. American Journal of Public Health 2001; 91: 1783), O'Campo P (Invited commentary: advancing theory and methods for multilevel models of residential neighborhoods and health, American Journal of Epidemiology 2003; 157: 9), and Messer LC (Invited commentary: beyond the metrics for measuring neighborhood effects. American Journal of Epidemiology 2007; 166: 868).

30. Roux AVD, Mujahid MS, Morenoff JD, Raghunathan T. Mujahid *et al*. respond to 'Beyond the metrics for measuring neighbourhood effects'. American Journal of Epidemiology 2007; 166: 872.

15

Methods of Collecting Data

During the planning phase of the study it is necessary to decide on the methods to be used for collecting information. These methods may be broadly classified as follows:

1. *Observation*, i.e. the use of techniques varying from simple visual observation to those requiring special skills (e.g. clinical examination) or sophisticated equipment or facilities (e.g. imaging procedures and biochemical and microbiological examinations).
2. *Interviews and self-administered questionnaires* (see Chapters 18 and 19).
3. The use of *documentary sources* – clinical records and other personal records, death certificates, published mortality statistics, census publications, etc. (see Chapter 21). Data derived from these sources are called *secondary*, as opposed to the *primary data* based on observation, interviews or questionnaires.

There are usually alternative methods of collecting the desired data. Information about hypertension, for example, may be obtained by measuring blood pressure (observation), by asking the subjects whether a doctor has ever told them they have 'high blood pressure' (interview), or by referring to medical records (documents). Furthermore, observational measurements of blood pressure may be made sitting or lying, with or without a prior rest period, by intra-arterial pressure measurements, ordinary indirect sphygmomanometry, an electronic gadget, etc. Diet may be studied by weighing the food eaten, by asking questions, or by using written records in which the subject has noted the amounts and types of foodstuffs eaten. If questions are asked, they may refer to the food eaten in the last 24 hours or in the last 48 hours, or the frequency with which different food items are usually consumed, etc. Exposure to tobacco smoke can be studied by asking questions about the smoking habits of the subjects or the people with whom they live or work. It can also be studied by measuring the concentration of carbon monoxide in expired air or of thiocyanate or cotinine in the saliva or other body fluids or (for passive smoking) nicotine in the hair.[1] If attitudes, feelings, values or motivations are to be measured, they will usually be inferred from the responses to questions, a large variety of which can be devised; sometimes, they may be inferred from observations or documentary records of actions, or from the responses to projective tests (in which the subject is required to react to a picture or other stimulus).

Different methods may yield very different information. The prevalence of chronic diseases, for example, may be studied by interviews, or by conducting examinations or

Research Methods in Community Medicine: Surveys, Epidemiological Research, Programme Evaluation, Clinical Trials J. H. Abramson and Z. H. Abramson Copyright © 2008, John Wiley & Sons Ltd

using existing clinical records. Most comparisons have shown very little correspondence between information obtained from interview surveys and that obtained by medical examinations. There is usually considerable underreporting of chronic diseases in interviews. Laymen are not physicians, and cannot be expected to supply the same information. They differ in what they know, and they differ in their language and concepts ('kidney trouble' is by no means the same thing as 'renal disease'). On the other hand, neither are physicians laymen, and interviews are preferable to medical sources when information is sought on symptoms or degree of disability or impact on quality of life, or on mild short-term diseases that are unlikely to bring the patient to a doctor or to be present at the time of an examination conducted in the course of a survey. As far as 'general health' is concerned, it has been said that 'the bulk of the research evidence can be interpreted as indicating that a clinical assessment of general health and the responses to survey questions about health are only slightly correlated phenomena'.[2]

A health appraisal by a clinician is not necessarily more useful than a self-appraisal. Numerous studies have shown that unfavourable responses to a question like 'In general, would you say your health at present is excellent, very good, good, fair, or poor?' are predictive of subsequent mortality.[3] Mortality has been found to be higher for elderly people who rate their health as unfavourable than for those who rate their health as favourable, independently of the physician's rating of their health. In at least one of these studies, mortality was more closely related to the subjective rating than to an objective rating.

Different medical sources may also yield differing information. Death certificates or autopsies will not reveal cases who have survived; official notifications of disease may not cover all cases; clinical records will tell us nothing about patients who have not attended for care or have attended and been misdiagnosed; and ordinary examinations will not reveal myocardial infarcts that have healed, leaving no symptoms or electrocardiographic traces, although ample evidence of the disease may be found in previous clinical records. In fact, any morbidity survey using information from only one source is likely to be incomplete.

The choice of method of data collection is largely based on the accuracy and relevance of the information they will yield – will the method provide sufficiently precise measures of the variables the investigator wishes to study, taking account of the purposes and objectives of the study? Two aspects of accuracy, i.e. reliability and validity, will be discussed in Chapters 16 and 17.

The selection of a method is also based on practical considerations, such as:

1. The need for personnel, skills, equipment, etc. in relation to what is available, and the urgency with which results are needed.
2. The subjects' preparedness and capacity to participate, as influenced by, for example, the 'friendliness' of the procedures (absence of undue inconvenience or unpleasantness or untoward consequences) and their requirements for literacy or numeracy skills or special motivation. If laboratory tests require prolonged fasting or the collection of all urine passed during a 24-hour period, they may be difficult to perform in a survey of apparently healthy people living at home, although the tests may be practicable in a hospital situation.

3. The probability that the method will provide a good coverage, i.e. will supply the required information about all or almost all members of the population or sample. If many people will not know the answer to a question, the question is not an appropriate one. If many of the clinical records of a factory health service do not show blood pressure, the use of these records is not a very practicable way of studying blood pressure.

4. The investigator's familiarity with a study procedure may be a valid consideration, but keep the 'Law of the Hammer' in mind: 'Give a small boy a hammer, and he will find that everything he encounters needs pounding. It comes as no particular surprise to discover that a scientist formulates problems in a way which requires for their solution just those techniques in which he himself is especially skilled'.[4]

These practical aspects should be considered not only in relation to the measurement of each separate variable, but also in relation to the methods of data collection as a whole. Each of a long series of questions or clinical tests may itself be a 'practicable' one; but, put together, they may make up a 3-hour interview or examination, which may be impracticable in terms of the time available to the study personnel, or be unacceptable to the subjects.

Accuracy and 'practicability' are often inversely correlated. A method providing more satisfactory information will often be more elaborate, expensive or inconvenient. Clinical examinations provide more accurate information on chronic diseases than do interviews, but they are more expensive, require medical or paramedical personnel, and are less acceptable to the subjects and, hence, associated with a higher refusal rate. Accuracy must be balanced against practical considerations, by choosing a method that will provide the required accuracy within the bounds of the investigator's resources and other practical limitations. In making this choice, account must be taken of the importance of the data, in the light of the purposes and objectives of the study. If the information is not very important, then a simple although less accurate method may suffice; if more accurate information is essential, then an elaborate or inconvenient method may be unavoidable. The aim is not 100% accuracy, but the maximal accuracy required for the purposes of the study and consistent with practical possibilities. Rapid epidemiological methods that sacrifice some accuracy in the interests of practicability will be discussed in Chapter 31.

Information on the accuracy and practicability of the proposed methods can often be obtained from previous methodological studies or from experiences in other investigations. In reading the literature on the study topic, the investigator should pay especial attention to methodological aspects.

Usually, however, it is found that there is a need to test at least some of the projected methods. It may be necessary to determine, for example, how long an interview or examination will take, how acceptable it is, whether questions are clearly intelligible and unambiguous, or whether the requisite data are available in clinical records. (Such 'pretests' are discussed in Chapter 24.) There may be a need for specific tests of reliability and validity (Chapters 16 and 17). Even if use is made of 'ready-made' questionnaires or other procedures developed elsewhere, it may be necessary to test them in the context of the planned study.

Blind Methods

Use is often made of 'blind' methods – i.e. the concealment of facts from observers, interviewers, the study subjects, people extracting information from documents, or anyone else who may influence the results – where such concealment may increase accuracy by avoiding bias. This applies to nonexperimental studies as well as to trials.

The terms 'single blind', 'double blind', and 'triple blind' are often used. But these terms may be ambiguous, and it is preferable to specify from precisely whom the facts are concealed. A *single-blind* experiment (or a *single-masked* one, to use a term preferred by researchers on eye diseases),[5] for example, may refer to one in which the researcher makes observations without knowing whether the subject is in the treatment or control group, or to one where this information is kept from the subjects. A *double-blind*[6] experiment generally means one where neither observers nor subjects know to which group the subjects belong, as in a double-blind experiment to test the efficacy of prayer, where some patients were prayed for and others not; the patients were not told of the prayers, and the physicians appraising their clinical progress did not know for which cases divine intercession had been requested.[7] If the processing and analysis or monitoring of data are also done 'blind', then an experiment may be called *triple blind*; but precise explanations are to be preferred.

Blinding is not always possible, and it often fails. Keeping subjects blind to their treatment generally requires a placebo or alternative treatment that cannot be identified by its appearance, taste, smell or effects. Elaborate stratagems may be needed to maintain the secret, such as the production of special pharmaceutical preparations and the use of containers identified only by symbols or numbers. Even then, the truth will often out. To test for breakdowns of secrecy it is helpful to ask subjects or physicians to guess the treatments, so as to see whether correct guesses outnumber what might be expected by chance. In a double-blind trial of the prevention and treatment of colds by vitamin C, half the subjects said they knew whether they were getting vitamin C or placebo – and were generally right (many admitted opening and tasting the capsules). Colds were reported to be milder and of shorter duration in the vitamin C treatment group, but only among subjects who thought they knew what capsules they were having – there was no apparent effect among other subjects.[8]

If it is essential for the doctors who treat the subjects of a clinical trial to know what their patients are receiving, or if there is no way of hiding this information, it may be decided to base the assessment of effects on appraisals made by independent 'blinded' investigators. This reduces the chance of biased assessments, but does not control any effects the physician's awareness of the treatment may have on the patient's progress.

In nonexperimental studies, 'blind' methods may prevent bias caused by the observer's or interviewer's knowledge that the subject is a case or a control (*exposure suspicion bias*, p. 264), or that there has or has not been exposure to the causal factor under study (*diagnostic suspicion bias*), or in other situations where the findings may be influenced by a 'halo effect' due to the observer's prior impression of the individual being studied. In a methodological study of the validity of wives' reports of their husbands' circumcision status, foreskins should be sought without knowledge of the wives' tales. The effect of prior knowledge may be especially troublesome in a longitudinal study in which subjects are examined repeatedly. In such a study, it may be advisable to plan a record system that ensures that the examiner will not see the previous findings.[9]

A 'double-blind' method may be used in nonexperimental studies. This was done in a case-control study of the relationship of childhood leukaemia to parents' exposure to diagnostic X-rays (the mother before or during pregnancy and the father before conception).[10] The interviewer was not told whether a leukaemic patient's or control's household was being visited, and the questions that might reveal this were left to the end of the schedule. The person interviewed was told that this was a health survey, but did not know it had to do with leukaemia. When blinding is not possible, efforts are often made to conceal the specific hypotheses from both interviewers and subjects, in so far as this is feasible and ethical.

In studies that evaluate screening and diagnostic tests (see pp. 171–173), blinding may be important if the result of a test (either the test under study, or the 'gold standard' test) may be influenced by knowledge of the patient's history, examination findings, or previous test results. This kind of observer bias ('*incorporation bias*') is especially likely in imaging tests. It may also be a problem in studies where the 'gold standard' is a final diagnosis (sometimes made by a panel of physicians) based on all available information about the patient; it has been suggested that in such instances, two judgements of the final diagnosis should be made, one using and one not using the result of the test under study. Blinding to previous findings is of course contraindicated in studies that aim to find whether a test *adds* to the certainty of diagnosis.[11]

Qualitative Research[12]

Some study methods are *qualitative* rather than quantitative, i.e. they are not based on measures of quantity or frequency – their findings are described in words rather than numbers. Many investigators pooh-pooh qualitative studies, and research is often considered real and serious only if it is quantitative. But what has been called 'our love affair with numbers'[13] should not blind us to the fact that in some situations qualitative methods are more appropriate than quantitative methods, and in others a combination of qualitative and quantitative methods offers advantages.

Qualitative methods are widely used in studies of concepts of health and disease and other cultural factors affecting health and health care. They are especially useful in investigations of beliefs, perceptions and practices regarding health, the prevention and treatment of illness, and the utilization of traditional and other health care. A qualitative study of patients who had a heart attack, for example, pinpointed the misconceptions (about heart-attack symptoms) that contributed to delay in calling for medical help.[14] In London, qualitative interviews led to the conclusion that women who have seen successful breastfeeding as part of their daily lives are more likely to breastfeed, leading to a recommendation that pregnant women hoping to breastfeed should be 'apprenticed' to a breastfeeding mother from her social network.[15]

Qualitative research provides 'culture specific maps [that] can help to improve the "fit" of programmes to people' – maps that show the presence of beliefs and behaviours, but not their numerical prevalence in the population (which can be investigated in a subsequent quantitative survey).[16] Proponents of the use of qualitative methods in evaluations of health care point out that they involve the researcher in new and close relationships with informants, open up dialogues on basic questions of health and health care, and 'can help to extend public health beyond an exclusively biomedical model'.[17]

Qualitative and quantitative approaches may often be regarded as complementary.[18] In a study of the reasons for incomplete immunization in Haiti, for example, qualitative methods were used to identify barriers to the use of preventive services, and these were then measured in a quantitative survey.[19] Qualitative methods can also be used as a follow-up to a quantitative study, to explain and expand the findings, and they may be a fruitful source of hypotheses for quantitative testing. Qualitative inquiries can also uncover and explain deficiencies in the manner of collection of quantitative data.[13]

Qualitative methods[12] encompass 'field studies' (observations of 'ongoing social life in its natural setting'), including observations in health-care facilities and the community at large; participant observation[20] (where the researcher is personally involved in the action being observed); interviews and conversations with key informants and other members of the community, in which people can express their attitudes, perceptions, motivations, feelings and behaviour; focus group interviews,[21] in which a small group of informants talk freely and spontaneously about themes considered important to the investigator; the study of case histories; and other methods.

If done properly, qualitative research is as rigorous as quantitative research, and the need for accuracy and for reaching conclusions that a repeated study (were it feasible) would replicate is as important as for quantitative research. Methods available for these purposes include *triangulation* (the use of more than one qualitative method, to ascertain their common conclusions) and independent analyses of data by more than one investigator. Three suggested questions for use in appraising the conclusions of a qualitative study of beliefs and practices are:

1. How well do the conclusions explain why people behave in the way they do?
2. How comprehensible would this explanation be to a thoughtful participant in the setting?
3. How well does it cohere with what we already know?[22]

A proposed hierarchy of qualitative health-related studies (especially interview studies) has four levels:[23]

1. (Least useful.) Single-case studies.
2. Descriptive studies of a sample, providing a series of illustrative quotations.
3. Conceptual studies, e.g. that attitudes are influenced by age, or that the method of acquiring AIDS may influence patients' views, in which the views of the participants or groups of participants are described.

4. (Most useful.) Generalizable studies in which the selection of participants is guided by a conceptual framework, data collection is described clearly, explanations are offered for the differences found between groups, and the applicability of the findings is given consideration.

Full-blown qualitative research requires professional training, and this book discusses only a few simpler applications, such as 'rapid ethnographic assessment' procedures (see p. 318), the Nominal Group technique (Chapter 20), and the use of qualitative methods in exploratory studies (see p. 27) and as part of the process by which a practitioner of community medicine 'gets to know' a community (Chapter 34).

Notes and References

1. Nafstad P, Botten G, Hagen JA, Zahlsen K, Nilsen OG, Silsand T, Kongerud J. Comparison of three methods for estimating environmental tobacco smoke exposure among children aged between 12 and 36 months. International Journal of Epidemiology 1995; 24: 88.
2. Feldman J. The household interview survey as a technique for the collection of morbidity data. Journal of Chronic Diseases 1960; 11: 535.
3. Idler EL, Benyamini Y. Self-rated health and mortality: a review of twenty-seven community studies. Journal of Health and Social Behavior 1997; 38: 21. See note 11, Chapter 11.
4. Kaplan A. The conduct of inquiry. New York, NY: Harper & Row; 1964.
5. The term *double masked* is recommended by Ederer F (Practical problems in collaborative trials. American Journal of Epidemiology 1975; 102: 111), who goes on to say 'Carrying out masking successfully is usually more easily said than done …. One ophthalmologist measured patients' visual acuity with their bodies draped with a cloth and their heads covered with a hood'. Ingelfinger FJ (Blind as a clinical investigator. New England Journal of Medicine 1973; 288: 1299) criticizes the term 'blind' ('The sections were read blindly under high-powered magnification'), especially if it supersedes a detailed account of the precautions taken to prevent bias (in such instances, he suggests that 'double purblind' might be a good term!).

   The statement, in a report of a follow-up study that showed an association between heartburn in pregnancy and the newborn baby's hairiness, that photographs of the babies 'were provided to two blind coders' may leave literally minded readers with doubts about the validity of the appraisals (Costigari KA, Sipsma HL, DiPietro JA. Pregnancy folklore revisited: the case of heartburn and hair. Birth 2006; 33: 311).
6. 'A fascinating instance of the blind leading the blind. With this, neither the physician nor the patient knows whether a drug or a placebo is being given – until, that is, the patient either recovers or expires. Some think this technique was borrowed from Russian roulette' (Armour R. It all started with Hippocrates: a mercifully brief history of medicine. New York, NY: Bantam Books; 1971. p. 132).
7. Joyce CRB, Welldon RMC. The objective efficacy of prayer. Journal of Chronic Diseases 1965; 18: 367.
8. Lewis TL, Karlowski TR, Kapikian AZ, Lynch JM, Shaffer GW, George DA. A controlled clinical trial of ascorbic acid for the common cold. Annals of the New York Academy of Sciences 1975; 258: 505.
9. Ignorance of the previous findings may also have disadvantages (Feinstein AR. Clinimetrics. New Haven, CT: Yale University Press; 1987. p. 98. Guyatt GH, Berman LB, Townsend M, Taylor DW. Should study subjects see their previous response? Journal of Chronic Diseases 1985; 38: 003).

10. Bross IDJ, Natajaran N. Genetic damage from diagnostic radiation. Journal of the American Medical Association 1977; 237: 2399.

11. Moons KGM, Grobbee DE. When should we remain blind and when should our eyes remain open in diagnostic studies? Journal of Clinical Epidemiology 2002; 55: 633.

12. *Qualitative research*: Pope C, Mays N. Qualitative research in health care, 3rd edn. Blackwell Publishing; 2006. Gantley M. An introduction to qualitative methods for health. Royal College of General Practitioners; 1999.
    See also Kiefer CW (Doing health anthropology: research methods for health scientists. Springer; 2006), a book that focuses on studies of cultural factors.

13. Black N. Editorial: Why we need qualitative research. Journal of Epidemiology and Community Health 1994; 48: 425.

14. Ruston A, Clayton J, Calnan M. Patients' action during their cardiac event: qualitative study exploring differences and modifiable factors. British Medical Journal 1998; 316: 1060.

15. Hoddinott P, Pill R. Qualitative study of decisions about infant feeding women in East End of London. British Medical Journal 1999; 318: 30.

16. Scrimshaw SCM, Hurtado E. Rapid assessment procedures for nutrition and primary health care: anthropological approaches to improving programme effectiveness. Los Angeles, CA: UCLA Latin American Center Publications; 1987.

17. See Beattie A (Evaluation in community development for health: an opportunity for dialogue. Health Education Journal 1995; 54: 465. Reprinted in: Sidell M, Jones L, Katz J, Peberdy A. Debates and dilemmas in promoting health: a reader. Houndmills: MacMillan Press; 1997), who lists the evaluation methods used in community development for health projects in the United Kingdom and describes some of the features of *pluralistic evaluation*, which combines different approaches.

18. Kroeger A. Anthropological and socio-medical health care research in developing countries. Social Science and Medicine 1983; 17: 147. Kroeger A. Health interview surveys in developing countries: a review of the methods and results. International Journal of Epidemiology 1983; 12: 465.

19. Coreil J, Augustin A, Holt E, Halsey NA. Use of ethnographic research for instrument development in a case-control study of immunization use in Haiti. International Journal of Epidemiology 1989; 18: S33.

20. *Participant observation* is a technique widely used in anthropology but little used in health research. An example would be a study of doctor–patient relationships, carried out by the physician or patient participating in the relationships. The hazards of this method are that the observer may influence the action, and may have a biased viewpoint.

21. *Focus groups.* See Powell RA, Single HM (Focus groups. International Journal of Quality in Health Care 1996; 8: 499), Khan ME, Anker M, Patel BC, Barge S, Sadhwani H, Kohle R (The use of focus groups in social and behavioural research: some methodological issues. World Health Statistics Quarterly 1991; 44: 145), Bowling A (Research methods in health: investigating health and health services. Buckingham: Open University Press; 1997. pp. 352–355).
    'If the desired answer is a number then the question does not indicate the use of focus groups as the method of choice ... The goal ... is 'transferability' rather than statistical generalisability ... theoretical insights which possess a sufficient degree of generality or universality to allow their projection to other contexts...' (Barbour RS. Making sense of focus groups. Medical Education 2005; 39: 742).

22. Pope C, Mays N (2006; see note 12).

23. Daly J, Willis K, Small R, Green J, Welch N, Kealy M, Hughes E. A hierarchy of evidence for assessing qualitative health research. Journal of Clinical Epidemiology 2007; 60: 43.

16

Reliability

Reliability (also termed *reproducibility* or *repeatability*) refers to the stability or consistency of information, i.e. the extent to which similar information is obtained when a measurement is performed more than once. We may be concerned either with the reliability of the information obtained about a particular variable (using a single measurement procedure or different measurement procedures), or with the reliability of a specific measurement procedure or a specific observer. The reliability of a measurement procedure is equivalent to an archer's capacity to hit the same spot each time, irrespective of whether or not this spot is the bull's-eye.

The concept is best explained by case illustrations:

1. A film was prepared, portraying the measuring of the blood pressures of seven subjects; it showed the mercury column in the sphygmomanometer, while the sound track played the accompanying sounds. When nurses were shown the film and asked to read the subjects' blood pressures, there was much variation between the pressures recorded by different nurses. The same film was later used to test physicians, with similar results ('some of the best results have been achieved by statisticians who had never taken a blood pressure before but who had been trained in objective and accurate recording of data').[1]
2. In a study of the utilization of hospital beds, panels of four physicians made appraisals of whether randomly selected beds were being appropriately used, i.e. whether the patient required hospital care on the day of observation. All four agreed in only 75% of cases.[2]
3. In Taiwan, two highly skilled ophthalmologists examined the same population sample, seeking evidence of trachoma, an infective disease of the eye often leading to disfigurement and sometimes to blindness. They used the same criteria (physical signs) and the same examination procedure; both had exceptionally keen vision. One found 122 cases of active trachoma, and the other found 136; but these included only 75 who were diagnosed by both experts; the other 108 were diagnosed by only one or other of them.[3]
4. The same chest X-ray films were examined independently by five experts in order to determine the presence of tuberculosis. Of 131 films which were recorded as positive by at least one reader, there were only 27 where all five observers agreed; in 17 cases, four observers gave a 'positive' verdict; in another 17, three said 'positive'

Research Methods in Community Medicine: Surveys, Epidemiological Research, Programme Evaluation, Clinical Trials   J. H. Abramson and Z. H. Abramson   Copyright © 2008, John Wiley & Sons Ltd

and two said 'negative'; in 23, two said 'positive'; and in 47, one said 'positive' and four said 'negative'. The films were later reread by the same observers, and there were many reversals of verdict.[4]

5. Material with a known concentration of haemoglobin (9.8 g per 100 ml) was sent to a number of hospital laboratories, and a separate determination of haemoglobin was performed in each laboratory; the results ranged from 8 to 15.5 g per 100 ml.[5]

6. A standard suspension of red blood cells was examined in a number of laboratories; when visual counting was performed the red blood cell counts ranged from 2.2×10^6 to 4.5×10^6 cells/mm^3; when electronic cell counters were used the range was from 0.7×10^6 to 4.7×10^6 cells/mm^3.[6]

7. A number of studies have shown that if children are measured during the morning they are, on average, taller, by 0.5 cm or more, than if they are measured in the afternoon.[7]

High reliability does not necessarily mean that a procedure is a satisfactory one – measurements that are 'far from the bull's-eye' may not provide the investigator with helpful information (what is more reliable – or less useful – than a broken watch?). On the other hand, it is obvious that the less reliable the procedure, the less useful it will be. The problem of reliability is especially acute in longitudinal studies where an attempt is being made to assess change, since the findings may express variability in the measurements rather than a real change in the attribute that is measured (see p. 74). In a study designed to measure the incidence rate of new cases of a chronic disease, performed by repeating a diagnostic procedure after a period of time, unreliability will tend to produce an unduly high estimate of incidence. This is because people who are falsely diagnosed as new cases on the second occasion, and ill people falsely diagnosed as being healthy on the first occasion, will usually outnumber new cases that are missed, while well people misdiagnosed as ill at the first examination will be excluded from the population at risk of developing the disease, thus further increasing the calculated incidence.

Tests performed by a laboratory may be unreliable because different technicians, or different instruments, yield different results. If, when duplicate tests are performed by two of its technicians, one consistently yields lower readings than the other, a comparison of their reports will show *systematic* or *one-sided variation*.

If the variation is random in direction, or if variations in the two directions cancel each other out, this is *nonsystematic variation*. In a large study in England and Wales, for example, it was found that in only 65% of the cases where death was ascribed to arteriosclerotic heart disease by the treating physician was the assignment to this cause confirmed by autopsy. However, there were other cases that were diagnosed on autopsy only, so that the total numbers of deaths ascribed to this disease by clinicians and pathologists were fairly similar.[8] In a study in which some deaths were certified by physicians and others by pathologists, the information about causes of death would clearly be unreliable.

The fact that variation is nonsystematic offers no guarantee against erroneous conclusions. If our marksperson's arrows are widely scattered, but centred around the bull's-eye, then the average or overall measurement may indeed be accurate. But it is obvious that the individual measurements cannot all be correct. If we use an unreliable measure we are likely – whether the variation is systematic or nonsystematic – to obtain incorrect information and (if the scale is categorical) to *misclassify* individuals (as sick or well, smokers or nonsmokers, etc.) and, hence, to obtain deceptive information about relationships between characteristics (see p. 163). Moreover, even if variation is on the whole nonsystematic, it is never easy to be sure that one-sided variation is not present in some part of the study population, since the balance between the opposing tendencies may differ in different strata. In the above study, for example, the findings varied in different age groups. Among people aged 45–64 years, slightly more deaths were ascribed to arteriosclerotic heart disease by clinicians than by pathologists; however, among people aged 75 and more, 22% fewer cases were ascribed to this cause by clinicians.

The term *error* should preferably not be used to describe variation (although it often is), unless there is definite knowledge that a particular value is correct.

Sources of Variation

Variation between measurements may have three different (although often interrelated) sources:

1. Changes in the characteristic being measured (a lack of stability or constancy), i.e. within-subject variation.
2. The measuring instrument, i.e. variation between readings by the same instrument (intra-instrument or within-instrument variation) or between instruments (inter-instrument or between-instrument variation); 'measuring instruments' refer here not only to mechanical devices, but to biochemical and other tests, questions, questionnaires, and the measuring procedure as a whole.
3. The observer, the person collecting the information – variation between measurements by the same observer (within-observer or intra-observer variation) or by different observers (between-observer or inter-observer variation).

For example, if two clinicians measure the same subject's blood pressure and record different readings, the possible explanations are: (1) that the blood pressure altered between the two measurements; (2) that the sphygmomanometer or the measuring procedure as a whole provides variable results or, if different sphygmomanometers or procedures were used, that these provide different results; and (3) that the clinicians differ in the way they read or record blood pressure measurements.

Variation in the characteristic being measured may be caused by variation in any of the whole complex of factors that determine the characteristic. These factors include the measuring procedure and the observer. For example, blood pressure may be affected by the conditions under which the measurement is performed – the subject's posture and emotional state – and by the clinician's demeanour, sex and pulchritude. The response to a question may be affected (and *response instability* thus produced) by the respondent's motivations, the degree of fatigue or boredom, the circumstances of the interview (at home or in hospital, the presence of other persons, etc.), the interviewer's sex, appearance and manner, etc. Dietary or other behaviour may be changed by the subject's awareness of being studied. In a clinical trial, the subject's condition may be influenced both by awareness of being studied and by knowing (correctly or not) whether they are receiving an active treatment or a placebo.

The *persons collecting the information* (clinicians or other observers, interviewers, or persons extracting data from documentary sources) may vary in what they perceive, in their skill, integrity, propensity to make mistakes, etc. They may be influenced, consciously or unconsciously, by their preconceptions and motivations.

Observer variation

Observer variation is a term that, strictly speaking, refers to variation arising from the persons making the observations, not from changes in the characteristic being measured or from the measuring instrument. In practice, it is often extremely difficult to separate these aspects completely, and the term is commonly used to indicate any differences between observations by different observers (*inter-observer variation*) or by the same observer on different occasions (*intra-observer variation*). Observer variation in blood pressure measurements may reflect the clinicians' influence (e.g. by their demeanour) on the subjects, or differences in the procedure of measurement (the rate at which the cuff is deflated, the level at which the cuff is placed, etc.), or the way in which they make the reading.

Inter-interviewer variation may be due not only to the way in which the interviewers perceive, interpret and record what the respondents say, but also to the way they ask questions, and their influence on the respondent.

In clinical examinations, observer variation is often due to the fact that different clinicians use different definitions of what they are measuring. This is one reason for the unreliability of diagnoses that besets studies in psychiatric epidemiology.[9] Clinicians may also be influenced by what they have come to regard as 'normal'. A physician working in a malnourished population may regard as well-nourished a child who, if seen by a physician accustomed to a better nourished population, would be appraised as malnourished.

There may also be a tendency for the observer to find what they *expect* to find. In a longitudinal study, a measurement may be influenced by knowledge of the previous measurement; and in a clinical trial, an investigator's awareness of whether the subject is in the experimental or control group may bias their observations. This effect of expectation has been demonstrated repeatedly. For example, in a study in which auscultatory measurements of the fetal heart rate were compared with the electronically recorded rate, it was found that when the true rate was under 130 beats per minute the hospital staff tended to overestimate it, and when it was over 150 they tended to underestimate it.[10] Experimenters who compared groups of rats that they had been told came from 'clever' and 'stupid' strains found that the 'clever' rats were much better at learning to negotiate mazes – although in fact the two groups were genetically identical (or maybe this was a *Pygmalion effect?*).[11]

Measuring Reliability

Although efforts should obviously be made to collect reliable information, it must be stressed that complete reliability is not essential. The measurement of a phenomenon should not be given up simply because there is some degree of unreliability. 'There is a danger in studies of reliability of permitting the perfect to become the enemy of the good or committing the error of errorlessness'.[12] It is important, however, to know *how much* unreliability there is, particularly with regard to the variables that play an important part in the investigation – how much variation arises from the method of measurement, as compared with the variation between the individuals or groups being studied? Unless this is known, it may be difficult to avoid reaching unwarranted conclusions. Sometimes, previous methodological studies may provide a sufficient guide. However, it is often necessary to measure reliability, either before embarking on the study, e.g. by performing a pretest (see Chapter 24), or by building reliability tests into the study itself.

Reliability is assessed by performing two or more independent measurements and comparing the findings, using an appropriate statistical index, such as *kappa*[13] for a measure of a categorical variable, or a suitable coefficient[14] for an interval- or ratio-scale measure. The comparison may be based on observations by different observers or interviews by different observers, on repeated measurements or interviews using the same instrument or questionnaire (the *test–retest* method), or on measurements with different instruments. Replicate tests may be made on the same blood specimens. A question may be repeated in the same questionnaire, or differently worded questions asking for the same information may be included.

The results of a test–retest comparison depend on the interval between the tests. A questionnaire-based measure of overall health, for example, was found to have a test–retest reliability of about 0.85 (this was the proportion of variance not attributable to random variation) over a 1-month period, but only about 0.56 over a 3-year interval.[15] The purpose of the measurement should be kept in mind when reliability is tested. Long-term reliability is appropriate if the aim is to measure a fairly stable attribute, such as a personality trait, but not if the aim is to measure transient or changeable characteristics. Tests of an 'anxiety inventory' demonstrated that test–retest reliability (for intervals of 1 hour to 104 days) was much higher for questions designed to measure 'anxiety trait' ('how you feel in general') than for those designed to measure 'anxiety state' ('how you feel right now').[16]

It is often advisable to appraise reliability in different subgroups of the sample. The test–retest reliability of the anxiety-state questionnaire, for example, was much higher for men than for women. The Minnesota Leisure Time Physical Activity Questionnaire has a high test–retest reliability (5-week interval), but reliability is somewhat lower among people who report more activity.[17] For investigators using a set of questions on the frequency of consumption of various foods, it would be important to know that test–retest reliability (over a 9-month period) was unaffected by age or relative weight.[18]

Reliability may, of course, differ for different items in an examination or interview. Repeated questioning of a sample of postmenopausal women, for example, revealed a high degree of concordance for a history of hysterectomy and a family history of breast cancer, but many disagreements with respect to a history of hot flushes.[19]

Sometimes it is impracticable or inadvisable to make repeated measurements of the same persons. In a test of an interview schedule, for instance, the two sets of responses may not be independent. The first interview may lead the respondent to give more thought to the survey topic, and give a different answer the second time; or the respondent may be less careful to give accurate answers the second time of asking, etc. Under such conditions, reliability may be tested by randomly dividing the subjects among a number of observers or interviewers, in order to see whether the differences between the groups are greater than are likely to be produced by the random allocation itself. If repeated measurements are made on the same subjects although there is reason to believe that their sequence may affect the findings, the order in which subjects are examined by different observers or interviewers or with different instruments should be determined by random allocation (see p. 328) or a satisfactory equivalent method.

Intra-observer variation may be particularly difficult to study in instances where the measurements are made by direct observations on human subjects, since the observer may remember the subjects and attempt (consciously or unconsciously) to be consistent. This difficulty is possibly less acute when the observations are based on X-ray plates, electrocardiogram tracings, etc., which may be less distinctive than faces and personalities.

If reliability is low, then the possible role of each possible source of variation should in principle be measured, by testing each source separately. For example, in studying the reliability of haemoglobin determinations, one factor at a time may be varied while the rest of the procedure is kept constant. In this way, separate attention can be given to the effect of the time of day that blood is sampled, the effect of using capillary or venous blood, the effect of using a tourniquet, the effect of delay in examining the specimen, the differences between biochemical methods, instruments, or technicians, the variation of results from a single photometer or technician, etc. Such tests can provide a rational basis for solutions; that is, they may indicate methods of correcting or allowing for the variation produced by each source. It may be difficult and sometimes impossible, however, to separate the different sources of error; moreover, this kind of methodological study is a formidable undertaking. In small-scale investigations, what is usually done instead is to make assumptions concerning the probable major sources of variation and to take arbitrary steps aimed at counteracting them.

The reliability of a combination score – one that combines the scores of component items in order to measure a composite variable (see p. 135) – can be measured not only by the test–retest and other methods described above, but also by appraising internal consistency. If the items in a scale are measures of the same attribute, then the extent to which they give the same result is a function of their reliability. Cronbach's *alpha* (see p. 137) is often called a measure of consistency-reliability and is commonly used for this purpose (but if the items are heterogeneous, *alpha* usually underestimates the true reliability).[20] It is customary to use more than one index of reliability.[21] Internal consistency is sometimes measured by the *split-half* method, in which a questionnaire that measures a single attribute is divided, purposively or randomly, into two parts and the findings they yield are compared; if there is little variation, then this is taken as evidence of consistency.

Enhancing Reliability

Steps should be taken not to attain complete reliability, but to reduce variation to reasonable limits.

To this end, clearly defined standardized procedures are required. The variables should have clear operational definitions, a standard procedure of examination should be used, and standard questions should be asked in a standard way. There should be detailed step-by-step descriptions of the methods (but remember that 'a carefully detailed manual of methods, however massive, is not good for much if ignored by the fieldworkers').[22]

The instrument should be one that supplies relatively consistent measurements. In particular, the variation associated with the instrument should be small in relation to the total range of variation of the attribute being measured; a ruler with coarse calibrations is sufficient if a large expanse is to be measured, but one with finer calibrations is needed if a short length is to be measured (an instrument or test meeting this requirement may be called *precise* or of high *discrimination*). If more than one measuring device is used, then they should be of the same model and/or standardized against each other. Equipment should be tested from time to time. Quality control procedures should be undertaken, e.g. chemical tests on a standard reference solution and comparisons of replicate tests of the same specimen.

The use of scores based on a number of related items generally increases reliability. In this context it may be noted that disease diagnoses based on a combination of manifestations are often of higher reliability than the data on the separate items. The use of repeated measures may also increase reliability – with quantitative measurements that show appreciable variation, the mean of two or more readings may be used.

If the procedure is one requiring special skill, then the necessary training should be provided. If there is more than one observer, then they should attune their methods, possibly by working together for a while. Where necessary, they should have standard reference pictures, such as colour photographs of different stages of a skin disorder, or X-ray plates showing radiological abnormalities.

If it is not possible to use a single observer, and much inter-observer variation is expected, then each subject should if possible be independently examined by more than one examiner. An advantage of this is that the disagreements can be exploited to produce a more discriminatory scale of measurement.[23] For example, if the severity of a disease is graded as 1 (mild), 2 (moderate) or 3 (severe), it may be assumed that subjects allocated to grade 1 by one clinician and to grade 2 by another lie close to the borderline between grades 1 and 2; such cases could be placed in an intermediate category, 1.5, lying between grades 1 and 2 in the ordinal scale. Alternatively, when there is disagreement, the cases may be re-examined and discussed until agreement is reached, or a referee may be called in for a casting vote; these latter procedures have been criticized, however, on the grounds that this may not mean a correct decision, but submission to the more experienced or forceful of the observers. Parallel observations of this kind are facilitated if there are permanent records of the observations, such as electrocardiogram tracings or retinal photographs.

Notes and References

1. Wilcox J. Observer factors in the measurement of blood pressure. Journal of the American Medical Association 1962; 179: 53. Rose GA, Holland WW, Crowley EA. A sphygmomanometer for epidemiologists. Lancet 1964; i: 296.
2. Zimmer JG. An evaluation of observer variability in a hospital bed utilization study. Medical Care 1967; 5: 221.
3. Assaad FA, Maxwell-Lyons F. Systematic observer variation in trachoma studies. Bulletin of the World Health Organization 1967; 36: 885.
4. Birkelo CC, Chamberlain WE, Phelps PS, Schools PE, Zacks D, Yerushalmy J. Tuberculosis case finding: a comparison of the effectiveness of various roentgenographic and photofluorographic methods. Journal of the American Medical Association 1947; 133: 359.
5. Belk WP, Sunderman FW. A survey of the accuracy of chemical analyses in clinical laboratories. American Journal of Clinical Pathology 1947; 17: 853.

   The rate of 'unacceptable' clinical chemistry laboratory results (discrepancies of seven standard deviations or more) was 162,000 per million tests according to the results reported in this study, but has since decreased to 447 per million, according to Witte DL, van Ness SA, Angstadt DS, Pennell BJ (Errors, mistakes, blunders, outliers, or unacceptable results: how many? Clinical Chemistry 1997; 43: 1352).
6. Lewis SM, Burgess BJ. Quality control in haematology: report of interlaboratory trials in Britain. British Medical Journal 1969; iv: 253.
7. Baker IA, Hughes J, Jones M. Temporal variation in the height of children during the day. Lancet 1978; 1: 1320.
8. Heasman LA, Lipworth L. Accuracy of certification of causes of death. General Register Officer, Studies on Medical and Population Subjects no 20. London: HMSO; 1966. pp. 84, 118.
9. See note 12, Chapter 12.
10. Day E, Maddern L, Wood C. Auscultation of foetal heart rate: an assessment of its error and significance. British Medical Journal 1968; ii: 422.
11. Rosenthal R (Experimenter effects in behavioral research. New York, NY: Appleton; 1966) found that if teachers were told that certain (randomly chosen) first- and second-grade children were particularly bright, up to twice as much improvement in IQ occurred in those children as in others. He called this ('reality can be influenced by the expectations of others') the *Pygmalion effect*, after the Bernard Shaw play in which Professor Henry Higgins's confidence in the talents of the Cockney flower girl Eliza Doolittle led to her becoming a lady. It is often called the *Rosenthal effect*.
12. Elison J. In: Levine S, Reeder L G, Freeman H E (eds) Handbook of medical sociology, 2nd edn. Englewood Cliffs, NJ: Prentice Hall; 1972. p. 493.
13. The simple *percentage agreement* (the proportion of cases placed in the same categories by independent determinations) may be misleading, since agreement may occur by chance. *Kappa* is a better index for categorical measures, since it makes allowance for the contribution of chance agreement; see Fleiss JL, Levin B, Paik MC. (Statistical methods for rates and proportions, 3rd edn. New York, NY: Wiley; 2003. Chapter 18). For example, in a study in which three trained

physiotherapists applied clinical criteria for osteoarthritis of the knee, the percentage agreement was 82%, but *kappa* was only 18% (Wood L, Peat G, Wilkie R, Hay E, Thomas E, Sim J A study of the noninstrumented physical examination of the knee found high observer variability. Journal of Clinical Epidemiology 2006; 59: 512).

A *kappa* of 75% or more may be taken to represent excellent agreement, and values of 40–74% indicate fair to good agreement; most comparisons of clinical examinations, as well as interpretations of X-rays, electrocardiograms and microscopic specimens yield values of 40–74%.

Kappa may be affected by disparity in the prevalences of the categories and by systematic variation between the ratings (Byrt T, Bishop J, Carlin JB. Bias, prevalence and kappa. Journal of Clinical Epidemiology 1993; 46: 423), and adjustments may be made for these effects.

For software, see Appendix C.

14. Mathematical models express *reliability* as the variance of the true scores as a proportion of the observed variance (which includes error components). Reliability theory is summarized by Guilford JP, Fruchter B (Fundamental statistics in psychology and education, 6th edn. Auckland: McGraw-Hill, 1986. Chapter 17).

Various *measures of reliability* or *agreement* for use with interval-scale and ratio-scale variables. appropriate for different purposes and for different kinds of data, are provided by statistical programs, whose manuals explain and reference the measures and describe their uses (see Appendix C for software).

The measures include several intraclass correlation coefficients, Lin's concordance correlation coefficient, repeatability coefficients, the standard error of measurement, the confidence interval for the 'true value' corresponding to an observed measurement, Spearman–Brown coefficients of reliability, St Laurent's correlation coefficient, and 95% limits of agreement.

The term *reliability coefficient* generally refers to an intraclass correlation coefficient.

A distinction may be made between measures of *reliability* (such as intraclass correlation coefficients) that give an idea of how well subjects in a particular sample can be distinguished from each other, and measures of *agreement* between repeated measurements of the same subjects (such as the 95% limits of agreement), which are important in studies that aim to measure change (De Vet HCW, Terwee CB, Knol DL, Bouter LM. When to use agreement versus reliability measures. Journal of Clinical Epidemiology 2006; 59: 1033).

15. Ware JE Jr. Methodological considerations in the selection of health status assessment procedures. In: Wenger NK, Mattson ME, Furberg CD, Elinson J (eds), Assessment of quality of life in clinical trials of cardiovascular therapies. LeJacq Publishing; 1984. pp. 87–111.

16. Spielberger CD, Gorsuch RI, Lushene RE. Manual for the state-trait anxiety inventory. Palo Alto, CA: Consulting Psychologists Press; 1970. Cited by Siegel JM, Feinstein LG, Stone AJ (Personality and cardiovascular disease: measurement of personality variables. In: Ostfeld AM, Eaker ED (eds) Measuring psychosocial variables in epidemiologic studies of cardiovascular disease. NIH publication no 85-2270. National Institutes of Health, US Department of Health and Human Services; 1985. pp. 367–401).

17. Folsom AR, Jacobs DR Jr, Caspersen CJ, Gomez-Martin O, Knudsen J. Test–retest reliability of the Minnesota Leisure Time Physical Activity Questionnaire. Journal of Chronic Diseases 1986; 39: 505.

18. Colditz GA, Willett WC, Stampfer MJ *et al*. The influence of age, relative weight, smoking and alcohol intake on the reproducibility of a dietary questionnaire. International Journal of Epidemiology 1987; 16: 392.

19. Horwitz RI, Yu EC. Problems and proposals for interview data in epidemiological research. International Journal of Epidemiology 1985; 14: 463.

20. Lord FM, Novick R. Statistical theories of mental test scores. New York, NY: McGraw Hill; 1968.

21. As an example, the findings of an appraisal in Sheffield of the reliability of eight combination scores provided by the SF-36 health survey questionnaire (readministered after 2 weeks)
were: reliability coefficients, 0.74 to 0.93; correlation coefficients, 0.60 to 0.81; mean difference
(on 100-point scale) 0.1 to 0.7 (regarded as 'of no practical significance'); Cronbach's alpha,
0.73 to 0.96. The authors concluded that the findings supported the internal consistency of the
questionnaire and that 'since an instrument with a high discriminatory power may be unreliable it was reassuring to find that test–retest reliability was excellent' (Brazier JE, Harper R,
Jones NMB, O'Cathain A, Thomas KJ, Usherwood T, Westlake L. Validating the SF-36 health
survey questionnaire: new outcome measure for primary care. British Medical Journal 1992;
305: 160).
22. Anderson DW, Mantel N. On epidemiologic surveys. American Journal of Epidemiology 1983;
118: 613.
23. Fletcher CK, Oldham PD. Diagnosis in group research. In: Witts LJ (ed.), Medical surveys and
clinical trials, 2nd edn. London: Oxford University Press; 1964. pp. 25–49.

17

Validity

This chapter deals with the *validity of measures*. The *validity of studies*, i.e. their capacity to produce sound conclusions, will be covered in later chapters. We will consider the ways in which validity can be appraised, and the evaluation of screening and diagnostic tests and risk markers.

The *validity of a measure* refers to the adequacy with which the method of measurement does its job – how well does it measure the characteristic that the investigator wants to measure? It is equivalent to an archer's capacity to hit the bull's-eye – if all arrows hit the bull's-eye (Robin Hood style) the measure is reliable as well as valid.

Clearly, if a measure is not reliable (see Chapter 16) this must reduce its validity; if the shots are scattered, they cannot all hit the bull's-eye. If reliability is high, then the measure is not necessarily valid – the shots may all hit the same innocent bystander. ('Just because it's reliable doesn't mean that you can use it'.[1]) But if reliability is low, the measure cannot have a high validity.

If we wish to know how much sugar a man consumes, we may obtain more valid information by asking how many spoons of sugar he puts in his tea or coffee and how many cups he drinks a day, than by merely asking him whether he has 'a sweet tooth'. The data will be still more valid if we obtain information about everything he eats or drinks, and calculate his sugar intake by using tables showing the average sugar content of various foodstuffs; and they will be even more valid if, instead of using these tables, we perform laboratory analyses of samples of the foods and drinks he actually consumes.

There is little point in considering whether a measurement is valid in relation to the *operational* definition of the variable being measured. If the operational definition is a good one, it will be phrased in terms of observable facts. These facts are hence automatically ('by definition') valid as a measure of the variable, as operationally defined. If prematurity is defined in terms of birth weight, as recorded in hospital records, then the recorded information on birth weight must constitute a valid measure of prematurity, so defined. If intelligence is defined as 'what is measured by an intelligence test', then an intelligence test must obviously be a valid measure of intelligence. To appraise validity meaningfully, it must be considered in relation to the *conceptual* definition of the variable.

In planning a study we should satisfy ourselves that every variable is measured as validly as its importance in the study requires, taking account of available resources and other practical constraints. If validity is low, then the measure will be a poor proxy

Research Methods in Community Medicine: Surveys, Epidemiological Research, Programme Evaluation, Clinical Trials J. H. Abramson and Z. H. Abramson Copyright © 2008, John Wiley & Sons Ltd

for the characteristic that we want to measure. Serum triglyceride estimations based on blood samples taken from people who have recently had a meal may be a reflection of what they ate rather than of the metabolic pattern that interests us. If the presence of a hernia is reported by only 54% of men who turn out to have obvious bulging inguinal hernias, and if hernias are also reported by men who have none,[2] then the misclassification of study subjects by interview data is likely to produce a biased picture of prevalence, the direction of the bias depending on the balance between false nonreports and false reports. This is an example of *information bias* (bias attributable to shortcomings in the way information is obtained or handled).

Appraising Validity

There are various ways of appraising validity. Some are essentially based on *judgement* alone (face, content and consensual validity), the issue being whether the operational definition of the variable being measured appears to be an appropriate rendering of its conceptual definition. Others are based on *checks against data*, permitting a judgement to be made about how well the measure does its job in the particular context represented by a specific sample or samples. The check may be against data that are available at the time the measure is used (sometimes called *concurrent validity*, or may pertain to the future (*predictive validity*)). The aspects of validity listed and discussed below express the various approaches to the question 'How valid is the measure?' They are not 'types of validity', but types of evidence.

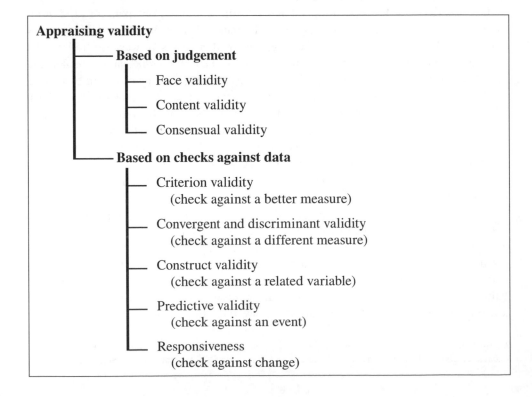

Appraising validity

Based on judgement

    Face validity

    Content validity

    Consensual validity

Based on checks against data

    Criterion validity
    (check against a better measure)

    Convergent and discriminant validity
    (check against a different measure)

    Construct validity
    (check against a related variable)

    Predictive validity
    (check against an event)

    Responsiveness
    (check against change)

Common sense is the first requisite. Feinstein speaks of a measure's sensibility (not to be confused with sensitivity); that is, How sensible is the measure? Does it make good sense? This requires consideration not only of face and content validity, but also of the measure's purpose (what is it supposed to do, and is it needed?), its comprehensibility (is it simple and transparent?), its replicability (are the instructions for its use clear enough?), the suitability of the scale (is it logical, comprehensive and sufficiently discriminatory?), and its ease of use.[3]

No measure should be used unless its validity has been appraised – a reasonable degree of face validity is a *sine qua non*. If validity is uncertain and the variable is of more than peripheral interest in the study, then a check against data should be considered. This may be done in a pretest or during the data-collection phase (in a sample of the study population), or even (if doubts arise only later) by collecting new data during the analysis phase. In some instances a simple tryout may be enough to raise or dispel doubts about the capacity of the measure to yield 'reasonable' and full responses. Appraisals of validity may influence the choice of study methods and, at a later stage, the interpretation of the findings.

Sometimes the results of previous tests of validity are available. These may be very helpful, but it is important to realize that the validity of a measure may differ in different groups or populations or in different circumstances. The significance of the WHO definition of low birth weight (less than 2500 g), for example, will differ in populations whose neonates, like their adults, are large or small for genetic reasons. A measure of chronic bronchitis based on the prevalence of cough and phlegm may be of high validity in one population, but less so in another where there is a low prevalence of chronic bronchitis and a high prevalence of other diseases (such as pulmonary tuberculosis) that may cause cough and phlegm. Indirect sphygmomanometer readings are a better index of intra-arterial blood pressure in leaner than in fatter people. The validity of simple questionnaires and tests for identifying people with presenile or senile dementia is seriously impaired by the effect of educational level on the responses.[4] In surveys in the United States, underreporting of hospitalization varied in different ethnic groups.[5] In Boston, mothers tended to underreport their children's attendances at outpatient clinics if there had been many such attendances, and to overreport them if there had been few.[6]

This possibility of *differential validity* should always be kept in mind – it is often advisable to test validity in different subgroups of the study population. If the validity of measures is not uniform then this can easily produce deceptive information about associations between variables. Suppose we want to compare the prevalence of a disease in two groups, using a measure that makes errors when classifying people as well or ill (here we can use the term *misclassification*). Patients will be 'diluted' with healthy people, and/or healthy people will be 'contaminated' by patients.

It has been shown that if a measure has the same validity in the two groups we are comparing (*nondifferential validity*), then the misclassification will tend to reduce the apparent difference between the prevalence in the two groups, or may even make it dwindle to vanishing point.[7] But if the measure is of different validity in the two groups, then the difference may be lessened, obscured or increased, or its direction may change; also, a difference may be seen when really there is none. The possibility of a spurious association exists whenever differential validity is suspected; if women who have borne deformed babies are for this reason especially prone to recall and report minor injuries that occurred during early pregnancy,[8] then a retrospective comparison with mothers of normal babies may produce deceptive evidence of an association between deformities and these injuries. The direction of the bias (are relationships spuriously strengthened or attenuated?) is especially difficult to predict if both the variables involved in an association (e.g. disease and personality type) are subject to misclassification – any kind of distortion may then occur. This is not an uncommon situation.

Possible differential validity should also be considered if we plan to use a study method that others have developed and tested – we should satisfy ourselves of its validity in our own study, performing a test if necessary. The earlier validation suffices only if we are reasonably sure that the study populations and circumstances are so similar that the method will be valid here too. Problems are especially likely if a questionnaire has to be translated from another language[9] or into terms that will be understood by a specific study population.

Face validity

The relevance of a measurement may appear obvious to the investigator. This is referred to as *face validity* (or *logical validity*). It may be obvious, for instance, that the dates of birth recorded on birth certificates provide a valid measure of age, or that weights will have a low validity if the scales used for weighing are inaccurate.[10] In choosing between different measures, common sense may indicate that some are more valid than others. It may be self-evident that the records kept in an obstetrics ward will provide a more valid indication of birth weights than information obtained by questioning mothers, or that an appraisal of the neurological status of neonates will provide a more valid measure of prematurity (as the investigator conceives it) than information on birth weights.

In formulating the questions to be included in a questionnaire, a prime consideration is whether they have face validity – do they seem likely to yield information of real relevance to what the investigator wants to measure? It must be remembered, however, that face validity may be deceptive. The question 'Do you have frequent headaches?', for example, may not necessarily provide a valid measure of the occurrence of frequent headaches. A positive response may reflect a general propensity to complain, or a state of emotional ill health, and have little relevance to headaches per se.

Sometimes the findings (of a pretest or the study itself) point to poor face validity. If there are many 'don't know' answers to a question, this is *ipso facto* evidence that the question does not supply the information the investigator needs. 'Unreasonable' findings – their nonconformity with expectations – may be evidence of poor validity: if the prevalence of acne in adolescents turns out to be only 1%, the measure is probably invalid. *Digit preference* points to impaired validity. For instance, if the question 'How old are you?' yields an undue number of replies of '20', '30', '40', etc., compared with the number of replies ending in digits other than zero, this may be taken as evidence of low face validity; in this instance it would probably be decided to use grouped ages, rather than single years, as the scale of measurement, and not to use ages ending in zero when defining the categories (i.e. to use '25–34', '35–44', etc., rather than '20–29', '30–39', etc.). Similarly, a question on the date of the first day of the last menstrual period, put to pregnant women, has been found to yield unduly high numbers of certain dates – the 1st, 10th, 15th, 20th and 25th days of the month.[11] In Canada, 90% of newborn babies have weights (in grams) that end with '0' and 16% have weights ending with '00';[12] and in a questionnaire survey in Yemen, 55% of reported birth weights were multiples of 500, and 23% were clustered at 2500 g[13] (low birth weight is defined by WHO as <2500 g). A question concerning the number of days since the onset of symptoms, put to patients seeking care for infectious diseases, may yield high numbers of replies of 1, 2, 3, 4, 7, 10, and 14 days. In the measurement of blood pressures, digit preference – usually a high proportion of readings ending in zero – is a well known phenomenon, and one that makes it more difficult to assess associations between blood pressure and other variables.[14]

Content validity

If the variable to be measured is a composite one, then one way of appraising validity is to see whether all the component elements of the variable (as conceived) are measured. This is *content validity*. Like face validity, this is a judgement of whether the conceptual definition has been appropriately translated into operational terms.

A composite scale for measuring satisfaction with medical care, for example, should specifically include attitudes to all important features of medical care, such as the way doctors and nurses relate with patients, the technical quality of care, convenience, cost, the efficacy of care, continuity of care, the physical environment, and the availability of facilities and care providers;[15] questions about specific aspects are more likely to tap dissatisfaction than general questions.[16] Thyrotoxicosis will be measured more validly if metabolic and biochemical tests are used as well as symptoms and clinical signs.

Consensual validity

When a number of experts agree that a measure is valid, this is *consensual validity*. Many experts agree, for example, that the British Registrar-General's classification (p. 110) is a valid measure of social class, or that a specific index based on the presence, frequency and duration of cough and phlegm is a valid indicator of chronic bronchitis. It must be remembered, however, that different groups of experts may differ in their consensus of opinion, and that a consensus may change – expert committees frequently recommend changes in diagnostic criteria (see p. 120).

Criterion validity

The best and most obvious way of appraising validity is to find a criterion (a reference standard or, in epidemiological jargon, a 'gold standard') that is known or believed to be close to the truth, and to compare the results of the measure with this criterion (*criterion validity*).

The ideal criterion is the 'true value' of the attribute that is being measured. A perfectly valid measure is one that correlates completely with 'God's opinion' concerning the attribute.[17] As 'God's opinion' is difficult to determine, the best criterion is a measure that has higher face validity than the measure being tested, or that has been tested previously and found to be of high criterion validity. Examples are legion. Questionnaire data on birth weights may be checked against the weights recorded in obstetric records, self-reports of overweight against weight and height measurements, and self-reported use of health-care services with medical billing records. Blood pressure measured by indirect sphygmomanometry can be checked against direct intra-arterial pressure measurements; the causes of death recorded on death certificates may be compared with those inferred from post-mortem examinations, and automated readings of electrocardiogram tracings with the appraisals made by a panel of experts; biochemical results may be checked by using standard solutions whose composition has been measured by tests of established accuracy. The responses to a 'yes–no' question on stiffness in the joints or muscles on waking in the morning (one of the diagnostic criteria of rheumatoid arthritis) may be validated by comparing them with the responses elicited by a skilled interviewer who asks additional questions to ensure that the sensation is really one of stiffness, and not of 'pins and needles' or general lassitude, etc. Similarly, the validity of a simple dietary questionnaire may be tested by a comparison with the findings obtained by a Burke research dietary history, a method involving very detailed questioning, with built-in cross-checks, by an experienced interviewer.[18] The validity of a new blood test for the diagnosis of a disease may be tested by comparisons with diagnoses established by clinicians after comprehensive examinations, using their own individual diagnostic criteria (which have face validity), generally accepted diagnostic criteria (which have consensual validity), or diagnostic criteria that have themselves been tested against some criterion.

If an unquestionably 'more valid' measure of the characteristic is available for use as a criterion, then the comparison can provide convincing evidence of validity. It must be kept in mind, however, that validity measured in this way may not be quite as well founded as it appears, since (like face validity) it is in the last resort based on judgement – if only the judgement that the criterion is of higher validity than the measure that is being tested.

It is often impossible to use the above approach. For one thing, there may be no measure that can be unequivocally regarded as more valid. If we wish to test the validity of a composite measure of social class, based on occupation, education and income, what unquestionably 'more valid' measure can we find? If we wish to test the validity of information on an attitude – a man's attitude to his work or his wife or whether he approves of contraceptive practices – how can we come close to the 'true value' of the attitude for use as a criterion of validity? Furthermore, even when a 'more valid' measure is theoretically available, the information required may not be available in fact, e.g. if it requires a biopsy or autopsy.

Table 17.1   Results of a 'yes–no' measure of a 'yes–no' attribute

	Attribute present	Attribute absent
Positive finding	TP	FP
Negative finding	FN	TN

The criterion validity of a 'yes–no' measure of a 'yes–no' attribute (e.g. the presence of a disease) is often expressed in terms of *sensitivity* and *specificity*. The findings may be shown in a simple table (Table 17.1) representing the observations in two samples, namely 'Attribute present' and 'Attribute absent'. TP represents the true positives, FP the false positives, FN the false negatives, and TN the true negatives. The measure's *sensitivity* is the proportion with a positive result, among people who truly have the attribute (e.g. the disease), i.e. TP/(TP + FN). The *specificity* of the measure is the proportion with a negative result, among people who truly do not have the attribute, i.e. TN/(FP + TN). The *false positive rate* is FP/(FP + TN), and the *false negative rate* is FN/(TP + *FN*).

If both sensitivity and specificity are high, then the measure is of high validity. Sensitivity and specificity must be considered together; separately, neither is very meaningful; the presence of a nose is a highly sensitive measure of kwashiorkor (100% of cases have noses) but its specificity is 0% (no individuals free of kwashiorkor are noseless); conversely, a bright green coloration of the ears (with purple stripes) is a highly specific index of kwashiorkor (100%), because it is absent in 100% of individuals without kwashiorkor, but its sensitivity is 0%.

If the measure (of, say, a disease) is not dichotomous, but has responses expressed on an ordinal, interval or ratio scale, its sensitivity, etc., can be computed for different cut-points; that is, at each of a number of selected points the scale is converted to a dichotomy (e.g. 120 or more equals a positive test, below 120 equals a negative test) and true and false positives and negatives are counted. Sensitivity can then be plotted against the false positive rate to produce a *receiver operating characteristics (ROC) curve*,[19] and the *area under the ROC curve* can be computed and used as an overall index that expresses the probability that the measure will correctly rank two randomly chosen persons, one with and one without the disease.

Other commonly used measures of validity of a 'yes–no' measure are mentioned below (under 'Evaluation of screening and diagnostic tests').

It must again be stressed that the validity of a measure may vary in different situations. A combination of signs and symptoms used as an index of a disease, for example, may have a higher sensitivity in a population where the disease tends to take a severe form than in one where the disease is generally mild. For example, sensitivity may be higher in hospital patients than in diseased persons found in a household survey. On the other hand, specificity may be lower in a hospital population, where patients free of this disease are more likely to have other diseases producing the same manifestations.

Convergent and discriminant validity

Convergent validity is based on a comparison with other measures – not necessarily better ones – of the same variable or a closely related one. A new measure of social class, for example, could be checked against other measures of social class. If it is uncertain whether the other measure is superior to the one under test, then convergent validity is being tested rather than criterion validity. Validation studies of the SF-36 health survey questionnaire, for example, included comparisons with quality-of-life scales and the Nottingham Health Profile.[20]

This approach is generally used for measures of composite variables. A new measure of mental health would be expected to show a strong correlation with other mental health measures (but if the correlation is too high then the need for the new measure may be questioned, unless there are practical advantages unrelated to validity). If it is a valid measure of mental health then it would not be expected to show such a strong correlation with a measure of physical health. This latter aspect, i.e. not showing a strong correlation with measures of variables that are not closely related, is called *discriminant validity*. Convergent and discriminant validity can be examined simultaneously by the *multitrait–multimethod matrix* technique.[21]

Qualitative research methods are commonly validated by *triangulation*, i.e. by seeing whether the results are confirmed when other methods are used or when investigations are repeated.

Construct validity

Another way of appraising validity is to see whether there are associations with other variables that there is reason to believe *should* be linked with the characteristic under study. This is *construct validity* – 'the extent to which a particular measure relates to other measures consistent with theoretically derived hypotheses concerning the concepts (or constructs) that are being measured'.[22] The usual question here is whether the measure discriminates between groups who are thought to differ with respect to the attribute that (it is hoped) it measures.

Examples abound. A measure of job satisfaction might be compared with information on what the subjects actually do (absenteeism, frequency of disputes at work, etc.), since it is reasonable to predicate some degree of association – although certainly not a one-to-one relationship – between these activities and the 'true' attitude to work. A scale measuring reported satisfaction with medical care might be validated in a similar way, using such criteria as the changing of doctors, the abandonment of health insurance, or the submission of formal complaints about the care received. If there are theoretical reasons for believing that satisfaction with medical care is correlated with income or ethnic group or emotional health, then evidence of such correlations might be taken as indirect evidence of validity. Tests of physical fitness might be used to validate a questionnaire on habitual physical activity, and habitual physical activity has been used to validate an index of physical health.[23] A study of the Rose questionnaire for angina pectoris validated it against the thickness of carotid artery walls (measured by ultrasound imaging), on the assumption that atherosclerosis of the coronary and carotid arteries are correlated.[24] Age is often used; 20 operational definitions of benign prostatic hyperplasia, for example, were rejected because they did not show an increased prevalence with age.[25]

One way of checking construct validity is to see how well the measure discriminates between groups that there is reason to believe should differ in the characteristic under study. In a validation study of the SF-36 health survey questionnaire, for example, these groups were selected on the assumptions that poorer perceived health was to be expected in women than in men, in older people than in younger people, in people in social classes IV and V than in higher social classes, and in users of health services than in nonusers.[26]

Construct validity is obviously less convincing than criterion validity. The value of this approach depends not only on how well the measure does its job, but on the validity of the underlying hypotheses leading to the selection of variables or groups.

Predictive validity

If the measure under consideration is to be used as a predictor of a future event, then the occurrence of this event is an appropriate gauge of validity: the prophetic value of the measure is examined. This is *predictive validity*, a particularly convincing way of testing validity. (As Niels Bohr said, 'prediction is very difficult, especially about the future'.)

As an example, the validity of a nine-item mortality risk indicator was tested in a nested case-control study that compared elderly men who were and were not alive 5 years after the start of a cohort study. The risk of dying was found to be fivefold in men whom this measure identified as being at high risk.[27] The indicator's validity was subsequently confirmed by testing it in women, although the relative risk was not as high.

This approach may also be used in other instances, when prediction is not the measure's primary aim. For example, the validity of measures of prematurity (birth weight, gestation period, neurological maturity, etc.) may be tested by examining their association with death or survival during the first month of life, on the assumption that, since prematurity is associated with neonatal mortality, the more strongly the measure is associated with neonatal mortality, the more valid it is (using the construct validity approach). The validity of various minor ECG abnormalities as measures of coronary heart disease may be tested by examining their relationship to the subsequent occurrence of myocardial infarction. The validity of measures of social support may be appraised by examining their capacity to predict mortality, psychiatric symptoms, and other adverse health outcomes,[28] and the validity of clinical appraisals of disease severity by their capacity to predict a fatal outcome.[29]

Responsiveness

Some measures are used to gauge within-person change with time, and are required to be sufficiently *responsive* (sensitive to change) to serve this purpose. A measure of the effect of a treatment, for example, should ideally detect and measure any clinically meaningful change, however small. A measure may be a valid indicator of the presence and intensity of an attribute, and useful for comparing individuals or groups, without being very responsive. For example, it was concluded from a study of patients with asthma and chronic obstructive pulmonary disease that the Nottingham Health Profile (a well-validated measure of perceived health status) was appropriate for comparing groups of these patients, or for comparing them with other patient populations, but not to measure changes in their health status.[30]

One way of appraising responsiveness is to compare findings before and after treatment. For example, administration of the SF-36 questionnaire to patients with migraine before treatment and a month later revealed differences in the responsiveness of the various scores derived from the questionnaire. The pain score decreased more than the other scores, one of which (the score for the impact of emotional problems on role performance) showed no significant change. The pain score also showed a change 6 months after treatment for back pain, whereas the general health score did not. The SF-36 health scores were more responsive to changes after treatment for asthma if the questions related to the previous week rather than to the previous 4 weeks.[31] In patients treated for lower back pain, measures of disability and pain were much more responsive than measures of physical impairment.[32]

Another method is to compare the changes observed in groups of patients who differ in their progress (according to an external criterion). This was done in tests of two measures of functional status, the Barthel Index and the Rehabilitation Activities Profile, which were administered to hospitalized patients 2 weeks after a stroke and repeated after various periods. The criterion of improvement was that the patient was living at home 26 weeks after the stroke. The change in scores (2-week scores were compared with 12-week and 26-week scores) in the two groups of patients showed that responsiveness was high for both measures, but more so for the Rehabilitation Activities Profile.[33]

Consequences of use

The above types of evidence should enable us to come to an adequate assessment of validity. But another (and as yet debatable) aspect has been incorporated in the latest *Standards for Educational and Psychological Testing*, prepared by educational and psychological pundits.[34] On the grounds that the essential question of test validity is how well a test does the job it was employed to do, attention is extended to appraisal of the consequences of test use – both intended and unintended, and often adverse – as part of the validation of the test. Important though such an appraisal is, its inclusion in the assessment of validity remains controversial, even in educational and psychological circles.[35]

The *Standards* say:

> Tests are commonly administered in the expectation that some benefit will be realized from the intended use of the scores. A few of the many possible benefits are selection of efficacious treatments for therapy, placement of workers in suitable jobs, prevention

of unqualified individuals from entering a profession, or improvement of classroom instructional practices. A fundamental purpose of validation is to indicate whether these specific benefits are likely to be realized.[34]

Evaluation of Screening and Diagnostic Tests

The testing of validity plays a central role in the evaluation of tests used to detect diseases. This applies both to *screening tests*, which are simple tests to identify people who are particularly likely to have the disease and who, therefore, merit fuller examination, and to *diagnostic tests*, which establish the presence or absence of diseases more definitively.

Numerous indices of validity are available,[36] but the key ones are *sensitivity* (the test's capacity to identify people who have the disease correctly) and *specificity* (its capacity to identify people free of the disease correctly). If both sensitivity and specificity are high, then the test is unquestionably a valid indicator of the disease (it has a high *discriminatory capacity*). Frequently, however, they are inversely related. A positive sputum culture, for example, is a very specific test for pulmonary tuberculosis but one of low sensitivity, whereas radiological examination is more sensitive but less specific.

The sensitivity and specificity of a test may vary in different circumstances, e.g. when it is used in apparently healthy people, or in hospital patients, or in patients with specific characteristics, signs, symptoms, or results of previous tests. Validity should, therefore, be measured whenever possible in a specific group or population, a spectrum of subjects similar to those in whom it is proposed to use the test – will it be used in a mass programme for the examination of apparently healthy people, or as a component of periodic health examinations, or as a routine test for all patients who seek medical care, or for patients in a defined high-risk group, or is it for use only in the presence of symptoms or other evidence suggestive of the disease?

The possibility of *work-up bias* when a test is appraised deserves mention. If a more valid test (often an elaborate or expensive one) that is used as a gold standard to indicate the presence of a disease is applied mainly to patients whose initial ('screening') test is positive, as part of their clinical work-up, and not to those with a negative test, this will inflate the proportions with positive screening tests in Table 17.1 (i.e. it will inflate the TP and FP proportions) and thereby exaggerate sensitivity and underestimate specificity.

It is often helpful to estimate the *predictive value*[36] of a positive or negative result and (in clinical contexts) the *gain in certainty*,[36] which expresses the change that the test can be expected to make in the estimated likelihood that the disease is present or absent. These indices, too, vary in different populations or subgroups of patients. They are influenced not only by sensitivity and specificity, but also by the prevalence of the disease in the specific population or subgroup.

As an example, a test of d-dimer measurement as an indicator of deep-vein thrombosis (using repeated leg ultrasound as the gold standard) might be conducted on patients suspected of having deep-vein thrombosis. The analysis would then compare the probability of disease presence when based only on the history and physical examination with its probability when the d-dimer measurement is used as well.[37]

Full information about the subjects in whom a test's validity was tested is, therefore, essential if the results are to be useful in practice. A checklist and flowchart are available for use in reporting these studies, together with a discussion of the sources of variability and possible bias.[38] Blinding to previous findings may be important in studies (e.g. of imaging tests) where observer bias may be a problem (see p. 146).

Consideration should be given to the purpose of the test as a diagnostic aid – discovery of a disease, confirmation of its suspected presence, or exclusion of its presence.[39] Some tests are used for only one of these purposes, some for two, and some for all three. A *discovery test*, used when there is no special reason to suspect the presence of the disease, may be a screening test or a diagnostic one. The aim is usually to find as many of the cases as possible; therefore, high sensitivity is of special importance. But specificity cannot be ignored, since a screening test with a low specificity will yield an unduly large number of 'false positive' cases requiring further examination.

A *confirmation test* is one used when the presence of disease is suspected. Its purpose is to verify this suspicion. The presence of tubercle bacilli in the sputum, for example, will confirm a diagnosis of tuberculosis (but their absence does not exclude the diagnosis). For this purpose, specificity must be high; sensitivity is less important. The specificity of the test should be measured in patients in whom the disease is suspected, but who turn out to be free of the disease.

An *exclusion test* has the purpose of 'ruling out' the presence of a suspected disease. Some exclusion tests are elaborate procedures, such as computerized tomography or magnetic resonance imaging. Their essential feature for this purpose is an extremely high sensitivity; there must be very few false negative results.

Validity is not the only consideration when evaluating screening and diagnostic tests, since their ultimate aim (it is to be hoped) is not only to establish a diagnosis, but also to influence decisions on care, and improve health status. It is important, therefore, to investigate the benefit or harm resulting from performance of the test and the action that it sets in motion. Simple questions about eyesight, for example, are valid tests for visual impairment; but a meta-analysis of randomized control trials of these tests in people aged 65 or more yielded no evidence that they led to a reduction in the prevalence of impaired vision.[40] Another example is the controversy about the value of the prostate-specific antigen screening test, which can detect most cases of early prostate cancer but may lead to unnecessary treatment and harm.[41] A further illustration is the consensus that possible benefits are enough to warrant repeated measurements of blood pressure during pregnancy as a screening test for pre-eclampsia, despite low sensitivity and specificity.[42]

Assessment of the effects of tests on health requires a longitudinal approach (a cohort study, or even a trial). It has been suggested that interest should be extended from assessment of diagnostic accuracy to the assessment of the accuracy of prognoses based on tests (the tests' dia-prognostic impact).[43]

Applying the basic evaluation scheme shown on p. 50, the following are the kinds of question that are usually asked:

1. *Requisiteness*. Is the test needed? Are other satisfactory tests not available? How important is it to detect the disease? What is the impact of the disease on the

individual (shortening of life, disability, pain and discomfort, cost of care), on the individual's family, and on the community (mortality, morbidity rate, reduced productivity, cost of care)? Is effective intervention possible, and how good is the evidence for this? Does early detection make treatment easier? Does it make it more effective?

2. *Quality.* How well does the test achieve its desired effects, i.e. how valid is it as a diagnostic tool (sensitivity, specificity, etc.) and does its performance lead to an improvement in health? Are there potential or actual adverse effects? May the 'labelling' of symptom-free people as 'diseased' have undesirable effects? What is the impact of false positive results (false 'labelling')?

3. *Efficiency.* What is the cost per test and per case found, in comparison with other tests? What is the cost compared with the cost of not detecting the disease? What resources are needed – are highly trained personnel required? What is the cost effectiveness of the test, using, say, the detection of one case or the prevention of one death as a measure of effectiveness?

4. *Satisfaction.* How acceptable is the test? What is the level of compliance? Is there a demand – is there dissatisfaction if the test is not done?

5. *Differential value.* How do the size of the problem, the need for the test, and the acceptability of the test vary in different groups or populations? Is the validity of the test consistent in different groups?

Evaluation of Risk Markers

The same questions should be asked in the evaluation of a *risk marker,* which aims to identify individuals or groups who are especially likely to develop a given disorder in the future (see p. 40). A high level of predictive validity is not enough. There must also be good reason to think that the detection of vulnerability is likely to be beneficial, i.e. that techniques and resources are available for reducing the risk and that the expected benefit outweighs any harm that may be done by 'labelling' and intervention. The use of the marker must also be practical in terms of cost, resources, acceptability and convenience. The most useful risk markers are probably those whose presence can be determined by questions, or simple procedures that can be built into ordinary clinical care.

With respect to validity, the primary requirement is a high sensitivity, since the usual aim is to find as many of the vulnerable individuals as possible. Account must also be taken of false positives; if these are numerous the predictive value of a positive test will be low, and the more intensive care recommended for vulnerable people will often be given unnecessarily.

An important consideration is the prevalence of the risk marker. This may be high either because the disorder it predicts is a very common one, or (if the disorder is less common) because the risk marker has a low specificity. If the marker puts over half the children in a practice into a high-risk group needing special attention, then it may be decided that the risk marker is of little value, since modification of the care programme so as to give extra attention to all children may be a more efficient and effective solution.

Women who are innately left-handed have been found to have twice the risk of premenopausal breast cancer.[44] Left-handedness is obviously not a cause, but could be used as a risk marker. Yet the investigators, and others who have discussed their findings, have not suggested that young left-handed women should undergo regular screening for breast cancer. (About 11% of women are left-handed, and the absolute risk of premenopausal breast cancer is not high.)

Notes and References

1. Baer DM. Reviewer's comment: 'Just because it's reliable doesn't mean that you can use it'. Journal of Applied Behavior Analysis 1977; 10: 117.
2. Abramson JH, Gofin J, Hopp C, Makler A, Epstein LM. Epidemiology of inguinal hernia: a survey in western Jerusalem. Journal of Epidemiology and Community Health 1978; 32: 59.
3. Feinstein AR. Clinimetrics. New Haven, CT: Yale University Press; 1987. Chapter 10.
4. The results of tests for dementia can be adjusted so as to remove the effect of education, but the role of education or education-related factors in the aetiology of dementia is then difficult to study. See Kittner SJ, White LR, Farmer ME *et al.* (Methodological issues in screening for dementia: the problem of education adjustment. Journal of Chronic Diseases 1986; 39: 163) and Berkman LF (The association between educational attainment and mental status examinations: of etiological significance for senile dementias or not? Journal of Chronic Diseases 1986; 39: 171).
5. National Center for Health Statistics. Reporting of hospitalization in the Health Interview Survey, and comparison of hospitalization reporting in three survey procedures. Vital and Health Statistics, series 2, nos 6, 8. Washington, DC: Public Health Service; 1965.
6. Kosa J, Alpert JJ, Haggerty RJ. On the reliability of family health information: a comparative study of mothers' reports on illness and related behavior. Social Science and Medicine 1967; 1: 165.
7. If a measure is wrong more often than it is right (false positive rate plus false negative rate exceeds 100%) then spurious associations may be produced even if misclassification is nondifferential. Validity as low as this is unusual. The effects of misclassification are described by Fleiss JL (Statistical methods for rates and proportions, 2nd edn. New York, NY: Wiley; 1981. pp. 188–200) and Kleinbaum DG, Kupper LL, Morgenstern H (Epidemiologic research: principles and quantitative methods. Belmont, CA: Lifetime Learning Publications; 1982. Chapter 12); see also Abramson JH (Making sense of data: a self-instruction manual on the interpretation of epidemiological data, 2nd edn. New York, NY: Oxford University Press; 1994. Units C3–C6. See also note 16, Chapter 27.
8. A study in Boston of the reporting of events during pregnancy, in comparison with antenatal records, showed that the mothers of malformed infants reported urinary tract and yeast infections, and the use of birth control after conception, much more fully than the mothers of normal children. There were slight or no differences in the completeness of reports of other events (Werler MM, Pober BR, Nelson K, Holmes LB. Reporting accuracy among mothers of malformed and nonmalformed infants. American Journal of Epidemiology 1989; 129: 415).
9. *Translation of questionnaires.* After a questionnaire has been translated to another language, it should be translated back for comparison with the original version. Modification of some questions may be unavoidable, and response categories such as 'excellent/very good/good/fair/poor' may not have exact equivalents. Concepts, and not only languages, are likely to differ

in different cultures. Basic concepts of mental wellbeing and other dimensions of health are not universal; the distinction between 'family' and 'friends', we are told, is not clear-cut in all Asian and African cultures; and 'check up' has no conceptual equivalent in any Chinese language.

Moreover, the translations are often so linguistically accurate that they are too literary for most people to understand. Questions phrased by schoolchildren may be preferable to translations by experts.

It may be unrealistic to expect full functional equivalence, i.e. to expect the questionnaire to do what it is supposed to do equally well in the other culture, despite conceptual, semantic and other differences.

A suggested 'state-of-the-art' procedure is:
  (a) translation of items by a team of bilinguals
  (b) comparison of translations
  (c) negotiation of 'best' items
  (d) consultations with people who are monolingual in the target language
  (e) item refinement
  (f) field testing with monolinguals
  (g) refinement as needed
  (h) testing for face, content, construct, and criterion validity
  (i) testing for reliability and responsiveness

(Hunt SM, Bhopal R. Self report in clinical and epidemiological studies with non-English speakers: the challenge of language and culture. Journal of Epidemiology and Community Health 2006; 58: 618).

The items in the SF-36 Health Survey that were most difficult to translate (from American English to nine European languages and Japanese) were those about moderate physical activity, 'such as moving a table, vacuuming, bowling', feeling full of pep, feeling blue, and the interference of health problems with social activities.

Typical minor adaptations (from original physical health questions in American English) are: 'bowling or playing golf' became 'walks in the forest or gardening' (in Swedish); 'walking one block' became 'walking 100 yards' (in British English) or 'going for a walk in the vicinity of your home' (in Hebrew); and 'scrubbing floors' became 'lifting and beating carpets or scraping and painting walls' (in Hebrew).

See Bowden A, Fox-Rushby JA (A systematic and critical review of the process of translation and adaptation of generic health-related quality of life measures in Africa, Asia, Eastern Europe, the Middle East, South America. Social Science and Medicine 2003; 57: 1289) and Bullinger M, Alonso J, Apolone G, Leplege A, Sullivan M, Wood-Dauphinee S, Gandek B, Wagner A, Aaronson N, Bech P, Fukuhara S, Kasa S, Ware JE Jr (Translating health status questionnaires and evaluating their quality: the IQOLA Project approach. Journal of Clinical Epidemiology 1998; 11: 913).

10. A check on physicians' scales in Kansas City found they were out by up to 9.5 lbs (4.3 kg) when the true weight was 150 lbs (68.3 kg). Scales that had been calibrated within the last year were significantly more accurate (Stein RJ, Haddock CK, Poston WSC, Catanese D, Spertus JA. Precision in weighing: a comparison of scales found in physician offices, fitness centers, and weight loss centers. Public Health Reports 2005; 120: 266).

11. Frazier TM. Error in reported date of last menstrual period. American Journal of Obstetrics and Gynecology 1959; 77: 915.

12. Edouard L, Senthilselvan A. Observer error and birthweight: digit preference in recording. Public Health 1997; 111: 77.

13. Boerma JT, Weinstein KI, Rutstein SO, Sommerfelt AE. Data birth weight in developing countries: can surveys help? Bulletin of the World Health Organization 1996; 74: 209.

14. Hessel PA. Terminal digit preference in blood pressure measurements: effects on epidemiological associations. International Journal of Epidemiology 1986; 15: 122.

15. This list of dimensions of satisfaction with care is by Ware JE, Snyder MK, Wright R, Davies AR (Defining and measuring patient satisfaction with medical care. Evaluation and Program Planning 1983; 6: 247).

16. Williams SJ, Calnan M. Convergence and divergence: assessing criteria of consumer satisfaction across general practice, dental, and hospital care settings. Social Science and Medicine 1991; 33: 707.

17. A concept attributed to AL Cochrane.

18. Burke BS. The dietary history as a tool in research. Journal of the American Dietetic Association 1947; 23: 1041

19. *ROC curves* (so named because they originated in studies of signal detection by radar operators): see Zweig MH, Campbell G (Receiver-operating characteristics (ROC) plots: a fundamental evaluation tool in clinical medicine. Clinical Chemistry 1993; 39: 561). For an example, see Armitage P, Berry G, Matthews JNS (Statistical methods in medical research, 4th edn. Blackwell Science; 2002. p. 697).

    The *area under the ROC curve* expresses the probability that the test will correctly rank a randomly chosen person with the disease (or other attribute) and a randomly chosen person free of it. Its value is 50% if the test does not discriminate.

    For software, see Appendix C.

20. Bullinger M (1998; see note 9); Brazier JE, Harper R, Jones NMB, O'Catham A, Thomas KJ, Usherwood T, Westlake L. Validating the SF-36 health survey questionnaire: new outcome measure for primary care. British Medical Journal 1992; 305: 160.

21. The *multitrait–multimethod matrix* (MTMM) requires measurement of two or more traits by two or more methods. A matrix of correlations provides a basis for assessments of convergent and discriminant validity (Campbell DT, Fiske DW. Convergent and discriminant validation by the multitrait–multimethod matrix. Psychological Bulletin 1959; 56: 81).

    For examples, see Brazier JE *et al.* (1992; see note 20).

22. Carmines EG, Zeller RA. Reliability and validity assessment. Beverly Hills, CA: Sage Publications; 1979. pp. 22–26.

23. Abramson JH, Ritter M, Gofin J, Kark JD. A simplified index of physical health for use in epidemiological studies. Journal of Clinical Epidemiology 1992; 45: 651.

24. Sorlie PD, Cooper L, Schreiner PJ, Rosamond W, Szklo M. Repeatability and validity of the Rose questionnaire for angina pectoris in the Atherosclerosis Risk in Communities study. Journal of Clinical Epidemiology 1995; 49: 719.

25. Bosch JL, Hop WC, Kirkels WJ, Schroder FH. Natural history of benign prostatic hyperplasia: appropriate case definition and estimation of its prevalence in the community. Urology 1995; 46(3 suppl. A): 34.

26. Brazier JE *et al.* (1992; see note 20).

27. Abramson JH, Gofin R, Peritz E. Risk markers for mortality among elderly men – a community study in Jerusalem. Journal of Chronic Diseases 1982; 35: 565.

28. Orth-Gomer K, Unden A-L. The measurement of social support in population surveys. Social Science and Medicine 1987; 24: 83.

29. Charlson M, Sax FL, MacKenzie R, Fields SD, Braham RL, Douglas RG Jr. Assessing illness severity: does clinical judgment work? Journal of Chronic Diseases 1987; 39: 439.

30. Jans MP, Schellevis FG, van Eijk JTH. The Nottingham Health Profile: score distribution, internal consistency and validity in asthma and COPD patients. Quality of Life Research 1999; 8: 501.

31. Bullinger M. (1998; see note 9); Keller SD, Bayliss MS, Ware JE Jr, Hsu MA, Damiano AM, Goss TF. Comparison of responses to SF-36 Health Survey questions with one-week and four-week recall periods. Health Services Research 1997; 32: 367.

32. Pengale, LHM, Refshauge KM, Maher CG. Responsiveness of pain, disability, and physical impairment outcomes in patients with lower back pain. Spine 2004; 29: 879.

33. Van Bennekom C, Jelles F, Lankhorst G, Bouter L. Responsiveness of the rehabilitation activities profile and the Barthel index. Journal of Clinical Epidemiology 1996; 49: 39.

34. American Educational Research Association, American Psychological Association, & National Council on Measurement in Education. Standards for educational and psychological testing. Washington, DC: American Psychological Association; 1999.

35. Goodwin LD, Leech NL. The meaning of validity in the new Standards for Educational and Psychological Testing: implications for measurement courses. Measurement and Evaluation in Counseling and Development 2003; 36: 181.

36. Indices used when appraising 'yes–no' screening and diagnostic tests for a disease or other attribute include *sensitivity, specificity, false negative* and *false positive* rates (defined in the text), the *likelihood ratios* for positive and negative test results, i.e. sensitivity%/(100 − specificity%) and (100 − sensitivity%)/specificity%, the *diagnostic odds ratio*, i.e. (TP × TN)/(TN × FN), and *Youden's index*, i.e. (sensitivity% + specificity% − 100). The *diagnostic odds ratio* is described by Glas AS, Liymer JG, Prins MH, Bonsel GJ, Bossuyt PMM. (The diagnostic odds ratio: a single indicator of test performance. Journal of Clinical Epidemiology 2003; 56: 1129).

    If the prevalence of the disease (its pre-test probability) in the population is known or assumed, TP, TN, FP and FN can be recalculated to express the expected proportions with these test results in the population. Use can then also be made of: the *predictive value* of positive and negative results, i.e. TP/(TP + FP) and TN/(FN + TN); *post-test probabilities* (the probability that the disease is present or conditional on the test result, i.e. TP/(TP + FP) and 1 − [TN/(FN + TN)] respectively; *gain in certainty* (the difference between the pre-test and post-test probabilities of the disease); the *percentage agreement*, i.e. [(TP + TN)/(TP + TN + FP + FN)] × 100; and *kappa* (which expresses the proportion of subjects whose test result coincides with their true status, after adjustment for chance agreement).

    When appraising a *screening or diagnostic test with a range of results*, use can be made of the computed *area under the ROC curve*, and of sensitivity, specificity, etc. (as above), at arbitrary cut-points.

    When appraising an *ordinal- or interval-scale measure of an ordinal- or interval-scale variable*, other indices can be used, e.g. the size and direction of the differences between the measure and the true value, and correlation and various other coefficients.

    For software, see Appendix C.

37. Moons KGM, Biesheuvel CJ, Grobbee DE. Clinical Chemistry 2004; 50: 473.

38. Bossuyt PM, Reitsma JB, Bruns DE, Gatsonis CA, Glasziou PP, Irwig LM, Lijmer JG, Moher D, Rennie D, deVet HCW. Towards complete and accurate reporting of studies of diagnostic accuracy: the STARD initiative, Clinical Chemistry 2003 49: 1. Bossuyt PM, Reitsma JB, Bruns DE, Gatsonis CA, Glasziou PP, Irwig LM, Moher D, Rennie D, deVet HCW, Lijmer JG. The STARD statement for reporting studies of diagnostic accuracy: explanation and elaboration. Clinical Chemistry 2003; 49: 7.

39. Feinstein AR. Clinical biostatistics. St Louis, MO: CV Mosby; 1977. Chapter 15.

40. Smeeth L, Iliffe S. Effectiveness of screening older people for impaired vision in community setting: systematic review of evidence from randomized controlled trials. British Medical Journal 1998; 316: 660.

41. In 2002, the US Preventive Services Task Force concluded that the evidence was insufficient to recommend for or against routine screening for prostate cancer using prostate specific antigen testing (US Preventive Services Task Force. Screening for Prostate Cancer: Recommendations and Rationale; statement available at http://www.ahrq.gov/clinic/3rduspstf/prostatescr/prostaterr.htm). The effect (if any) on mortality is very limited (Martin RM. Commentary:

prostate cancer is omnipresent, but should we screen for it? International Journal of Epidemiology 2007; 36: 278).

42. US Preventive Services Task Force. Guide to clinical preventive services, 2nd edn. Washington, DC: US Department of Health and Human Services; 1996. pp. 419–424.

43. Knottnerus JA. Challenges in dia-prognostic research. Journal of Epidemiology and Community Health 2002 56: 340. Knottnerus JA, Muris JW. Assessment of the accuracy of diagnostic tests: the cross-sectional study. Journal of Clinical Epidemiology 2003; 56: 1118.

44. See note 7, Chapter 4.

18

Interviews and Self-Administered Questionnaires

Interviews may be highly structured or less structured. A clinician uses a relatively un-structured interview – a flexible approach is used, leads are followed as they arise, and the content, wording and order of the questions vary from interview to interview. In the same way, a public health worker conducting interviews as part of the investigation of a local outbreak of disease has an idea of what information is wanted – the nature and time of onset of the symptoms, the patients' prior movements, their contacts with other ill persons, their recent meals, their milk and water supply, and so on – but does not decide in advance exactly what questions will be asked, or in what order.

In other situations, a more standardized technique may be used, the wording and order of the questions being decided in advance. This may take the form of a highly structured interview, in which the questions are asked orally, or a self-administered questionnaire, in which case the respondent reads the questions and enters answers or checkmarks or clicks a mouse (sometimes in the presence of an interviewer who 'stands by' to give assistance if necessary). For simplicity, we will use the term 'questionnaire' to indicate the list of questions prepared for either of these purposes. (In the behavioural sciences, a 'questionnaire' usually means a self-administered question-naire, and the term is not applied to the interview schedule used by an interviewer).

Standardized methods of asking questions are usually preferred in surveys and other research, since they provide more assurance that the data will be reproducible. But less structured interviews may be useful in a preliminary survey, where the purpose is to obtain information to help in the subsequent planning of a study rather than facts for analysis, and in studies of perceptions, attitudes, motivations and affective reactions. Unstructured ('free-style') interviews are characteristic of qualitative (nonquantitative) research (see p. 148).

Mode of Administration

The choice between a self-administered questionnaire and a highly structured inter-view may not be an easy one. The use of self-administered questionnaires is simpler and cheaper; self-administered questionnaires can be administered to many persons

Research Methods in Community Medicine: Surveys, Epidemiological Research, Programme Evaluation, Clinical Trials   J. H. Abramson and Z. H. Abramson   Copyright © 2008, John Wiley & Sons Ltd

simultaneously (e.g. to a class of schoolchildren) and, unlike interviews, can be sent by post or e-mail or displayed on a computer screen. On the other hand, they demand a certain level of education and skill on the part of the respondent.

Face-to-face or phone *interviews* have many advantages. A good interviewer can stimulate and maintain the respondent's interest, and can create a rapport and atmosphere conducive to the answering of questions.[1] If anxiety is aroused (e.g. 'Why am I being asked these questions? Have I an illness they haven't told me about?'), the interviewer can allay it. If a question is not understood, then an interviewer can repeat it and, if necessary (and in accordance with guidelines decided in advance), provide an explanation or alternative wording. Optional follow-up or probing questions that are to be asked only if prior responses are inconclusive or inconsistent cannot easily be built into paper questionnaires. A paper questionnaire is perforce restricted to simple questions with simple instructions, designed to elicit simple data. In a face-to-face interview, observations can be made as well; the so-called 'coronary-prone behaviour pattern', for example, was originally detected in interviews during which note was taken not only of what the subject said but of how they said it, whether they clenched their fists and teeth, etc.[2] Furthermore, the interviewer can use visual aids; cups and saucers of various sizes and models of food servings can be an invaluable aid in a quantitative dietary interview.

For most purposes, interviews would be preferable to self-administered questionnaires, if they were not so costly and time consuming. They elicit much fuller information about past diseases, especially for milder or transient conditions.[3] It is important, however, that they be conducted by skilled interviewers. Otherwise, there is much truth in the statement that 'to gain information by interview resembles the use of questionnaires, except that questionnaires only contain errors caused by the patient, but interviews include errors caused by the interviewer as well'.[4]

A drawback of interviews, however, is that in interviews there may be more reluctance to give 'socially undesirable' responses than in a situation perceived as being more impersonal, especially if anonymity is assured.[5] In a study of the use of seat restraints for children in cars, for example, nonuse of a restraint on the last trip was reported by only 18% of parents in face-to-face interviews, but by 26% in postal questionnaires and 30% in phone interviews.[6]

Self-administered questionnaires are widely and successfully used. They have been found to yield appreciably more reports of disability, pain and emotional disturbance than interviewer-administered questionnaires, and to increase significantly the numbers of sexual partners and sexually transmitted diseases reported by women. A decision on the use of a self-administered questionnaire may require a pretest to obtain information on the response rate, rates of unanswered items, and the validity of responses.

The main problems with *postal questionnaires* are that response rates tend to be relatively low and that there may be underrepresentation of less literate subjects. There may be more missing answers than in interviews. The questionnaires often find their way to wastepaper baskets, even if they are short and simple, attractively designed, accompanied by a persuasive covering letter and a stamped return envelope, preceded by a courteous 'pre-letter' and followed by one or more reminders by mail or by phone.[7] Response rates may be high, however, in surveys where subjects have a special motivation, as in the instance of questionnaires sent to patients or ex-patients by their own physicians or treating agencies, enquiring about their progress.

In terms of speed and cost, *e-mailed questionnaires* are an attractive substitute for postal questionnaires in colleges or other groups or organizations where everyone has e-mail facilities. Even there, response rates in most randomized trials have been lower than for mailed questionnaires.[8] With the current epidemic of spam, it is probably increasingly unlikely that unsolicited e-mails from unknown senders will be read, let alone replied to. A further problem is the lack of anonymity. A mixed-mode approach, benefiting from the advantages of e-mails but not relying solely on them, has been suggested. In one randomized trial, the use of e-mails, supplemented by mailed questionnaires for people without valid e-mail addresses, yielded the same response rate as a mailed questionnaire, but with the advantage of speed and fuller answers.[9]

Phone interviews are sometimes preferred to mailed questionnaires and face-to-face interviews. This choice depends on feasibility (e.g. the prevalence of telephones), costs, and the nature and purpose of the study. Some studies show little difference in cost or data quality between phone and personal interviews. Some questions are easier to ask on the telephone and others are easier to ask face to face, but the differences between these two interview modes are not consistent. Comparisons yield inconsistent findings.[10] Phone interviews sometimes elicit fewer reports of ill health than mailed questionnaires. In general, fewer problems are reported and more socially desirable responses are given. Phone surveys on drug use incite more refusals than face-to-face interviews, and more questions go unanswered. In one study, the proportion of respondents who admitted to 'nervousness, worry or depression or trouble sleeping' (symptoms that might be considered embarrassing) was somewhat lower in phone interviews than in mailed questionnaires.[11]

The future of phone interviews is uncertain. Nonresponse rates (due to refusals or to failure to make contact with a live person) appear to be rising, particularly in large cities,[12] possibly because of resentment of telemarketing and the increased use of new technologies (answering machines, paging, caller identification).

Mixed strategies are often used, e.g. trying mail or telephone first and then using home interviews only for persistent nonrespondents.[11]

Computer-assisted Interviews

Computer-aided interviewing (where the interviewer uses a computer) and self-administered computer questionnaires have become increasingly popular. The questions are shown on a computer screen, and the keyboard or mouse is used for entering the answers. Skipping and branching patterns (i.e. 'if so-and-so, go to question such-and-such') are built into the program, so that the screen automatically displays the appropriate question. Checks can be built in and an immediate warning given if a reply lies outside an acceptable range or is inconsistent with previous replies; revision of previous replies is permitted, with automatic return to the current question. The responses are entered directly on to the computer record, avoiding the need for subsequent coding and data entry. The technique may be especially helpful if question structure is complicated or there are many possible responses, as in a survey that required information about asthma medication, in terms of 486 possible combinations of drug, dose and delivery system.[13] The program can make an automatic selection of subjects who require additional procedures, such as special tests, supplementary questionnaires, or follow-up visits.

The advantages of the procedure are obvious, but consideration should also be given to its drawbacks. Apart from the need to write and test a computer program, there is also a possibility of errors, mainly caused by typing slips when entering the answers. In one careful comparison it was found that 2.0% of recorded responses were erroneous, as compared with 1.1% when a paper-and-pencil technique was used.[14] This is counterbalanced by the avoidance of errors that may occur during the transfer and entry of ordinary interview data. The automatic skip patterns can, however, lead to other and irremediable errors. Suppose that subjects are asked if they smoke and, if they say 'yes', are then asked about the number and kind of cigarettes smoked. In an ordinary interview, if the response to the first question is 'yes' but is erroneously entered as 'no', and the subsequent questions are (correctly) asked and answered, the inconsistency can be detected when the data are checked, and the reply to the first question can be corrected. In a computer-aided interview, if 'no' is entered by mistake the other questions will not be asked at all. Also, if the interviewer has to code responses before keying them in, then there is later no way of detecting coding errors, since there is no record of the actual responses. Other drawbacks are that the use of a computer lengthens the interview slightly, and that interviewers may find their work boring. Printed questionnaires must be available for emergency use; in one study using computer-aided personal interviews, printed forms were needed in 5% of instances.[14]

If the right software is available (see Appendix C) the preparations generally present no technical problems.

The various methods of computer-assisted interviewing (CAI) have catchy nicknames. For example, CAPI is computer-assisted personal interviewing (face to face); CATI is computer-assisted telephone interviewing (the interviewer uses both a phone and a computer); and CASI is computer- assisted self-interviewing, alias CSAQ (computerized self-administered questionnaire). All these are contrasted with PAPI, or paper-and-pen interviewing.

The use of self-administered computer questionnaires is sure to increase. Like self-administered paper questionnaires, they apparently boost willingness to report socially undesirable behaviours.[15] In a randomized trial in a study of drinking habits in Edinburgh, men who entered their own responses reported the consumption of 30% more alcohol than men asked the same questions in face-to-face interviews.[16] In controlled comparisons, more responses suggesting the possibility of HIV infection were provided by self-administered computer questionnaires than by self-administered paper questionnaires and face-to-face interviews, and adolescents reported more alcohol use, illicit drug use, and psychological distress than in paper questionnaires.[17]

Audio-CASI (or ACASI), with audio playback of the questions shown on the screen, is a promising enhancement, and a multimedia approach, embracing pictures as well, has been warmly advocated: 'Computers can conduct personalized, in-depth interviews without interviewers; provide standardized data collection with appropriate levels of probing; automate data entry; encourage subjects to review and correct inconsistent data; and ensure that responses are complete. Interactive multimedia tools can motivate subjects and improve participation. Visual and aural cues may stimulate recall and improve data quality. CASI is appropriate for use in populations in which literacy is low and in multiple ethnic groups'.[18] In a study of drug users, behaviours carrying a stigma were reported more freely in audio-CASI than in face-to-face interviews; but reports of psychological distress were more frequent in the face-to-face interviews.[19]

Palmtop-assisted self-interviewing (PASI) has now been reported to be as effective as ACASI and self-administered paper questionnaires for collecting sensitive behavioral data, and better than face-to-face interiews.[20]

Validity

Information obtained by interviewing and questioning is often referred to as 'soft' data, as opposed to the presumably 'hard' data[21] derived from observations. A man who says he has heart disease may have a noncardiac disease, or none at all. A youth who says he has, or has not, been circumcised may be wrong.[22] In a study of questionnaire responses by registered nurses in the United States, only 74% of cases of cancer of the uterus reported in questionnaires were confirmed by medical records.[23] In a Californian study, the proportions of various chronic diseases (recorded in medical records) that were not reported in interviews ranged from 15 to 79%, and the over-reporting rate from 1 to 83%.[24] A person who says they do not have a disease may be unaware that they have it, or may have forgotten, or may be unwilling (on a conscious or unconscious level) to admit its presence – particularly if the disease carries a stigma (this has been called 'unacceptable disease bias'). In a survey in which comparisons were made with cancer registry data, it was found that only 51% of men with a previous diagnosis of cancer of the lip reported this condition when asked about previous illnesses, and only another 13% reported it when they were specifically asked about cancer.[25] When a survey shows that more reports of severe sexual abuse in childhood are provided by depressed women than by nondepressed women,[26] it is legitimate to ask whether this reflects differential validity rather than an aftermath of sexual abuse. If patients with herpes zoster are much more likely than controls to report that they had a blow at the site of the rash in the month before its appearance, does this necessarily prove an association between trauma and herpes zoster?[27] When a large-scale case-control study found a relationship after 10 years or more of cell-phone use between the side on which brain tumours occurred and the side on which the cell-phone was said to be held, the possibility could not be excluded that this was an artefact resulting from the patients' awareness of the hypothesis being tested.[28]

People may be reluctant to admit to induced abortions, drug abuse, overindulgence in alcohol or tobacco, or other socially undesirable behaviour – a study in Holland showed that a question-based survey of alcoholism would miss over half the known problem drinkers.[29] This effect was demonstrated in a study in which the personality trait of social desirability ('the defensive tendency of individuals to portray themselves in keeping with perceived cultural norms') and physical activity (using objective meta-bolic measurements) were measured, and it was found that the social desirability trait was associated with overreporting of physical activity.[30] Self-reported weight may tend to be an underestimate, and self-reported height an overestimate; in one study, the prevalence of obesity (using a definition based on weight and height) was 50% higher when based on actual measurements than when based on reported weights and heights.[31] A mother reporting that her children have an abundance of milk, fruit, veg-etables and meat may be saying this only to put herself into a favourable light, whereas a mother reporting that her children have none of these foodstuffs may be trying to elicit sympathy or welfare assistance.

Interviews conducted at home and in a clinic may elicit different information, and the responses may depend on who else is present. Suspicions about the interviewers' motives may influence responses. Different answers may be given to an interviewer who is older than, younger than, or the same age as the respondent, or who is of the same, a higher or lower social class, or of the same or a different ethnic group. Doctors and lay interviewers may obtain different responses to the same questions – the easiest way to ensure a high degree of satisfaction with medical care is to base the appraisal on interviews conducted by the treating physicians themselves.

A tactic sometimes used is to have the interviewer make an appraisal of the respond-ent's 'reliability' (trustworthiness), based on impressions gained during the interview. This appraisal may be aided by asking additional informal questions (preferably after the structured part of the interview) that plumb consistency and accuracy. These appraisals can be taken into account when the data are analysed, e.g. by comparing the results for 'reliable' and 'unreliable' informants. In the study of cell-phone use and brain tumours referred to above,[28] the association with the side on which the cell-phone was used became weaker and statistically nonsignificant when the analysis was confined to subjects who, in the interviewers' opinion, recalled their cell-phone use 'very well'.

The interviewer, as well as the respondent, may be a source of bias – their expecta-tions or preferences may influence the answers or the way they are interpreted and recorded. An interviewer who knows the study hypothesis may tend to get responses that fit in with their view of the correctness of the hypothesis. Bias of this sort is least likely to occur in cohort studies in which the interviewer is unaware of the subject's prior exposure to the causal factors under study, and is most likely to occur in a case-control study in which the interviewer knows whether the subject is a case or a control.

Answers may also be influenced by the wording of the questions (see Chapter 19). A greater number of surgical procedures may be reported in reply to a question about 'stitches' or 'sutures' than to one about 'operations'. In one study, 'How old were you when you had our first child?' was found to be a much more reliable question (*kappa* = 88%) than 'How old is your eldest child?' (*kappa* = 66%).[32] The sequence of the ques-tions may also affect the responses.

Memory is fallible, and recall bias often occurs. Mild injuries and illnesses, brief stays in hospital, and other past episodes and experiences that made little impact on the respondent may be forgotten and not reported, especially if the time lapse is long. On the other hand, if the question refers to the recent past (say the last month), episodes that occurred longer ago may also be reported (telescoping bias). As a compromise, questions about acute illnesses and injuries are usually confined to the previous 2 weeks. Test–retest reliability of interview data on 'simple' events (such as hysterectomy) is high, but it is lower for more complicated data, such as age at occurrence of menopause, or the reasons for starting or stopping drug treatment.[33] When there is an option it is preferable to ask for current rather than historical information. Population studies of age at menarche or menopause and duration of breast-feeding, for example, are more accurate if they use current status than if they rely on 'When did you …' questions.[34]

Cues may be needed to tickle the memory. When mothers were asked about the taking of prescription drugs during pregnancy, for example, specific mention of headache, nausea, and various other symptoms increased the number of reports of having taken drugs by 32–58%, and mentioning the drugs by name increased the reports by an extra 6–40%.[35] The number of chronic diseases reported can be doubled if a checklist (phrased in lay terms) is shown or read to the respondents,[36] and can be further increased by using an extensive questionnaire that provides multiple cues and includes probing questions.[37] Reporting of symptoms may be doubled if a checklist is shown to the respondents.[38] Responses become more accurate in studies in which respondents can use memory aids, such as health diaries or wall calendars maintained for this purpose (see p. 219); in a randomized controlled study, 50% more symptom episodes were reported by subjects who had been given wall calendars for the recording of symptoms.[39]

'Simple memory failure' of this sort can produce biased estimates of prevalence or incidence and (if groups are being compared) can make it more difficult to detect differences that actually exist. Other effects may occur if there is 'differential memory failure', i.e. where the validity of what is recalled varies in the groups that are compared (see differential validity, p. 163). True differences between the groups may then be diminished, magnified or masked, and spurious differences may be produced. Precautions can be taken to detect and deal with this form of recall bias.[40] For example, in a case-control study where an association with a specific drug is postulated and it is believed that taking of the drug may be overreported by cases and/or underreported by controls, questions may be asked about other drugs (or other factors) known to be unrelated to the disease, to see whether they are reported more frequently by cases than by controls. These results will provide an indication of the degree of recall bias, and can be taken into account when analysing or interpreting the study findings. Also, at the end of the interview the subjects may be asked about their beliefs concerning the cause of the disorder – recall bias is especially likely if the respondents suspect the drug under study to be a cause.

The replies to questions also depend on who is asked. *Proxy informants* may be inaccurate. Husbands and wives tend to report more illness for themselves than for their spouses ('the health of the nation improves markedly when proxy respondents are used; differences are even more noticeable when the respondent for a family is Uncle Joe').[41] Respondents may be unaware of most of the diseases suffered by their brothers and sisters, may not correctly report the causes of their relatives' deaths, and may be more likely to report that family members have a given disease if they themselves have the disease.[42] Details of a man's drinking and smoking habits may be reported differently by himself and his wife,[43] and agreement between parents and children with respect to information about the children varies from excellent (e.g. for eye and hair colour) to very poor (e.g. for a history of peeling sunburn).[44] The taking of medications may be reported quite differently by patients and their doctors.[45]

Whatever the variable we are trying to measure, we are dealing with statements, not with direct measurements. This applies as much to attitudes, for which there are no more direct methods of measurement, as to any other variable. If a respondent says they feel well, we have not necessarily learnt their self-perception of their health, but only their reported self-perception of their health – which, however useful it may be as a datum in its own right, is not quite the same thing.

The validity of responses may be appraised by the methods described in Chapter 17. Many studies have compared interview responses with presumably accurate medical records. These found that only 30–53% of documented diagnoses were reported; most hospital admissions and operations were reported, but diagnostic X-ray examinations and many medications were poorly reported.[46] Comparisons with old records may permit tests of the validity of interview data about long-past events or experiences; the validity of such data is sometimes surprisingly high.[47]

Observational data that can be used as criteria are sometimes available. A comparison with angiographic findings, for example, showed that the sensitivity of the WHO questionnaire on intermittent claudication, as an indicator of severe grades of peripheral arterial disease, was 50% and its specificity was over 98%.[48] Self-reports of the taking of vitamin and mineral supplements were validated by blood and urine assays,[49] and the question 'Do you have a hearing loss?' by audiometry.[50]

Where suitable criteria are not available, construct validity (see p. 168) may be examined. A questionnaire on habitual physical activity, for example, was validated by finding the expected associations with age, sex, kind of job, self-appraisals of physical activity, caloric intake, maximal oxygen intake, body fatness, and exposure to health-promotion programmes.[51] When possible, differential validity in different subgroups of the study population should be examined.

Interview Technique

The accuracy of interview data can be boosted not only by the choice of an appropriate mode of administration, the use of memory aids, and careful attention to the construction of the questionnaire and the selection and wording of questions, but also by proper interview technique.[1] It is important, but not sufficient, to follow the 'golden rule of survey research':[52] 'Do unto your respondents as you would have them do unto you' (thank them at the start and end of the interview, be sensitive to their needs, and watch for signs of discomfort).

In the interests of accuracy, the main requirement is that the interviewer should beware of influencing the responses. Questions should be asked precisely as they were written, and reworded or supplemented by explanations only when this is absolutely necessary. The questions should be asked in a neutral manner, without showing (by words, inflection or expression) a preference for any particular response. Agreement, disagreement or surprise should not be shown, and the precise answers should be recorded, without sifting or interpreting them. This, like the ability to encourage the respondents' participation and other necessary skills, demands training and practical experience. Good interviewers are made, not born (although some people are congenitally incapable of becoming good interviewers).

It may be noted that physicians, nurses and social workers often make poor interviewers in a research setting. They have been trained to see their role as the provision of help to patients or clients, and often have difficulty in accepting or fulfilling the different role of collecting standardized data. They may be incapable of merely reading out questions, but insist on rephrasing them or altering their order. They are often skilled interviewers, but have been trained to conduct interviews of a different type, in which selective information is sought to clarify a specific case problem, and efforts are made to exert influence by providing advice, directions, information or reassurance; these habits are not easily unlearned.

Notes and References

1. For useful practical advice on *the art of interviewing*, see Bowling A (Research methods in health: investigating health and health services. Buckingham: Open University Press, 1997. Chapter 13), Kornhauser A, Sheatsley PB (Questionnaire construction and interview procedure. In: Selltiz C, Wrightsman LS, Cook SW (eds), Research methods in social relations, 3rd edn. New York, NY: Holt, Rinehart & Winston, 1976), or Britten N (Qualitative research: qualitative interviews in medical research. British Medical Journal 1995; 311: 251.

2. Friedman M, Rosenman R. Type A behavior and your heart. New York, NY: Knopf; 1974.

3. Bergmann MM, Jacobs EJ, Hoffman K, Boeing E. Agreement of self-reported medical history: comparison of an in-person interview with a self-administered questionnaire. European Journal of Epidemiology 2004; 19: 411.

4. Glaser EM. Volunteers, controls, placebos and questionnaires in clinical trials. In: Witts LJ (ed.), Medical surveys and clinical trials. Oxford: Oxford University Press; 1964. pp. 115–129.

5. *Comparisons of self-administered and interviewer-administered questionnaires*: Picavet HSJ, Van den Bos GAM (Comparing survey data on functional disability: the impact of some methodological differences. Journal of Epidemiology and Community Health 1996; 50: 86), Grootendorst PV, Feeny DH, Furlong W (Does it matter whom and how you ask? Inter- and intra-rater agreement in the Ontario Health Survey. Journal of Clinical Epidemiology 1997; 50: 127), De Leeuw ED (Data quality in mail, telephone and face-to-face surveys. Amsterdam: TT-Publikaties; 1993), Tourangeau, R, Rasinski K, Jobe JB, Smith TW, Pratt WF (Sources of error in a survey on sexual behavior. Journal of Official Statistics 1997; 13: 341), Okamoto K, Ohsuka K, Shiraishi T, Hukazawa E, Wakasugi S, Furuta K (Comparability of epidemiological information between self- and interviewer-administered questionnaires. Journal of Clinical Epidemiology 2002; 55: 505).

6. Pless IB, Miller JR. Apparent validity of alternative survey methods. Journal of Community Health 1979; 5: 22.

7. *Response to postal questionnaires*. According to a systematic review, response may be improved by repeated mailings, telephone reminders, and use of a short questionnaire; incentives

do not help (Nakash RA, Hutton JL, Jorstad-Stein EC, Gates S, Lamb SE. Maximising response to postal questionnaires – a systematic review of randomized trials in health research. BMC Medical Research Technology 2006; 6: 5).

The effect of *incentives* varies. Cash incentives improved response in a study of physicians in Hong Kong (Leung GM, Ho LM, Chan MF, Johnston JM, Wong FK. The effects of cash and lottery incentives on mailed surveys to physicians: a randomized trial. Journal of Clinical Epidemiology 2002; 35: 801). In studies in the UK and the USA, enclosing a pen or pencil had a significant effect; in other studies this had no effect (Sharp L, Cochran C, Cotton SC, Gray NM, Gallagher ME. Journal of Clinical Epidemiology 2006; 59: 747. White E, Garney PA, Kolar AS. Increasing response to mailed questionnaires by including a pencil/pen. American Journal of Epidemiology 2005; 162: 261).

According to a meta-analysis, *personally addressed hand-signed letters* increase response (Scott P, Edwards P. Personally addressed hand-signed letters increase questionnaire response: a meta-analysis of randomised controlled trials. BMC Health Services Research 2006; 6: 111). In a study of obstetricians and gynaecologists, hand-written signatures had no effect (McKenzie-McHarg K, Tully L, Gates S, Ayers S, Brocklehurst P. Effect on survey response rate of hand written versus printed signature on a covering letter: randomized controlled trial. BMC Health Services Research 2995; 5: 52).

In an Australian study, *hand delivery* (by project staff) produced a better response than postal delivery (Mond JM, Rodgers B, Hay PJ, Owen C, Beaumont PJV. Mode of delivery, but not questionnaire length, affected response in an epidemiological study of eating-disordered behavior. Journal of Clinical Epidemiology 2004; 57: 1167).

In a study of physicians in the USA, *questionnaire length* had a threshold effect. The response rate was 38% if there were over 10,000 words, and 59% if there were fewer (Jepson C, Asch DA, Hershey JC, Ubel PA. In a mailed physician survey, questionnaire length had a threshold effect on the response rate. Journal of Clinical Epidemiology 2005; 58: 103).

8. Couper MP, Blair J, Triplett T. 1999 A comparison of mail and e-mail for a survey of employees in U.S. statistical agencies. Journal of Official Statistics 2005; 15: 39. Akl EA, Maroun N, Klocke RA, Montori V, Schunemann HJ. Electronic mail was not better than postal mail for surveying residents and faculty. Journal of Clinical Epidemiology 2005; 58: 425.

9. The *mixed-mode* strategy was tested by Schaeffer DR, Dillman DA (Development of a standard e-mail methodology: results of an experiment. Public Opinion Quarterly 1998; 52: 378). They personalized the e-mail messages, and did not use their e-mail program's 'carbon copy' ('cc') or 'blind carbon copy' ('bcc') options, which reveal that the recipient is part of a mailing list.

10. Recent studies of *phone interviews* include: Beehe TJ, McRae JA Jr, Harrison PA, Davern ME, Quinlan KB (Mail surveys resulted in more reports of substance use than telephone surveys. Journal of Clinical Epidemiology 2005; 58: 421), Hocking JS, Lim MS C, Read T, Hellard ME (Postal surveys of physicians gave superior response rates over telephone interviews in a randomized trial. Journal of Clinical Epidemiology 2006; 59: 521), and a Danish study by Feveile H, Olsen O, Hugh A (A randomized trial of mailed questionnaires versus telephone interviews: response patterns in a survey. BMC Medical Research Methodology 2007; 7: 27), which found that people interviewed by phone tended to report better health.

11. Siemiatycki J. A comparison of mail, telephone and home interview strategies for household health surveys. American Journal of Public Health 1979; 69: 238.

12. Steeh C, Kirgis N, Cannon B, De Witt J. Are they as bad as they seem? Nonresponse rates at the end of the twentieth century. Journal of Official Statistics 2001; 17: 227.

13. Anie KA, Jones PW, Hilton SR, Anderson HR. A computer-assisted telephone interview technique for assessment of asthma morbidity and drug use in adult asthma. Journal of Clinical Epidemiology 1996; 49: 653.

14. Birkett NJ. Computer-aided personal interviewing: a new technique for data collection in epidemiologic surveys. American Journal of Epidemiology 1988; 127: 684.

15. A meta-analysis has shown that CASI reduces social desirability bias, but suggests that this effect may be weaker than it was in earlier years (unpublished study by Weisband S, Kiesler S; cited by De Leeuw E, Nicholls W II. Technological innovations in data collection: acceptance, data quality and costs. Sociological Research Online 1996; 1: 4).

16. Waterton J, Duffy JC. A comparison of computer interviewing techniques and traditional methods in the collection of self-report alcohol consumption data in a field survey. International Statistical Review 1984; 52: 173.

17. Locke SE, Kowaloff HB, Hoff RG *et al.* Computer interview for screening blood donors for risk of HIV transmission. MD Computing 1994; 11: 26. Wright DL, Aquilino WS, Supple AJ. A comparison of computer-assisted and paper-and-pencil self-administered questionnaires in a survey on smoking, alcohol, and drug use. Public Opinion Quarterly 1998; 62: 331.

18. Kohlmeier L, Mendez M, McDuffie J, Miller M. Computer-assisted self-interviewing: a multimedia approach to dietary assessment. American Journal of Clinical Nutrition 1997; 65(4 suppl.): 1275S.

19. Newman JC, Des Jerlais DC, Turner CF, Gribble J, Cooley DP, Paone, D. The differential effects of face-to-face and computer interview modes. American Journal of Public Health 2002; 92: 294.

20. Van Griensven F, Naorat S, Kilmarx PH, Jeeyapant S, Manopalboon C, Chalkummao S, Jenkins RA, Uthalvoravit W, Wasinrapee P, Mock PA, Tappero JW. Palmtop-assisted self-interviewing for the collection of sensitive behavioral data: randomized trial with drug use urine testing. American Journal of Epidemiology 2005; 163: 271.

21. In a review of what *hard data* means, Feinstein AR (An additional basic science for clinical medicine: IV. The development of clinimetrics. Annals of Internal Medicine 1983; 99: 843) considers five attributes, i.e. preservability, objectivity, dimensionality, accuracy (criterion validity) and consistency, and, after citing examples of data that are not regarded as 'soft' although they are ephemeral, subjective, nondimensional, or inaccurate, concludes that the fundamental quality of 'hard' data is their consistency – they are 'repeatable by the same observer and reproducible by another'.

22. In a Texas study in which adolescents were asked if they had been circumcised, 5% gave wrong answers and another 40% said they did not know (Risser JMH, Risser WL, Elssa MA, Cromwell PF, Barratt MS, Bortot A. Self-assessment of circumcision status by adolescents. American Journal of Epidemiology 2004; 159: 1095).

23. Colditz GA, Martin P, Stampfer MJ *et al.* Validation of questionnaire information on risk factors and disease outcomes in a prospective cohort study of women. American Journal of Epidemiology 1986; 123: 894.

24. Madow WG. Net differences in interview data on chronic conditions and information derived from medical records. Vital and Health Statistics, series 2: 57. Washington, DC: Public Health Service.

25. Chambers LW, Spitzer WO, Hill GB, Helliwell BE. Underreporting of cancer in medical surveys: a source of systematic error in cancer research. American Journal of Epidemiology 1976; 104: 141.

26. Cheasty M, Clare AW, Collins C. Relation between sexual abuse in childhood and adult depression: case-control study. British Medical Journal 1998; 316: 198.

27. Thomas SL, Wheeler JG, Hall AJ. Case-control study of the effect of mechanical trauma on the risk of herpes zoster. British Medical Journal 200; 328: 439.

28. Lahkola A, Auvinen A, Raitanen J, Schoemaker MJ, Christensen HC, Feychting M, Johansen C, Klæboe L, Lönn S, Swerdlow AJ, Tynes T, Salminen T. Mobile phone use and risk of glioma in 5 North European countries. International Journal of Cancer 2007; 120: 1769.

29. Mulder PGH, Garretsen HFL. Are epidemiological and sociological surveys a proper instrument for detecting true problem drinkers? International Journal of Epidemiology 1983; 12: 442.

30. Adams SA, Matthews CE, Ebbeling CB, Moore CG, Cunningham JE, Fulton J, Hebert JR. The effect of social desirability and social approval on self-reports of physical activity. American Journal of Epidemiology 2005; 161: 389.

31. Stewart AW, Jackson RT, Ford MA, Beaglehole R. 1987 Underestimation of relative weight by use of self-reported height. American Journal of Epidemiology 1987; 125: 122.

32. Yorkshire Breast Cancer Group. Observer variation in recording clinical data from women presenting with breast lesions. British Medical Journal 1977; 2: 1196.

33. When interviews of postmenopausal women were repeated after 2–22 months, *kappa* values were 89–93% for data on hysterectomy, a family history of breast cancer, hot flushes, and other 'simple' variables; in 22% there were discrepancies of over 2 years in reported age at menopause (Horwitz RI, Yu EC. Problems and proposals for interview data in epidemiological research. International Journal of Epidemiology 1985; 14: 463).

34. This requires probit analysis. As an example, data on current breast-feeding status were converted to an estimate of the average duration of breast-feeding by Ferreira MU, Cardoso MA, Santos AL, Ferreira CS, Szarfarc SC (Rapid epidemiologic assessment of breastfeeding practices: probit analysis of current status data. Journal of Tropical Pediatrics 1996; 42: 50).

35. Mitchell AA, Cottler LB, Shapiro S. Effect of questionnaire design on recall of drug exposure in pregnancy. American Journal of Epidemiology 1986; 123: 670.

36. Linder FE. National health interview surveys. In: Trends in the study of morbidity and mortality. Public Health Papers 27. Geneva: WHO; 1965. p. 78.

37. National Center for Health Statistics. Reporting health events in household interviews: effects of an extensive questionnaire and a diary procedure. Vital and Health Statistics, series 2, no 49. Washington, DC: Public Health Service; 1972.

38. Spilker A, Kessler J. Comparison of symptoms elicited by checklist and fill-in-the-blank questionnaires. Pharmaco-Epidemiology Newsletter 1987; 3: 8.

39. Marcus AC. Memory aids in longitudinal health surveys: results from a field experiment. American Journal of Public Health 1982; 72: 567.

40. Raphael K. Recall bias: a proposal for assessment and control. International Journal of Epidemiology 1987; 16: 167. Also, see Coughlin SS (Recall bias in epidemiologic studies. Journal of Clinical Epidemiology 1990; 43: 87).

41. Kirscht JP. Social and psychological problems of surveys in health and illness. Social Science and Medicine 1971; 5: 519.

42. *Family histories* of disease should be used with caution. Diseases of relatives tend to be underreported (Grootendorst PV, Feeny DH, Furlong W. Does it matter whom and how you ask? Inter- and intra-rater agreement in the Ontario Health Survey. Journal of Clinical Epidemiology 1997; 50: 127), and reported causes of death often differ from the certified causes (Napier JA, Metzner H, Johnson BC. Limitations of morbidity and mortality data obtained from family histories – a report from the Tecumseh Community Health Study. American Journal of Public Health 1972; 62: 30).

When people with rheumatoid arthritis were questioned, 27% reported that their parents were free of arthritis; but when their unaffected siblings were questioned, 50% reported that the same parents were free of arthritis (Schull WJ, Cobb S. The intrafamilial transmission of rheumatoid arthritis. Journal of Chronic Diseases 1969; 22: 217).

Children aged 10 or more can accurately report their parents' smoking status (Barnett T, O'Loughlin J, Paradis G, Renaud L. Reliability of proxy reports of parental smoking by elementary schoolchildren. Annals of Epidemiology 1997; 7: 396), and women's current use of contraceptives can be accurately reported by their husbands, less so by their mothers and sisters (Poulter NR Chang CI, Farley TMM, Marmot MG. Reliability of data from proxy respondents in an international case-control study of cardiovascular disease and oral contraceptives. Journal of Epidemiology and Community Health 1996; 50: 674).

In a study in Lebanon, husbands' and wives' reports of wife beating were fairly congruent (Khajawa M, Tewtel-Salem M. Agreement between husband and wife reports of domestic violence: evidence from poor refugee communities in Lebanon. International Journal of Epidemiology 2004; 33: 526).

43. Passaro KT, Noss J, Savitz DA, Little RE, ALSPAC Study Team. Agreement between self and partner reports of paternal drinking and smoking. International Journal of Epidemiology 1997; 26: 315.

44. Whiteman D, Green A. Wherein lies the truth? Assessment of agreement between parent proxy and child respondents. International Journal of Epidemiology 1997; 26: 855.

45. Hulka BS, Kupper LL, Cassel JC, Efird EL, Burdette JA. Medication use and misuse: physician-patient discrepancies. Journal of Chronic Diseases 1975; 28: 7.

46. Harlow SD, Linet MS. Agreement between questionnaire data and medical records: the evidence for accuracy of recall. American Journal of Epidemiology 1989; 129: 233.

47. *Interview data about the remote past* can sometimes be compared with old records. A study in Iowa found that the reported birth weights of adolescents were accurate enough to permit inferences about relationships with other factors (Burns TL, Moll PP, Rost CA, Lauer RM. Mothers remember birth weights of adolescent children: the Muscatine Ponderosity Family Study. International Journal of Epidemiology 1987; 16: 550). In Pittsburgh, birth weights were recalled accurately after an average of 57 years (Catov JM, Newman AB, Kelsey SF, Roberts JM, Sutton-Tyrrell KC, Garcia, M, Ayonayon HN, Tylavsky F, Ness RB. Accuracy and reliability of maternal recall of infant birth weight among older women. Annals of Epidemiology 2006; 16: 429). In Jerusalem, mothers were found to provide valid information (kappa = 80%) about the breast-feeding of army recruits (in their infancy of course) (Kark JD, Troya G, Friedlander Y, Slater PE, Stein Y. Validity of maternal reporting of breast feeding history and the association with blood lipids in 17 year olds. Journal of Epidemiology and Community Health 1984; 38: 218).

Elderly college-educated US women who had breast-fed a child for a short time 49–66 years previously tended to overreport the duration of breast-feeding, and those who had breast-fed for a long time tended to underreport it (Promislow JHE, Gladen BC, Sandler DP. Maternal recall of breastfeeding duration by elderly women. American Journal of Epidemiology 2005; 161: 289).

Records of a cohort study showed that 8% of 36-year-old men who said they had never smoked regularly had reported regular smoking when questioned at younger ages (Britten N. Validity of claims to lifelong nonsmoking at age 36 in a longitudinal study. International Journal of Epidemiology 1988; 17: 525.

Careful interviews gave 'usefully accurate' information about social circumstances 50 years earlier (father's occupation, number of rooms, etc.), but not about illnesses and diet in childhood (Berney IR, Blane DB. Collecting retrospective data: accuracy of recall after 50 years judged against historical records. Social Science and Medicine 1997; 45: 1519).

The current diet exerts a strong influence on the recall of past diet, and probes and memory aids may be needed to obtain more accurate information about the past (Friedenreich CM, Slimani N, Riboli E. Measurement of past diet: review of previous and proposed methods. Epidemiologic Reviews 1992; 14: 1770).

48. Fowkes FGR. The measurement of atherosclerotic peripheral arterial disease in epidemiological surveys. International Journal of Epidemiology 1988; 17: 248.

49. Satia-Abouta J, Patterson RE, King IB, Stratton KL, Shattuck AL, Kristal AR, Potter JD, Thornquist MD, White E. Reliability and validity of self-report and mineral supplement use in the Vitamins and Lifestyle Study. American Journal of Epidemiology 2003; 157: 944.

50. Sindhusake D, Mitchell P, Smith W, Golding M, Newall P, Hartley D, Rubin G. Validation of self-reported hearing loss. International Journal of Epidemiology 2001; 30: 1371.

51. Blair SN, Haskell WL, Ho P *et al.* Assessment of habitual physical activity by a 7-day recall in a community survey and controlled experiments. American Journal of Epidemiology 1985; 122: 794.
52. The golden rule according to Trochim WMK (1997. Question placement and sequence. Previously available on the Internet). See also: Matthew 7: 12.

19

Constructing a Questionnaire

Before a questionnaire is constructed, the variables it is designed to measure should be listed (see Chapter 10). This done, suitable questions should be formulated, i.e. questions that have (at least) face validity (see p. 164) as measures of these variables, and that also meet the other requirements listed below.

It may be decided to ask multiple questions to measure some variables, both because reliance on a single question may increase the chances of inaccuracy due to misunderstanding or other factors, and because it may not be possible to cover all facets in a single question. For example, even if it is known that a single question asking for a self-rating of health status (e.g. 'Would you say that your health in general is excellent, very good, good, fair, poor, or very poor?') has been validated and found useful in many studies, it may be decided to complement it with more specific questions about physical health, mental health, disabilities, and other dimensions of health.[1] Multiple questions can be brought together in a composite scale of measurement (see Chapter 14), and (by a comparison of responses) they permit an appraisal of reliability.

To enhance comparability with other studies, questions may be borrowed from other sources rather than creating them anew. 'Something old, something new, something borrowed, something blue' – apart maybe from the last ingredient, this is the recipe for most questionnaires. The use of borrowed questions or 'standard' questionnaires has the advantage that they have already been tested and found to be serviceable. But comparability is sometimes an illusion, since the same questions may differ in their validity in different kinds of population, different languages[2] or cultures, or in different circumstances. The investigator should always consider the possible need to revalidate the questions or questionnaire. A decision on what to borrow is not always easy. A researcher wanting to measure social support, for example, can choose between many different questionnaires, varying in their conceptual framework, content, convenience, applicability, and validity.[3]

This chapter will deal with open and closed questions, the requirements that a question should meet, ways of dealing with sensitive topics, and the structure of the questionnaire as a whole.

Research Methods in Community Medicine: Surveys, Epidemiological Research, Programme Evaluation, Clinical Trials J. H. Abramson and Z. H. Abramson Copyright © 2008, John Wiley & Sons Ltd

Open or Closed?

Questions may take two general forms: they may be 'open-ended' (or 'free-response') questions, which the subject answers in their own words, or 'closed' (or 'fixed-alternative') questions, which are answered by choosing from a number of fixed alternative responses.

Open-ended questions often produce difficulties when it comes to interpreting the responses. Suppose, for example, we were interested in knowing how many people had given up smoking for reasons connected with health. The question 'Why did you stop smoking? State your main reason' might elicit such responses as: 'I thought it was better not to smoke', 'I'd been smoking for 30 years, and decided it was time to give it up', and 'Because my wife said I should'. There is obvious difficulty in categorizing these answers; in all three instances, it is impossible to tell whether the main reason was connected with health. In a self-administered questionnaire, even a question like 'What is your marital status?' may be answered 'Unsatisfactory' or 'Ask my wife'; a closed question ('Are you at present single, married, widowed or divorced?') is preferable (in the hope that the reply will not be 'Yes').

There is, of course, no difficulty in the use of open-ended questions in instances where the responses can be easily handled, e.g. 'In what country were you born?' or 'How old were you at your last birthday?' (although even here an answer such as 'very' might be given). Open-ended questions have an important role in exploratory surveys, where they indicate the range of likely replies and provide a guide to the formulation of alternative responses to closed questions. They may also be used to provide colourful case illustrations to brighten up an otherwise dull report. If followed by 'probe' questions, open-ended questions have certain advantages in the study of complicated or ill-formed opinions or attitudes. Qualitative research (see p. 148) uses open-ended rather than closed questions.

Closed questions make for greater uniformity and simplify the analysis, and, therefore, are preferred for most purposes, although they limit the variety and detail of responses. They may provide two responses (such as 'yes–no', 'agree–disagree') or more (such as 'never', 'seldom', 'occasionally', 'fairly frequently', and 'very often'). The range of responses is equivalent to the scale of measurement we have previously spoken of (Chapter 13); it should be comprehensive, and the categories should be mutually exclusive. An 'other (specify) ...' category is sometimes included, as insurance against oversights in the choice of categories; but respondents who mark 'other' very commonly fail to supply the added specific information requested.[4]

When there is a range of responses extending from one extreme to the opposite extreme (e.g. from 'strongly disagree' to 'strongly agree'), it may be decided to try to force the respondent to make a stand by presenting an even number of alternatives, with the same number (generally two or three) on each side. If an odd number are presented, there is a tendency to select the middle response; the offer of a central 'neutral', 'undecided' or 'no opinion' option is likely to reduce the nonresponse rate.

Except in simple instances such as 'yes–no' choices, the alternative responses should be read to the subject, or may be shown (e.g. on a card) or, in a self-administered questionnaire, specified after the question. If shown, they should be arranged one under the other, to avoid confusion, rather than side by side. Experience shows that, if the question is presented orally, respondents tend to choose one of the later answers in the list (*recency effect*), whereas they tend to choose one of the first answers if it is shown (*primacy effect*).[5]

To avoid the need to express all the alternative responses in words, use may be made of graphic rating (visual analogue) scales. The subject is shown a line or ladder, and asked to answer the question by indicating an appropriate point on the scale. Points along the scale may be shown by numbers (often 0 to 10 or 1 to 10), or a score can be obtained by measuring the position of the point marked by the respondent. The scale can be labelled at its ends with the two extreme responses (e.g. 'very satisfied' and 'completely dissatisfied'), and intermediate labels may also be printed.

The formulation of response categories for a question like 'What was your main reason for giving up smoking?' often needs careful thought. A misguided selection of alternatives may, like a Procrustean bed, achieve conformity at a considerable price. It is sometimes advisable to use an open-ended question first (in a pretest), so that free responses can be collected and used as a basis for the design of 'closed' categories. Another approach is to follow the closed question with a suitable open-ended one on the same topic; in a pretest, this may demonstrate flaws in the closed question; in the study itself, the combination provides the advantages of both types of question.

Sometimes more than one response is permitted, e.g. to the question 'Which of the following cereals do you eat?' In this instance, each item represents a separate 'yes–no' variable.

Requirements of Questions

Questions are very easy to write. Good questions are hard to write. They require skill and experience (or expert advice),[6] careful thought, and practical testing. The answers they elicit may vary widely, depending on precisely how the questions are constructed and worded. The proportion of elderly people who say they are 'unable to walk', for example, can range from 4 to 16%, depending on how the question is phrased – walking 'a block' or '400 metres', walking 'without help' or 'without standing still', and with or without the specification 'using a cane if necessary'.[7] The propensity of competing public opinion polls with differently worded questions to supply conflicting results is notorious.

The minimal requirement is, of course, that the question should have *face validity* as a measure of the variable it is wished to study. Implicit in this requirement is the obvious

---

Requirements of questions

1. Must have (at least) face validity
2. Respondents can be expected to know the answer
3. Must be clear and unambiguous
4. Must be 'user friendly' (not demanding undue effort)
5. Must not be offensive or embarrassing
6. Must be fair

but sometimes neglected principle that questions should be asked only if they are necessary. Ensuring that a question accurately reflects what the investigator wishes to know may demand rethinking of the conceptual definition. Is information on 'ability to walk', for example, being requested as a measure of physical capacity or of independence in daily living?

The questions should be ones to which the respondents can be *expected to know the answers*. There is little point in asking 'Did your grandmother have piles?' or (cited from an Internet questionnaire) 'As a baby, did you have milk scurf (itching and scratched weeping lesions)?', or in inviting opinions on a matter the respondent has never thought about, or asking the respondent to state attitudes or motivations of which they may not be aware. People who have not been told they have diabetes cannot report that they have the disease. There is little value in questions concerning events or experiences that had little impact and that many subjects will not recall, such as minor injuries or food eaten 3 days previously. Many mild illnesses not requiring medical care and not restricting activity fail to be reported after the lapse of 1 week, and many hospitalizations are not recalled after 1 year. Illnesses requiring a single consultation with a physician are reported more poorly than those requiring many consultations, and conditions requiring a long stay in hospital or involving surgery are reported more fully than other conditions.

It is often decided that since the respondents cannot be expected to supply the required information in a direct way, indirect questions will be asked, the desired information being inferred from the responses to questions on other matters. Instead of asking a subject if he is emotionally healthy, he may be asked about a series of symptoms from which his emotional health can be inferred. Instead of asking a mother to state her attitudes concerning permissiveness towards children, she may be asked whether she carries or carried out specific actions, or what she would do in a specific situation, or how she thinks other mothers would feel or act, or how she thinks mothers should act. Instead of (or as well as) asking respondents whether they are satisfied with their own medical care, they may be asked what they think of the medical care in their neighbourhood, or whether they agree or disagree with such statements as 'Most doctors take a real interest in their patients'.

The way in which questions are worded can 'make or break' a questionnaire. Questions must be *clear and unambiguous*. They must be phrased in language that it is believed the respondents will understand, and that all respondents will understand in the same way. This is more easily said than done – when a questionnaire is tested, unexpected double meanings are often found concealed in apparently crystal-clear questions. 'Single' may mean 'never married' to some people, and 'not married at present' to others; 'abortion' may mean different things to different people. 'Family' may be understood to mean the immediate family, or relatives in the same household, or the far-flung extended family, or forebears. To some people, 'family planning' means 'saving money for vacations'. The most everyday words may evoke different interpretations. In one methodological study it was found that when answering questions about 'usual' behaviour – where the intended meaning was 'in the ordinary course of events' – 20% of respondents gave it other interpretations, e.g. 'more often than not' or 'at regular (even if infrequent) intervals' or 'sometimes', and 19% disregarded the term completely and gave answers that were not constrained by it at all.[8] The word 'frequently' was found to connote from 36% to 72%, on average, in different studies, and the range for individual users extended beyond this range of means; similarly, the average frequency denoted by 'often' ranged from 42% to 71%.[9]

Medical terms, even those commonly used in everyday speech, may occasion much difficulty. 'Anaemia' and 'heart disease' may have different connotations for the layman and the physician; to many laymen, 'palpitation' means a feeling of breathlessness or of fright, and 'flatulence' means an acid taste in the mouth.[10] A question about 'menarche' may elicit a blank stare.

Questions should be as *user friendly* as possible, i.e. as easy and convenient as their purpose and content will permit. Intricate or demanding questions, and questions requiring complicated responses or a choice between complicated alternatives, should if at all possible be avoided. 'Double-barrelled' questions like 'Do you take your child to a doctor when he has a cold or diarrhoea?' may be difficult to answer (and the answers may be difficult to interpret), and should be split into separate questions. Questions requiring a 'yes' answer to indicate agreement with a negative statement may confuse respondents (e.g. 'Should a woman aged 50 not have regular breast X-rays?').

If closed questions are used, the possible responses should be clearly expressed, and stated at the end, not at the beginning; that is, not 'Do you very often, often, occasionally, hardly ever or never do the Highland fling?', but 'How often do you do the Highland fling – very often, often, occasionally, hardly ever or never?' Also, the need for responses should be reduced where possible; for example, to find out to which of a list of sources of stress the respondent feels exposed, it may be better to ask for a mark against those that apply (with an added 'none of the above' category), rather than to request a 'yes–no' response to each; the former approach, which assumes a 'no' for unchecked items, was found to reduce the nonresponse rates for items from 12–50% to 2%.[4]

As examples of questions that some respondents would find burdensome, here are two from Internet surveys.

1. What is your weight (in kilograms – multiply pounds by 0.45 to get kilograms)?

2. Suppose, in the future, a woman finds out that she carries a gene which greatly increases her chances of developing endometriosis. Her own brothers, sisters and children would have a 50% chance of carrying this gene. The doctor tells the woman that she should inform her female relatives about her situation to let them decide if they want to learn if they are also at increased risk of developing endometriosis. Women known to be at an increased risk for endometriosis may choose to have children earlier in life or take some kind of drug as a possible form of prevention. The woman refuses to tell them, because she says they will only worry. What do you think the doctor should do?
   - Go along with the woman's wishes and not tell the relatives?
   - Tell the relatives whether or not they ask about endometriosis?
   - Without talking specifically about the woman, recommend testing to relatives if they ask about endometriosis?
   - Without talking specifically about the woman, recommend testing to relatives even if they do not ask about endometriosis?

Short questions are generally regarded as preferable to long ones. But experiments have shown that length may sometimes be a virtue – longer questions may elicit fuller responses.[11] More symptoms or chronic disorders, for example, tend to be reported if longer questions are used. This may partly be because the additional material helps the respondent's recall. But a longer question may evoke a fuller response even if the added verbiage seems redundant. In one study, the question 'The next question is about medicines during the past 4 weeks. We want to ask you about this. What medicines, if any, did you take or use during the past 4 weeks?' yielded more information than the same question with the first two sentences removed. The reasons for this are not clear – maybe asking a longer question inclines the respondent to answer at equal length, or maybe the extra material simply gives the respondent more time to think. Short, terse questions appear to be preferable for the study of attitudes,[12] but longer ones may have advantages for symptoms, disorders, and practices. However, longer questions should be used with discrimination – 'if we larded all questions with "filler" phrases, a questionnaire would soon be bloated with too few, too fat questions'.[13]

Another recommendation is that interviews should be conducted at a slow pace, so that respondents have time to think.

It is wise to try to avoid questions that may *offend or embarrass* the respondent. If 'sensitive' questions of this sort *must* be asked, special care should be taken (see below).

The questions should be *fair*. They should not be phrased (or voiced) in a way that suggests a specific answer, and should not be loaded or one-sided. The question 'What are the main things that are wrong with the care you get from your doctor?' is an obviously unfair one. A format that 'begs the question' in this way (by assuming the truth of something not yet known) should be used, if at all, only in studies of attitudes in which it is felt that the best way to get a respondent to give voice to prejudices is to indicate that the questioner shares them.

'Sensitive' Questions

It may not be possible to avoid asking 'sensitive' questions that might offend or embarrass some respondents, e.g. requests for intimate or confidential information, questions that may seem to expose the respondent's ignorance, and questions that may elicit socially undesirable answers, such as admitting to a sexually transmitted disease or a shameful habit.

Simple solutions are sometimes feasible. For example, reluctance to disclose age or income may be countered by using broad categories of response (if these satisfy the needs of the study), such as '45–64 years', '65 or more', etc., instead of an open-ended question like 'How old are you?', and questions to measure level of knowledge can be presented as requests for an opinion ('Do you think that…?').

Possible offence or embarrassment can often be mitigated by including a statement designed to show that the questioner's interest is nonjudgemental: 'We know that all married couples sometimes quarrel with each other; how often does it happen that you quarrel with your husband?' Possible tactics, as amusingly described by Barton,[14] are:

1. *The everybody approach*. 'As you know, many people have been killing their wives these days. Do you happen to have killed yours?'
2. *The other people approach*. (a) 'Do you know any people who have murdered their wives?'(b) 'How about yourself?'
3. *The Kinsey technique*. Stare firmly into the respondent's eyes and ask in simple, clear-cut language such as that to which the respondent is accustomed, and with an air of assuming that everybody has done everything, 'Did you ever kill your wife?'

Self-administered questionnaires usually elicit a greater number of socially undesirable responses. But a study of reactions to questions concerning behaviour about which many people are reluctant to talk fully and honestly, in three large samples in the United States, showed that the effects of mode of administration (face to face, phone, or self-administered) were small, whereas the construction of the question made a great deal of difference.[15] In particular, there were two ploys that produced a two- to three-fold increase in the amount of reporting of behaviour. The first was the use of a long introduction to the question, and the second was the use of an open-ended question. In this study, the open-ended format was used only for questions about the amount or frequency of behaviour (How much liquor do you drink? How many times a week do you drink?), where the answers could be fairly easily coded. The findings suggested that long questions and an open-ended format should routinely be used when asking about the frequency of sensitive behaviour. The open-ended questions gave significantly higher frequencies for beer, wine and liquor drinking, petting, intercourse, and masturbation. A suggested reason is that the presence of low-frequency categories ('never, once a year or less, every few months, once a month, every few weeks ...') made people less willing to admit to higher frequencies.

Another recommended approach, which increased the reported frequencies of socially undesirable behaviour by about 15%, is the use of words familiar to the respondent. A suggested method is to let the respondent decide what term should be used, and then to use this in subsequent questions. For example, 'Different people use different words for sexual intercourse [or marijuana, masturbation, etc.]. What word do you think we should use?' It may also be helpful to ask whether the respondent has engaged in the socially undesirable behaviour in the past ('Did you ever, even once ...?'), before asking about current behaviour.[12]

Another simple technique is putting the possible responses on cards, so that the respondent need only point to the answer, without letting the offending words sully their lips.

Putting It All Together

A questionnaire should always have an introductory explanation, stating the purposes and sponsorship of the study. A statement about confidentiality should be included, but anonymity should not be guaranteed unless there is really no way of tracing which questionnaire belongs to whom. If the questionnaire is self-administered, then the introduction should include clear instructions and examples. If the questionnaire is to be used by an interviewer, then it may be preferred to put the explanation and instructions in an accompanying guide or manual. The instructions to the interviewer should be full and explicit.

The introductory explanation must be drafted with care, since it may markedly affect the responses to the questions. In surveys of the elderly in Holland, the reported prevalence of disability was much lower if the introduction emphasized that the questions referred to longstanding rather than temporary limitations. This reduced the prevalence of disability in mobility by 13.7 percentage points.[7]

In a questionnaire covering different topics, each new topic should have an introductory phrase (e.g. 'Now, about …') or explanation.

The first questions should be easy to answer, of obvious relevance to the topic of the study and (if possible) interesting. 'Sensitive' questions, which may engender embarrassment or resentment, should be left until later – even questions about age, education, ethnic group, etc. are sometimes left to the end for this reason. It may be inadvisable to start a postal questionnaire with an open-ended question.

The sequence of the questions needs careful attention. They should follow an order that the respondent will see as natural, with smooth movement from item to item. On the other hand, if the questionnaire is long it may be wise to have breaks in the continuity by switching topics or altering the format of questions, since 'changes of scenery' may prevent boredom. Long successions of questions that can elicit repeated identical responses (e.g. 'yes') should be avoided, as the respondent may fall into a rut (a 'response set') and continue to give the same response unthinkingly.

With proper sequencing, irrelevant questions can be bypassed. A 'sieve' or 'filter' question about drinking, for example, might screen out people who take no alcohol, so that subsequent detailed questions about the consumption of alcoholic beverages are skipped, or it might direct the respondent to an appropriate 'branch' (if, say, there are other questions for ex-drinkers). Skipping and branching patterns (indicated by 'go to …' instructions or arrows) are usually acceptable in a self-administered questionnaire, provided that they are simple; but multistep branching and skipping schemes may be confusing, and should be avoided.

When arranged in order, the questions should be gone through carefully ('put yourself in the respondent's boots') to examine the implications of the sequence. In particular, the answer to a prior question may influence the response to a later question (in which case the order should probably be reversed). If the questionnaire includes both specific and general questions about attitudes, the general question should come first, since specific questions tend to be answered in the same way wherever they are placed, whereas the response to a general question may be affected by prior specific questions. One study showed that the answer to a question about marital happiness was not influenced by a previous question about happiness in general, whereas the question on general happiness tended to be answered differently, depending on whether the marriage question was asked first.[16] Similarly, questions about general health and functional capacity should be put near the beginning of the questionnaire, unless the investigator wants the appraisal to be influenced by questions about specific illnesses, symptoms and disabilities. A run-through of the questionnaire may also reveal awkward sequences. For example, some women may resent being asked 'Are you married?' after giving a positive answer to 'Do you have children?'

When the questionnaire is reconsidered and discussed with colleagues, it is invariably found to need modification. Usually, more than one redraft is needed. The questionnaire should then be tested in practice – 'if you do not have the resources to pilot-test your questionnaire, don't do the study'.[11] It may be decided to try alternative wordings of the questions, in the same questionnaire or in questionnaires tested on different respondents. Pretests (see Chapter 24) are indispensable; they usually reveal a need for changes in the questions or their sequence or, very frequently, for shortening the questionnaire.

Notes and References

1. The use of sin*gle versus multiple questions*, with specific reference to self-ratings of health, is discussed by Bowling A (Just one question: if one question works, why ask several? Journal of Epidemiology and Community Health 2005; 59: 342).
2. *Translations of questionnaires* are discussed in note 9, Chapter 17.
3. Perrin KM, McDermott RJ. Instruments to measure *social support* and related constructs in pregnant adolescents: a review. Adolescence 1997; 32: 533.
4. Dengler R, Roberts H, Rushton L. Lifestyle surveys – the complete answer? Journal of Epidemiology and Community Health 1997; 51: 46.
5. Ayidiya SA, McClendon MJ. Response effects in mail surveys. Public Opinion Quarterly 1990; 54: 229.
6. For *advice on the formulation of questions*, see Choi CK, Pak AWR (A catalog of biases in questionnaires. Preventing Chronic Disease Jan 2005. Available at http://www.cdc.gov/pcd/isssues/200v/jan/04_0050.htm), Fink A (How to ask survey questions, 2nd edn. Beverly Hills, CA: Sage Publications; 2003), Fowler FJ Jr (Improving survey questions: design and evaluation. Beverly Hills, CA: Sage Publications; 1995), Kornhauser A, Sheatsley PB (Questionnaire construction and interview procedure. In: Selltiz C, Wrightsman L S, Cook SW (eds), Research methods in social relations, 3rd edn. New York, NY: Holt, Rinehart & Winston; 1981), Payne SL (The art of asking questions. Princeton, NJ: Princeton University Press; 1980), Converse JM, Presser S (Survey questions: handcrafting the standardized questionnaire. Beverly Hills, CA: Sage Publications; 1986), or Sudman S, Bradburn NM (Asking questions. San Francisco, CA: Jossey-Bass, 1983).
7. Picavet HSJ, Van den Bos GAM. Comparing survey data on functional disability: the impact of some methodological differences. Journal of Epidemiology and Community Health 1996; 50: 86.
8. Belson WA. The design and understanding of survey questions. Aldershot: Gower; 1981.
9. Aronson JK, Ferner RE. Clarification of terminology in drug safety. Drug Safety 2005; 28: 851. Aronson J. When I use a word: sometimes, never. British Medical Journal 2006; 333: 445. The latter paper adds: 'Perhaps when we use words like this we should remember what the German conductor Hans Richter supposedly once said: "Up with your damned nonsense will I put twice, or perhaps once, but sometimes always, by God, never".'

Nine learned articles in the journal Statistical Science (1990; 5: 2–34) debate the feasibility of ascribing numerical probabilities to fuzzy words like 'frequent' and 'occasionally'– words that (on average) the respondents in 20 studies defined as meaning 'on 61% of occasions' and 'on 22% of occasions' respectively. But not only are such terms used differently by different people, they are used and understood differently in different contexts. In studies cited by Clark HH (Statistical Science 1990; 5: 12), 'frequent' was judged to mean a relative frequency of 76% (on average) when Miss Sweden said that men frequently found her attractive, but only 29% when side effects with neomycin sulphate were reported to be frequent.

10. Boyle CM. Difference between patients' and doctors' interpretation of some common medical terms. British Medical Journal 1970; ii: 286.
11. Henson R, Cannell CF, Lawson SA. In: Cannell CF, Oksenberg L, Converse JM (eds), Experiments in interviewing techniques. Ann Arbor, MI: Institute for Social Research, 1979. Laurent A. Effects of question length on reporting behavior in the survey interview. Journal of the American Statistical Association 1972; 67: 298. Belson WA (1981; see note 8).
12. Sudman S, Bradburn NM (1983; see note 6).
13. Converse JM, Presser NM (1986; see note 6).
14. Barton AJ. Asking the embarrassing question. Public Opinion Quarterly 1958; 22: 67.
15. Bradburn NM, Sudman S et al. Improving interview method and questionnaire design. San Francisco, CA: Jossey-Bass; 1981.
16. Turner CF. Why do surveys disagree? Some preliminary hypotheses and some disagreeable examples. In: Turner CF, Martin E (eds), Surveying subjective phenomena, vol 2. New York, NY: Russell Sage; 1984.

20

Surveying the Opinions of a Panel: Consensus Methods

There is sometimes interest in learning the opinions of a group of people with special knowledge or interests, in order to ascertain their consensus (majority opinion) or, if there is no consensus, to map their main disagreements. The group may be a panel of experts who have skills and knowledge relevant to some field of health care, or of professionals or laymen who have a special interest in some situation or topic, such as a specific community and its problems. In the context of community-oriented primary care, they may be key informants – community members and others – who know the community well.

There may be two kinds of study objective:

1. To determine attitudes, concerns, appraisals of the relative importance of various factors or the desirability of various options, and the reasons for these judgements. When planning a health programme, for example, it may be helpful to know what knowledgeable people think are the chief problems and how they appraise the relative importance of these problems, or their opinions about the desirability, feasibility or pros and cons of various solutions. When a programme is to be evaluated, experts may be asked to choose criteria for the evaluation and to decide on the relative importance of these criteria, so that an appropriate weight can be allocated to each of them.
2. If objective facts about a situation are difficult or impossible to obtain, experts may be asked what they judge the facts to be. These 'guesstimates' may in some circumstances provide a basis for programme planning, on the assumption that an informed guess is better than no information at all. This use of experts' opinions may be especially appropriate in developing countries in instances where 'hard' data cannot be gathered. In studies of cost effectiveness, experts' estimates of the effectiveness of intervention procedures may be used as a substitute for objective measurements. In long-term planning, decisions may be based on experts' forecasts of the future situation.

Such surveys call for special methods. The main limitation of ordinary interview and questionnaire methods is that they permit no communication among the members of the

Research Methods in Community Medicine: Surveys, Epidemiological Research, Programme Evaluation, Clinical Trials   J. H. Abramson and Z. H. Abramson   Copyright © 2008, John Wiley & Sons Ltd

group, who have no opportunity to reach a modified judgement after appraising the opin-ions of others. On the other hand, group techniques that permit free communication – focus groups and other group discussions, committee meetings and conference telephone calls – permit too much interaction. The group's decisions may be heavily influenced by this interaction, and may be unduly affected by a chairperson's bossiness or ineffective-ness, dominance by verbose or forceful speakers, deference to authority, power, prestige or age, or friendships or antagonisms between participants.

These problems can be minimized by methods that avoid or restrict interaction between participants, but provide interim feedback of the opinions of the group as a whole, which each participant can take into account before giving a final judgement. This is then pooled with other contributions to yield a group decision.

The *nominal group technique* (NGT) is a simple method that may be used if the participants can be brought together at a meeting.

The *Delphi* technique needs more elaborate preparation and organization, but it does not require the members of the panel to come together. With both techniques, the find-ings depend, of course, on the selection of the participant experts. If these are not well chosen 'there is the danger of defining collective ignorance rather than wisdom'.[1] Both these consensus techniques are qualitative methods (see p. 148), although the results may be expressed in quantitative terms.

Nominal Group Technique

The NGT, which was developed by Van de Ven and Delbecq,[2] is so called because, although the participants sit together, discussion is permitted only during specified phases of the process. Hence, during most phases they are a group 'in name only'.

The technique may be used in a variety of situations requiring group decision-making. The participants may be any knowledgeable or concerned individuals, professional or lay. The technique was originally developed as a method of involving disadvantaged citizens in community action agencies, and it has been recommended for use in exploratory studies of citizens' or professionals' perceptions of health-care problems, and may be of special value in community-oriented primary care (see p. 360).[3] It has been used (for example) to learn why teenagers do or do not seek pre-ventive health care, to study beliefs about susceptibility to AIDS, to obtain general practitioners' consensus about the management of chronic fatigue syndrome, and to select outcome measures for use in clinical trials.[4]

The procedure[5] is simple. Five to nine participants (preferably not more than seven) sit round a table, together with a leader (facilitator). If there are more participants, then they are divided into small groups. A single session, which deals with a single ques-tion, usually takes at least 60–90 minutes (longer if the judgements of different groups are to be pooled).

For a typical meeting of a single small group, the following are the successive steps:

1. Silent generation of ideas in writing
2. 'Round-robin' feedback of ideas

3. Serial discussion of ideas
4. Preliminary vote
5. Discussion of preliminary vote
6. Final vote

1. *Silent generation of ideas in writing.* After making a welcoming statement, which stresses the importance of the task and of each member's contribution, the leader reads out the question that the participants are required to answer. This is usually an open-ended question that calls for a list of items, e.g. the elements of a specified problem or of a proposed programme for dealing with a problem. Each member is given a worksheet (at the top of which the question appears) and is asked to take 5 minutes to write their ideas in response to the question. The leader also does this. Discussion is not permitted.
2. *'Round-robin' feedback of ideas.* The leader goes round the table and asks each member in turn to contribute one of the ideas they have written, summarized in a few words. The leader also takes a turn in each round. Each idea is numbered and written on a large blackboard or on a flip pad, completed sheets of which are taped or pinned where they are visible to all members. Members are asked not to contribute ideas that they regard as complete duplicates. Members are encouraged to add ideas to their worksheets at any time; they may 'pass' in one round and contribute in a later one. The process goes on until no further ideas are forthcoming. Discussion is not permitted during this stage.
3. *Serial discussion of ideas.* Each of the ideas listed on the board or flip pad is discussed in turn. For each one, the group is asked whether there are questions, or whether anyone wishes to clarify the item, explain the logic behind it, or express a view about its relative importance. The object of the discussion is to obtain clarity and to air points of view, but not to resolve differences of opinion. If there is much overlap between items, then it may be desirable to modify the list after the serial discussion. One way of doing this is to rearrange the items so that variants of a single factor appear consecutively under a broad heading. Modest rewording may be undertaken if the group wishes to refine the list.
4. *Preliminary vote.* Each participant is asked to select a specified number (five to nine) of 'most important' items from the total list, and copy them on to cards. If six are to be chosen, each participant is asked to write '6' (underlined or circled) on the 'most important' card, then '1' on the least important, then '5' on the most important of the remaining four, then '2', and so on. The leader also ranks the items. The cards are then collected and shuffled to maintain anonymity, and the votes are read out and recorded on a tally-chart that shows all the items and the rank numbers allocated to each.
5. *Discussion of preliminary vote.* Brief discussion of the voting pattern is now permitted. Members are told that the purpose of this discussion is additional clarification, and not to pressure them to change their votes.
6. *Final vote.* Step 4 is then repeated. The most important items may again be ranked, or they may be given ratings on a scale from 0 (unimportant) to 10 or 100 (very important). The rank numbers or ratings allotted to each item may be averaged by summing them and dividing by the total number of participants. Other rating methods may be used. For example, members may be asked to assign 100 points to

the most important item and to give points to the other items in proportion to their relative importance, e.g. 50 points for an item half as important.[6]

If there are 10 or more participants then they should be divided into small groups, and steps 1 to 4 are performed separately in each group. There is then a break, during which the group leaders meet to prepare a master list of items, including the top five to nine priorities identified by each group. Where necessary, items are reworded or combined. The master list shows the aggregated votes relating to each of the items included. All the participants then gather in a single large group, and discuss each item in the master list in turn, for clarification. The preliminary vote is then discussed. At any member's request, items not included in the master list can be added. A final vote is then conducted.

Modifications of this procedure may be used.[1] For example, the first step can be conducted by post, followed by the face-to-face meeting; a detailed literature review can be provided as background material; or there can also be a nonparticipant observer collecting qualitative data about the group.

Delphi Technique

The Delphi technique (named after the oracle) is more elaborate. It was first used to forecast what atom bomb targets might be selected by a potential enemy of the United States and how many bombs would be needed. Since then its applications have broadened considerably. It has been defined as a 'method for structuring a group communication process so that the process is effective in allowing a group of individuals, as a whole, to deal with a complex problem'.[7] The method has been applied extensively in the health field,[8] e.g. to achieve a consensus on diagnostic criteria.[9]

Face-to-face contact between the participants is not required, although the 'Delphi' label is sometimes attached to procedures that include group discussion.[1] A series of mailed questionnaires is usually used, each one sent out after the results of the previous one have been analysed. The time taken by this process may be cut down considerably by the use of modern communications.

The elements that are usually included are an opportunity for individuals to contribute ideas or information, an assessment of the group judgement, clarification of reasons for differences, a chance for individuals to revise their views, and some degree of anonymity for the individual responses. Votes may be cast and results fed back repeatedly, until stability or consensus is reached.

The Delphi procedure is protean in its manifestations, and no simple prescription can be given.[10] A learned compendium on the technique states that 'if anything is true about Delphi today, it is that in its design and use Delphi is more of an art than a science'.[7]

Notes and References

1.   Jones J, Hunter D. Consensus methods for medical and health services research. British Medical Journal 1995; 311: 376. Also in: Mays N, Pope C (eds). Qualitative research in health care. London: BMJ Publishing Group; 1996.

2. Van de Ven AH, Delbecq AL. American Journal of Public Health 1972; 62: 337.
3. *Nominal group technique (examples)*. Gallagher M, Hares T, Spencer J, Bradshaw C, Webb I. The nominal group technique: a research tool for general practice? Family Practice 1993; 10: 76. Allen J, Dyas J, Jones M. Building consensus in health care: a guide to using the nominal group technique. British Journal of Community Nursing 2004; 9: 110. Lewis H, Rudolph M, White L. Rapid appraisal of the health promotion needs of the Hillbrow community, South Africa. International Journal of Healthcare Technology and Management 2003; 5(1–2): 20.
4. *Nominal group technique (more examples)*. Ginsburg KR, Menapace AS, Slap GB. Factors affecting the decision to seek health care: the voice of adolescents. Pediatrics 1997; 100: 922. Manning D, Balson PM, Barenberg N, Moore TM. Susceptibility to AIDS: what college students do and don't believe. Journal of the American College Health Association 1989; 38: 67. Raine R, Carter S, Sensky T, Black N. General practitioners' perceptions of chronic fatigue syndrome and beliefs about its management, compared with irritable bowel syndrome: qualitative study. British Medical Journal 2006; 328: 1354.
5. The *nominal group technique* is fully described by Delbecq AL, Van de Ven AH, Gustafson DH (Techniques for program planning: a guide to nominal group and Delphi processes. Glenview, IL: Scott, Foreman; 1975). The procedure described in the text is based on detailed instructions given in Chapter 3 of that book.

    The authors point out the importance of asking the right questions and the right people, likening the nominal group technique to a microscope and a vacuum cleaner: 'NGT is like a microscope. Properly focused by a good question, NGT can provide a great deal of conceptual detail about the matter of concern to you. Improperly focused by a poor or misleading question, it tells you a great deal about something in which you are not interested' (p. 75). 'NGT is like a vacuum. It is a powerful means to draw out the insight and information possessed by group members. However, if there is nothing to "draw out" even a powerful vacuum is useless' (p. 79).
6. If the total points are assigned to the referent item, it may be desirable to standardize the scores by expressing each one as a proportion or percentage of the sum of all the points allocated by the person. See Edwards W, Guttentag M, Snapper K (A decision-theoretic approach to evaluation research. In: Struening EL, Guttentag M (eds), Handbook of evaluation research. Beverly Hills, CA: Sage, 1975. p. 155).
7. Linstone HA, Turoff M (eds). The Delphi method: techniques and applications. Reading, MA: Addison-Wesley; 1975.
8. *Delphi method (examples)*. Combe B, Landewe R. EULAR recommendations for management of early arthritis. Annals of the Rheumatic Diseases 2005; 64(Suppl. 3): 60. Cabral D, Katz JN, Weinblatt ME, Ting G, Avorn J, Solomon DH. Development and assessment of indicators of rheumatic arthritis severity: results of a Delphi panel. Arthritis & Rheumatism 2005; 53: 61. Hunter DJW, McKee CM, Sanderson CFB, Black NA. Appropriate indications for prostatectomy in the UK: results of a consensus panel. Journal of Epidemiology and Community Health 1994; 48: 58. Attala JM, Gresley RS, McSweeney N, Jobe MA. Health needs of school-age children in two Midwestern counties. Issues in Comprehensive Paediatric Nursing 1993; 16: 51. Mertens AC, Cotter KL, Foster BM, Zebrack BJ, Hudson MM, Eshelman D, Lotis L, Sozio M, Oeffinger KC. Improving health care for adult survivors of childhood cancer: recommendations from a Delphi panel of health policy experts. Health Policy 2004; 69: 169.
9. Graham B, Regehr G, Wright JG. Delphi as a method to establish consensus for diagnostic criteria. Journal of Clinical Epidemiology 2003; 56: 1150. Ferguson ND, Davis AM, Slutsky AS, Stewart TE. Development of a clinical definition for acute respiratory distress syndrome using the Delphi technique. Journal of Critical Care 2005; 20: 147.
10. Interested readers may refer to Linstone and Turoff (1975; see note 7) for a number of detailed examples. Simple guidelines are provided by Jones and Hunter (1995; see note 1) and Delbecq *et al.* (1975; see note 5).

21

The Use of Documentary Sources

The use of documentary sources is attractive because it is a relatively easy way of obtaining data; documents can provide ready-made information both about the study population as a whole and about its individual members.

Documents may also constitute the best or only means of studying past events. ('There are two ways of telling the age of a rhinoceros. The first is to examine its teeth. The second is to collect the evidence of those who remember the beast when it was young, and may even have kept some newspaper cutting recording its birth.')[1]

The documents may be written, printed, or recorded electronically (e.g. in computer files, compact disks, or audio or video recordings). They include clinical records, 'vital records' (certificates of birth, death, marriage, etc.), other personal records (such as health diaries specially maintained for the purpose of a study), and registers, databases and archives containing aggregations of data on individuals. Use may also be made of documents that provide ready-made statistics and other information on populations (demography, mortality, morbidity, hospitalization rates, use of ambulatory medical services, etc.), sometimes derived from censuses or other surveys planned to collect this information, and sometimes based on data recorded in an ongoing way for administrative or other specific purposes.

Documents are frequently the only or the most convenient source of information at the investigator's disposal. But it must be remembered that if they were produced for clinical, administrative or fiscal ends rather than for research purposes, then questions of their validity for study purposes are very likely to arise. There may be no uniform definitions (of diseases and demographic or other variables), methods of investigation may be unstandardized or used differentially, and the records may not have been maintained with the obsessive care that would be expected in a planned investigation. A study of cases of abortion in a Danish national hospital register, for example, revealed that in over a third of cases the diagnostic code did not reflect the diagnosis in the discharge record.[2] In a hospital discharge data set in Kentucky, which contained 16 apparent cases of serious uncommon communicable diseases, six of these were coding errors and four were cases that had been suspected but not confirmed by subsequent workup.[3] Variables important to the investigator may be lacking; and even if uniform

Research Methods in Community Medicine: Surveys, Epidemiological Research, Programme Evaluation, Clinical Trials   J. H. Abramson and Z. H. Abramson   Copyright © 2008, John Wiley & Sons Ltd

definitions and careful procedures were used, they may not be consistent with the investigator's concepts, so that the data may be of low validity for the purposes of the study. Secondary data should always be used with circumspection.

The use of these records is, of course, also subject to practical constraints;[3] confidentiality or difficulty of access may present a problem, or the identifying information may be incomplete or inaccurate.

Clinical Records

Medical records may be very disappointing as a source of data, unless they have been planned and maintained as a basis for research. To quote Mainland:

> Most of the people responsible for hospital and clinic records are not trained investigators, and moreover the pressure of routine work is commonly heavy. From experience gained in the making of clinical records myself, from watching others making them, and in trying to use them, I have come to believe that the only records trustworthy for anything more than superficial impressions, or as hints for further research, are: (a) The records made meticulously by a physician regarding his own patients because he wishes to learn from them; (b) Records kept regarding a particular group of patients by a suitable and adequately instructed person, specially assigned to the task.[4]

There are generally problems of reliability and validity. The information may have been collected by more than one person, using different definitions. Since the data are second hand, it is possible that even if uniform definitions and procedures were used, these may not be consistent with the investigator's requirements. Moreover, recording may be patchy; occupations, body weights and blood pressures may be recorded in some instances, but not in others. If the presence of a symptom, sign or specific disease is not recorded, then this may mean that it was found to be absent, that no attempt was made to establish its presence, or that its presence was established but not recorded, whether by oversight or because it was regarded as unimportant or irrelevant.[5] In one study, mention of the presence or absence of urinary tract symptoms was found in the medical records of only 18% of a sample of older men, but 30% reported moderate to severe symptoms when questioned.[6] As an extreme example, only 2% of outpatients attending an African hospital were recorded as having avitaminoses or other deficiency states, although field surveys showed that most people in their neighbourhoods of residence had clinical evidence of malnutrition.

Special care must be taken not to make errors when the information is extracted from the records. These are especially likely to occur if handwritings are difficult to read or if the required information has to be hunted for, e.g. if it is not recorded in a standard place or is buried in long works of prose. A study of reliability, based on replicate extractions by carefully trained personnel from a set of hospital records, showed a good deal of interextractor and intraextractor variation; for example, in 23% of instances there was disagreement between extractors on the presence of a history of hypertension, and in 21% there were discrepancies between two extractions (6 months or more apart) by the same person. The main reasons for disagreements were failure to find information recorded in unexpected places, and errors (despite careful training) in the coding of data.[7]

In these days of computerized records, the potential research benefits of high-quality clinical databases are well recognized. The General Practice Research database and the Doctors' Independent Network database in the United Kingdom,[8] for example, have provided a basis for studies of drug safety, disease incidence and prevalence, resource utilization and disease treatment and prevention, and for case-control studies, as have databases maintained by health maintenance organizations. The requirements for a good database are, however, demanding – 'such databases must include individual data on all consecutive cases, use standard definitions of conditions and outcomes, ensure data are complete and accurate, and include data on all patient characteristics that affect outcome' – but there is generally 'a lack of interest on the part of clinicians, managers, and researchers'.[9]

However good the records and however carefully the data are extracted, it is important to remember that the information in these databases, as in all clinical records, is unlikely to be complete. Use is being made of the selected facts determined and recorded by clinicians concerning selected people who came for care. Moreover, the aim of most databases is usually to facilitate accounting or information retrieval at an individual level, rather than with an eye to statistical processing and epidemiological analysis. In a database of visits to a paediatric clinic, set up in part to generate claims for reimbursement for visits, only 77% of the diagnoses in the medical record were accurately coded in the database.[10]

Routine primary-care clinical records

Unless special care is taken, routine clinical records are generally of little value as a basis for research. This applies especially to routine general practice records, which may give only a very rough guide to morbidity patterns and the utilization of services. Not only may the quality of the diagnostic information be unsatisfactory, for lack of suitable diagnostic facilities and other reasons, but the records are seldom full or maintained in a manner that lends itself to analysis. Records of home visits are usually especially incomplete; a study of the clinical records maintained in a medical care plan in New York indicated that half the home visits (as opposed to one-sixth of the office visits) were not recorded, and that respiratory diseases were consequently underrepresented in the diagnostic data.[11]

However, routine records that include reasonably well recorded information of reasonable quality can be reasonably useful as a basis for investigations, and routine records from general practices and other primary-care services can be of immense value if pains are taken to collect and record information accurately, and especially if the records are computerized.[12] Not only do people who attend for primary medical care constitute a very much larger and more representative population group than patients treated in hospitals or specialty clinics, but the records of a primary-care service directed at a defined eligible population can sometimes provide data about all members of that population, including those who do not seek care. Moreover, primary-care records can yield data about mild illnesses as well as those that need specialized care, and in many instances can also provide information about incipient and potential illnesses and about factors that may endanger or promote health. They can provide a basis for research on the aetiology, natural history, prevention and care of common diseases and disabilities, processes of growth and development, and the effects of familial factors and social supports and pressures on health and health care.

The use of clinical records for epidemiological purposes is an essential element in community-oriented primary care (see Chapter 34). There are a number of tools and procedures that can help physicians to conduct epidemiological, operational and other research based on their own work.[13] These include age–sex registers of the practice population, 'minimum data sets', registers of patients with selected disorders or risk factors, and 'problem-oriented' and other improved records.

Medical Audit

In recent years, much attention has been paid to the development of techniques of evaluating the quality of clinical care by measuring the performance of diagnostic, therapeutic and other procedures. These 'medical audit' and related techniques[14] are usually based on an examination of clinical records. In order to enhance objectivity, use is generally made of explicit criteria. These may be *normative* standards, which express experts' opinions as to what procedures should be carried out in specific types of cases, or *empirical* standards, based on what is actually done in clinical facilities that are of an acceptable level.

The review may cover all cases cared for, a representative sample, or defined categories, such as patients with selected conditions. Attention may be concentrated on the performance of specific marker procedures chosen as indicators of the quality of care, as in a study in inner-city New York, which showed that 74% of children cared for by private physicians were not fully immunized, 80% were not screened for lead, and 83% were not screened for tuberculosis.[15] It is often especially helpful to review the past history of patients with poor outcomes, such as those with preventable disorders or complications. This may identify deficiencies not only in the care that was given, but also in compliance and in the availability and use of services.

Audit techniques have their main application in evaluative reviews (as opposed to trials) of clinical services. The audit is based on the assumption that the performance of certain procedures is likely to benefit patients, and care is favourably evaluated if the audit shows that these activities have been satisfactorily performed. The assumptions themselves are not tested. This means, of course, that the evaluation is valid only in so far as the assumptions are valid. Sceptics point out that evidence of the efficacy of the procedures is usually lacking; that is, there is seldom convincing proof of a cause–effect relationship between the recommended procedures and the outcome.[16]

An important advantage of an audit is said to be the ease with which the evaluation results can be translated into practical recommendations. If the audit shows that X is *not* being done, then the recommendation is made that X *should* be done. It may also be a useful educational tool – a new doctor or nurse in a clinic will rapidly learn that it is expected that X *will* be done. However, the actual effect of audit programmes on the quality of care remains controversial, despite many observational studies and a number of trials ('we will never really know … audit will always be an act of faith').[17] In some instances the procedures are chosen largely because information about them is easily obtainable rather than because they are the best markers of quality. In these instances, the danger exists (especially when audit results entail rewards or penalties) that practitioners will increase the performance of these procedures – improving their audit score but not necessarily the quality of care.

Audit systems in general practice are sometimes moderately effective, and sometimes ineffective.[18]

In some audit systems, account is taken of outcomes as well as performance. The outcomes that are measured include not only end results, but also intermediate outcomes, such as the establishment of correct diagnoses or changes in the patient's health behaviour. The assumption is made that satisfactory end results indicate that care was satisfactory. This is, of course, not necessarily true; but, if patients do well, there is at least no cause for concern.

A basic problem of medical audit is that the records may not provide the required information unless they are planned for this purpose, and unless pains are taken to keep full clinical notes (computerization does not necessarily solve these problems). Fuller notes may, of course, not mean better care. A comparison of the charts of patients treated for acute appendicitis, for example, revealed considerable disparity among three hospitals in the frequency of documentation of commonly sought symptoms and signs, yet at each hospital the disease was diagnosed with the same accuracy. Similarly, in cases with acute myocardial infarction, the documentation of elements of the history, physical examination and special tests bore no relationship to the outcome of care, such as the length of time lost from work, or the occurrence of new angina pectoris, a repeated infarction, or death. 'Outstanding clinicians may keep inadequate records, whereas others less competent may write profusely … The mere act of writing cannot improve a patient's outcome'.[19]

Administrative data accumulated as a by-product of health-service administration, reimbursement for services, etc. are, at present, of little value as a basis for assessing the quality of care. At best, they point to possible problem areas that may merit proper investigation.[20]

Hospital Statistics

Hospital records have come a long way since Florence Nightingale wrote 'In attempting to arrive at the truth, I have applied everywhere for information, but in scarcely an instance have I been able to obtain hospital records fit for any purposes of comparison'.[21]

In most hospitals today, most diagnoses regarded as important are recorded, despite the inaccuracies in clinical records, and most recorded diagnoses are reasonably well substantiated. Despite their shortcomings, hospital statistics provide a useful source of data on the morbidity pattern of a population. The same applies to diagnostic statistics based on the utilization of some health maintenance organizations and other medical care agencies.

Problems in the use of hospital statistics include the bias caused by selective factors influencing hospitalization, including possible Berksonian bias affecting associations between diseases and between diseases and other factors (see p. 65). Another problem is that diagnostic statistics based on hospital records are usually based on the selection of a single one of the patient's diagnoses. The WHO makes the following recommendation:[22]

> The condition to be used for single-condition morbidity analysis is the main condition treated or investigated during the relevant episode of health care. The main condition is defined as the condition, diagnosed at the end of the episode of health care, primarily responsible for the patient's need for treatment or investigation. If there is more than one such condition, the one held most responsible for the greatest use of resources should be selected. If no diagnosis was made, the main symptom, abnormal finding or problem should be selected as the main condition.

It may be a physician (often a junior one) who makes the choice, or a medical recorder, and there may be no certainty that the detailed guidelines provided by the WHO are followed, or indeed that any consistent method of selection is used. Diagnostic statistics based on hospital statistics should be treated with reserve, especially in studies of time trends. In the United States there was a substantial increase in reported hospitalizations for acute myocardial infarction between 1981 and 1986, caused by a change in the way diagnoses were selected.[23]

In some countries diagnosis-related groups (DRGs) are used for determining rates of payment for hospital care. This could provoke a tendency to record diagnoses and additional information entitling the hospital to higher reimbursement. A study of hospital diagnostic statistics in the United States before and after the introduction of payment by DRGs showed differences consistent with the hypothesis that 'within the range of accepted medical practice, diagnoses will be recorded which maximize hospital revenues'[24] (a possibility described by Simborg as 'DRG creep').[25] In a study of hospital diagnoses of stroke in two states in the United States in which the use of DRGs was introduced 2 years apart, its introduction in each state was seen to be followed by a steep change in the types of stroke recorded. The proportion of cerebral occlusion rose from 27–30% to 71–74%, and the proportion of acute ill-defined stroke decreased from 52% to 8%.[26]

Nevertheless, say the authors of one of these studies, 'while it is true that epidemiologists must operate in a world of imperfect information, they should not be paralyzed by this lack of knowledge; rather they must become as aware as possible of the nature and extent of these imperfections'.[24]

As Major Greenwood said: 'The scientific purist, who will wait for medical statistics until they are nosologically perfect, is no wiser than Horace's rustic waiting for the river to flow away'.[27]

Death Certificates and Mortality Statistics

Mortality statistics are based on the causes of death reported in death certificates. As shown in this excerpt (see Figure 21.1) from the international form, several causes may be entered. One of these is selected as the underlying cause of death; this is defined by the WHO as '(a) the disease or injury which initiated the train of events leading directly to death, or (b) the circumstances of the accident or violence which produced the fatal injury'. If the certificate has been filled in correctly, this is the last condition entered in part I of the certificate. What is written there is not automatically selected – if it seems highly improbable that it was, in fact, the underlying cause of death, then a different condition may be chosen, using a series of rules recommended by the WHO.[22] The wording chosen for the diagnosis (e.g. 'chronic ischaemic heart disease' or 'arteriosclerotic cardiovascular disease' – or 'cancer of the uterus' or 'cancer of the cervix') may determine the coding category to which the cause is allotted.[28] Sometimes additional information is requested, e.g. (in Finland)[29] a short case history.

There are a number of obvious sources of inaccuracy. As any physician who fills in death certificates knows, it is not always easy to complete the form accurately. The certifier may not be sure of the true cause or causes of death, either because there is insufficient clinical information, or because the clinical picture is a complicated one – and may yet feel bound to specify a cause of death, so as to avoid forensic complications or for other

Cause of death	
I	
Disease or condition directly leading to death*	(a) ....
	due to (or as a consequence of)
Antecedent causes: Morbid conditions, if any,	(b) ....
giving rise to the above cause, stating the	due to (or as a consequence of)
underlying condition last	(c) ....
II	
Other significant conditions	....
contributing to the death, but not related to	
the disease or condition causing it	....
*This does not mean the mode of dying, e.g. heart failure, respiratory failure. It means the disease, injury or complication that caused death.	

Figure 21.1   Part of the international form of the medical certificate of cause of death

reasons. It may not be easy to distinguish between direct, antecedent and contributory causes, or to determine a simple sequence of causes, as required by the certificate.[30] The physician may in any case regard the certificate as 'red tape' rather than a scientific document, and not attempt to complete it conscientiously. Even when an autopsy is performed, the certificate is often made out before the autopsy, and not modified in the light of the post-mortem findings. In one study of certificates, major errors in the way they were filled in occurred in 11% of cases, and minor errors in 28%.[31] Add to this the known unreliability of clinical diagnoses, and the possibility that coders may vary in their selection of an underlying cause (largely because of disagreements as to whether what the physician has written can be taken at its face value),[32] and it is clear that death certificate data and mortality statistics must be treated with some reserve.[33]

Numerous studies have demonstrated the inaccuracy of death certificate data. In a study in England and Wales, for example, the underlying causes of death determined by pathologists (using both autopsy and clinical findings) differed from the certified cause in 55% of cases. In half of these the difference was not in wording or opinion, but in 'fact' – either the clinician named an underlying cause that was not mentioned in the pathologist's certificate or notes, or the pathologist named one that the clinician did not mention even as a contributory cause or in the differential diagnosis that was appended to the certificate. Differences of 'fact' occurred in 16% in cases where the clinician had claimed reasonable certainty of the diagnosis.[34] In four US communities, death certificates overestimated mortality from coronary heart disease by about 20%.[35] In Finland, incorrect assignments to cerebrovascular disease ('false positives') amounted to 39%, and failure to assign deaths to cerebrovascular disease ('false negatives') to 50%, leading to an overall underestimation of this cause of death.[29]

Although death certificate data must be treated with reserve, this certainly does not nullify their usefulness, since they undoubtedly contain a sufficient core of hard fact, provided that their lack of complete accuracy and possible biases are taken into consideration. They can certainly be used to appraise time trends and geographical differences, if consideration is given to the possible effects of changes or differences in diagnostic methods and criteria and in coding methods. There is little justification for the pronouncement that their 'error rate ... is notorious ... Basically, they only record that there was a corpse at a certain time in a certain place ... Bad data do not make good studies'.[36] For one thing, the false positives and false negatives may, to an extent, cancel each other out; this was observed in the British autopsy study, although for some conditions there was a definite bias – clinicians tended to 'underdiagnose' chronic bronchitis, peptic ulcer and malignant neoplasms of the lung, and to 'overdiagnose' bronchopneumonia and cerebral haemorrhage.[34] A study in Finland found that, overall, the death certificate data for myocardial infarction were of reasonable validity; but in Belgium there was a tendency to underreport.[37] Second, there is less inaccuracy if mortality from broad groups of diseases, rather than specific diseases, are considered. In the British autopsy study,[34] for example, it was found that, while for specific neoplasms there were differences between the statistics based on clinicians' and pathologists' diagnoses, there was fair agreement on the total number of malignant neoplasms. Similarly, when all categories relating to pneumonia and bronchitis were combined, this eliminated the inconsistencies shown by specific conditions.

It must, of course, be remembered that whatever the validity of death certificate data as a reflection of *causes* of death, they have less validity as a measure of the *presence* of diseases at death,[38] and still less as a measure of prevalence among the living. Only half of the deaths of patients previously diagnosed as having prostatic carcinoma, for example, are caused by the carcinoma.[39] About one-half or less of diabetic decedents have diabetes mentioned on their death certificates, and much fewer as the underlying cause of death.[40]

Notifications

In most countries, physicians are required by law to notify the public health authority of cases of certain (mainly communicable) diseases; doctors, laboratories and others may also be requested to make voluntary reports of certain other diseases to public health or other agencies.

The main problem besetting the use of disease notifications and statistics based on them is that reporting is often far from complete, even where notification is mandatory. In the United States, the completeness of notification ranges from 9% (for invasive *pneumococcus pneumoniae* in Hawaii in 1998) to 99% (for tuberculosis notified by laboratories in Wisconsin in 1995), and is significantly higher for AIDS, sexually transmitted diseases, and tuberculosis as a group (79%) than for all other infectious diseases combined (49%).[41] It was estimated that for every 100 persons infected with *Shigella*, 76 became symptomatic, 28 consulted a physician, nine submitted stool cultures, seven had positive culture results, and six were reported to the local health department.[42]

Reporting is likely to be fuller when the physician feels that notification will benefit the patient or the community and less complete when it seems that it will bring no benefit, or may embarrass the patient. Furthermore, reporting may be selective; cases of sexually transmitted diseases treated in public clinics may be far more fully notified than those treated by private practitioners. Such selective factors may introduce biases, in social class or other characteristics, that must be taken into account when inferences are drawn from the data.

These shortcomings apply to all reporting systems, such as those set up for the surveillance of hospital infections, drug reactions, movements into or out of a neighbourhood, etc. The information collected tends to be far from complete, unless a great deal of trouble is taken to ensure full reporting.

Nevertheless, the number of notifications can be a useful rough guide to time trends in incidence, provided that notification practices have not altered greatly over the period studied. They can form a basis for studies of disease transmission and for ecological studies, e.g. of the relationship of incidence to ambient temperature.

Registers

Health services and other agencies often maintain registers of people who have specific disorders or have other specific features. These registers may list patients with cancer, tuberculosis, psychiatric or other diseases, people who are blind, housebound, or otherwise handicapped, pregnant women, infants, the elderly, twins, children or families who are at risk of disease, etc. The diagnostic index of a hospital or clinic may be used as a disease register. The registers may be simple lists, card indexes, or computerized. In many cases they fulfil important functions in the day-to-day provision of a service, e.g. by identifying patients who require care and by providing a check on the performance of procedures, apart from collecting data that can be analysed for epidemiological or evaluative purposes.

Registers, and the statistics based upon them, may provide valuable data. An investigator not connected with the responsible agency must remember, however, that the information is second hand or, very often, third hand – obtained by the agency from other sources – and should find out what definitions and procedures were used, in order to decide on the suitability of the data for the purpose of the study.

Registers of patients with chronic or other selected conditions can be especially valuable in primary-care settings, as a basis for the planning and conduct of organized programmes (see p. 362). The maintenance of such registers is, however, not easy, unless clinical records are computerized, which can avoid the need to record the diagnosis twice, both in the clinical record and in a separate register. A register is likely to be complete only if physicians are convinced that it is helpful in their work or research.

The *capture–recapture technique* can be used to compensate for underregistration, if two or more overlapping registers for the same condition are available. This is a method originally used for estimating the size of an animal population, by marking and releasing a batch of captured animals and then seeing how many are recaptured in the next batch caught, thus permitting estimation of the chance of being caught. Similarly, the total number of cases of a disease in the population can be estimated[43] from the numbers (totals and shared) in separate registers, which provide estimates of the 'chance of being caught' (the completeness of case ascertainment) in each register. In a study of childhood diabetes in Madrid, for example, 451 cases were identified – 432 by one procedure and 138 by another, with 119 common to both; the estimated total, computed from these figures, was 501.[44] In Glasgow, where 2,006 injecting drug users were ascertained from three sources, the computed 'ascertainment-corrected' total was 13,050, a number that the authors reduced to 9,424 to compensate for possible false positive reports.[45] The capture–recapture method can be used to correct for underascertainment in any case-finding survey, if an appropriate independent case register is available.

But capture–recapture results must be used with caution – the case totals may be underestimates, because registers or case-finding procedures are usually not independent, and cases ascertained by one may be especially likely to be identified by another. Conversely, they may be overestimates if cases ascertained by one method are likely to be missed by the other. Elaborate methods of computation can largely control these and other biases, but even they may not provide completely valid estimates. If, for example, cases of a certain kind are 'uncatchable', i.e. systematically missed by all procedures, then no manipulation can estimate their number; or if all cases have in fact been found, the computed total will be an overestimate.

Health Diaries and Calendars

In some studies, people are asked to record symptoms, illnesses or other events, physician contacts, self-medication, food consumption, or other data in diaries or calendars. These documents (which for convenience are mentioned in this chapter) can then be used as direct sources of data, or as memory aids in face-to-face or phone interviews. They generally lead to a considerable increase in the reporting of symptoms and minor illnesses and injuries.

A drawback of these methods is that not everyone is able or willing to maintain such a record. Nonresponse tends to be higher for poorly educated and elderly subjects. Even in uneducated populations, however, appropriate techniques may be devised; in a study in Bangladesh, for example, health calendars were prepared in which diarrhoea, scabies and conjunctivitis were indicated by appropriate drawings, and parents were asked to record episodes by putting the affected child's handprint in the appropriate space.[46]

Also, the value of the record tends to decline if it has to be maintained for more than a short period ('fatigue effect') – reported symptoms or illness rates tend to decline after a month, and sometimes during the first month. There is also evidence of a 'sensitization effect' – maintaining a health diary may make respondents more aware of health problems and may spur them to take greater care of their health; in a study in Detroit, the average number of days spent in bed because of illness increased during the 6 weeks in which the diary was maintained.[47]

Census Data

Census data may be invaluable, but possible shortcomings should not be ignored. Population censuses cannot be assumed to be completely accurate. There may be underenumeration, especially of illegal immigrants and their families, members of minority ethnic groups, young adults, infants, and the very old. The 1991 British census, for example, missed an estimated 10% of men in their twenties and 8% of those aged 85 or more.[48] Common inaccuracies in the information reported in censuses include a tendency of divorced men to describe themselves as single (never married) and a tendency for elderly people to overstate their age. 'Investigations into the causes of reported "superlongevity" invariably show that age mis-statement, rather than eating yoghurt, lies behind them'.[49] There may be disparities between census data and other records, pointing to inaccuracies in the one record or the other; for example, a comparison of death certificates in the United States with census records completed shortly before death showed that only 72% of White persons recorded as divorced on their census records were also recorded as divorced on their death certificates; 17% were recorded as widowed, 5% as single, and 6% as married.[50]

Special problems in the use of national census data face an investigator doing a survey in a small locality. Not only may the area be difficult to define in terms of the census tracts or sub-tracts, zip code (postcode) areas, or other geographical entities used in the census and its reports, but data for small areas may be difficult to access, or may not include the required variables, or (if the information was collected from a population sample) may be subject to marked random sampling variation. Census figures for a small area are particularly liable to be distorted by a failure to include or exclude people temporarily away from their homes, such as students and migrant workers. The data may also be out of date if population size or composition is changing rapidly, as in a fast-developing town or urban neighbourhood. The capture–recapture method (see above) has been used to estimate population size when more than one population register is available for a small community.[51]

In a longitudinal study, changes between censuses in the boundaries of census tracts may pose a problem.

Census figures should not be used as denominators for specific rates (by ethnic group, income level, etc.) without confirming that the definitions used are equivalent to those used for the numerator data.

Other Documentary Sources

A large variety of other documents may be useful as sources of information on morbidity or other characteristics – medical certificates, sick-absence records, medical insurance records, certificates of birth and fetal death, social welfare records, police records, school records, parish records, etc.

In each instance, the investigator should explore the possible limitations of the information provided. It is important, however, not to expect too much. These documents were designed for someone else's purposes, and it is no more than a happy chance if they meet the investigator's needs (see Finagle's Third Law).[52]

Record Linkage

With the advent of computers there has been increased interest in the bringing together of records from different sources to obtain a fuller picture than is provided by any single source (creating 'new data from old').[53]

Different records relating to the same person may be linked, such as records from various hospitals, or death certificates and hospital or census data. Alternatively, the linkage may be of records relating to different people, such as members of a family; this is a useful method in genetic research.

Record linkage presents considerable practical problems, especially arising from the inaccurate or incomplete recording of identifying information, and may be beset by the ethical problem of possible breaches of confidentiality. When practicable, it has extensive applications in epidemiological and other health research.

Notes and References

1. Morton JB. The best of Beachcomber. Harmondsworth: Penguin Books, 1966. p. 102. "'Fancy that", said the man who handed a rhinoceros to the pigeon fancier' (*ibid*. p. 219).

2. Sorensen HT, Sabroe S, Olsen J. A framework for evaluation of secondary data sources for epidemiological research. International Journal of Epidemiology 1996; 25: 435.

3. Finger R, Auslander MB. Results of a search for missed cases of reportable communicable diseases using hospital discharge data. Journal of the Kentucky Medical Association 1997; 95: 237.

4. Mainland D. Elementary medical statistics, 2nd edn. Philadelphia, PA: WB Saunders; 1963. p. 147.

5. A study at the Yale–New Haven Hospital showed that among postmenopausal women whose medical records provided no information on the presence or absence of certain phenomena, the proportion who reported the phenomenon on interview ranged from 72% for hot flashes, through 39% for benign breast disease, to 1% for the taking of beta-blockers or reserpine (Horwitz RI. Comparison of epidemiologic data from multiple sources. Journal of Chronic Diseases 1986; 39: 889).

6. Collins MF, Friedman RH, Ash A, Hall R, Moskowitz MA. Underdetection of clinical benign prostatic hyperplasia in a general medical practice. Journal of General Internal Medicine 1996; 11: 513.

7. Horwitz RI, Yu EC. Assessing the reliability of epidemiologic data obtained from medical records. Journal of Chronic Diseases 1984; 37: 825.

8. Hollowell J. The General Practice Research Database: quality of morbidity data. Population Trends 1997; 87: 36. Jick SS, Kaye JA, Vasilakis-Scaramozza C, Garcia Rodriguez LA, Ruigomez A, Meier CR, Schlienger RG, Black C, Jick H. Validity of the general practice research database. Pharmacotherapy 2003; 23: 686. Carey IM, Cooka DG, De Wildea S, Bremnera SA, Richards N, Caine S, Strachan DP, Hilton SR. Developing a large electronic primary care database (Doctors' Independent Network) for research. International Journal for Medical Informatics 2004; 73: 443. Bremner SA, Carey IM, DeWilde S, Richards N, Maier WC, Hilton SR, Strachan DP, Cook DG. Early-life exposure to antibacterials and the subsequent development of hayfever in childhood in the UK: case-control studies using the General Practice Research Database and the Doctors' Independent Network. Clinical & Experimental Allergy 2003; 33: 1518.

9. Black N. Editorial: Developing high quality clinical databases: the key to a new research paradigm. British Medical Journal 1997; 315: 381.

10. Woods CR. Impact of different definitions on estimates of accuracy of the diagnosis data in a clinical database. Journal of Clinical Epidemiology 2001; 54: 782.

11. Densen PM, Balamuth E, Deardorff NR. Medical care plan as a source of morbidity data: the prevalence of illness and associated volume of service. Milbank Memorial Fund Quarterly 1960; 38: 48.

12. Wood M, Mayo F, Marsland D (Practice-based recording as an epidemiological tool. Annual Review of Public Health 1986; 7: 357) review the reasons for using primary-care records in epidemiology, discuss methods and instruments, problems with diagnoses and their classification and problems with numerators (what is an illness episode?) and denominators, and give examples of collaborative and other research in primary-care settings.

13. Eimerl TS, Laidlaw AJ. A handbook for research in general practice. Edinburgh: Livingstone; 1969.

14. Medical audit and similar techniques for evaluating clinical care – 'self-audit', 'peer review' (by others), 'internal audit' (by colleagues in the same institution), 'external audit', 'medical care evaluation studies', 'nursing audit', etc. – may be based upon routine records, upon specially modified or designed records, or upon special investigations, including direct observations of practitioners at work.

15. Fairbrother G, Friedman S, DuMont K, Lobach KS. Markers for primary care: missed opportunities to immunize and screen for lead and tuberculosis by private physicians serving large numbers of inner-city Medicaid-eligible children. Pediatrics 1996; 87: 785.

16. Brook RH. Quality of care assessment: a comparison of five methods of peer review. DHEW Publication No HRA-74-3100. Rockville, MD: US Department of Health, Education, and Welfare; 1973.

17. Lord J, Littlejohns P. Evaluating healthcare policies: the case of clinical audit. British Medical Journal 1997; 315: 668. See also Forster DP (Leading article: Uncertainties in medical audit. Public Health 1997; 111: 67) and Robinson MB (Evaluation of medical audit. Journal of Epidemiology and Community Health 1994; 48: 435).

18. *Audits in general practice.* Holden JD. Systematic review of published multi-practice audits from British general practice. Journal of Evaluation in Clinical Practice 2004; 10: 247. Sandbaek A, Kragstrup J. Randomized controlled trial of the effect of medical audit on AIDS prevention in general practice. Family Practice 1999; 16: 510.

19. Fessel WJ, van Brunt EE. Assessing quality of care from the medical record. New England Journal of Medicine 1972; 286: 134.

20. Jezzoni LI. Assessing quality using administrative data. Annals of Internal Medicine 1997; 127: 666.

21. Nightingale, F. Notes on hospitals. 3rd edn. London: Longman, Green, Longman, Longman, Roberts, and Green; 1863.

22. World Health Organization. International statistical classification of diseases and related health problems: 10th revision, vol 2: Instruction manual, 2nd edn. Geneva: World Health Organization; 2004.

23. Statistics on hospitalizations for acute myocardial infarction in the United States were based on the 'first-listed' diagnosis until 1982, when it was decided that if this diagnosis was not the first one recorded, but occurred with other circulatory diagnoses, it would be moved to first place. As a result, the proportion of acute myocardial diagnoses that were regarded as the principal reason for hospitalization rose from 60% in 1981 to 87% in 1986 (Vital and Health Statistics series 13, no 96).

24. Cohen BB, Pokras S, Meads MS, Krushat WM. How will diagnosis-related groups affect epidemiologic research? American Journal of Public Health 1987; 126: 1.

25. Simborg DW. DRG creep: a new hospital-acquired disease. New England Journal of Medicine 1981; 304: 1602.

26. Derby CA, Lapane KL, Feldman HA, Carletom RA. Possible effect of DRGs on the classification of stroke: implications for epidemiological surveillance. Stroke 2001; 32: 1487.

27. Greenwood M. Medical statistics from Graunt to Farr. Cambridge: Cambridge University Press; 1948.

28. Nelson M, Farebrother M (The effect of inaccuracies in death certification and coding practices in the European Economic Community [EEC] on international cancer mortality statistics. International Journal of Epidemiology 1978; 16: 411) show how differences in certification and coding practices may affect international comparisons of cancers of the cervix and body of the uterus. Sorlie PD, Gold EB (The effect of physician terminology preference on coronary heart disease mortality; an artifact uncovered by the 9th Revision ICD. American Journal of Public Health 1987; 77: 148) show how the change in the 9th revision of the ICD, whereby 'arteriosclerotic cardiovascular disease' was no longer classified as 'ischemic heart disease', might account for part of the apparent decline in coronary heart disease mortality.

29. Lahti RA, Penttila A. The validity of death certificates: routine validation of death certification and its effects on mortality statistics. Forensic Science International 2001; 115: 15.

30. When 121 physicians filled in death certificates for four fictional decedents, the proportions agreeing on the underlying cause of death ranged from 31 to 91% (Lu T-H, Shih T-P, Lee M-C, Chou M-C, Lin C-K. Diversity in death certification: a case vignette approach. Journal of Clinical Epidemiology 2001; 54: 1086).

31. Shau WY, Shih TP, Lee MC, Chou MC, Lin CK. Factors associated with errors in death certificate completion A national study in Taiwan. Journal of Clinical Epidemiology 2001; 54: 232.

32. Lu T-H, Lee M-C, Chou M-C. Accuracy of cause-of-death coding in Taiwan: types of miscoding and effects on mortality statistics. International Journal of Epidemiology 2000; 29: 336.

33. Sirken MG, Rosenberg HM, Chevarley FM, Curtin LR (The quality of cause-of-death statistics. American Journal of Public Health 1987; 77: 137) stress the need for periodic assessment of the quality of cause-of-death statistics in the USA. Grubb GS, Fortney JA, Saleh S *et al.* (A comparison of two cause-of-death classification systems for deaths among women of reproductive age in Menoufia, Egypt. International Journal of Epidemiology 1988; 17: 385) show how the findings of a detailed local survey can reveal biases in official cause-of-death statistics in a developing country.

34. Heasman LA, Lipworth L. Accuracy of certification of cause of death. A report on a survey conducted in 1959 in hospitals of the National Health Service to obtain information on the extent of agreement between clinical and post-mortem diagnoses. General Register Office, Studies on Medical and Population Subjects no 20. London: HMSO; 1966.

35. Coady SA, Sorlie PD, Cooper LS, Folsom AR, Rosamond WD, Conwill DE. Validation of death certificate diagnosis for coronary heart disease the Atherosclerosis Risk in Communities (ARIC) Study. Journal of Clinical Epidemiology 2001; 54: 40.

36. Dressler D, Zettl UK, Rummel J, Wegener R. Bad data do not make good studies. Cerebrovascular Diseases 2004; 18: 254.

37. Madsen M, Davidsen M, Rasmussen S, Abildstrom SZ, Osler M. The validity of the diagnosis of acute myocardial infarction in routine statistics. A comparison of mortality and hospital discharge data with the Danish MONICA registry. Journal of Clinical Epidemiology 2003; 56: 124.

38. Beadenkopf WG, Abrams M, Daoud A, Marks RU. An assessment of certain medical aspects of death certificate data for epidemiologic study of arteriosclerotic heart disease. Journal of Chronic Diseases 1963; 16: 249. Abramson JH, Sacks MI, Cahana B. Death certificate data as an indication of the presence of certain common diseases at death. Journal of Chronic Diseases 1971; 24: 417.

39. Satariano WA, Ragland KE, Eeden SKVD. Cause of death in men diagnosed with prostate carcinoma. Cancer 1998; 83: 1180.

40. Will JC, Vinicor F, Stevenson J. Recording of diabetes on death certificates Has it improved? Journal of Clinical Epidemiology 2001; 54: 239. Coppell K, McBride K, Williams S. Underreporting of diabetes on death certificates among a population with diabetes in Otago Province, New Zealand. Journal of the New Zealand Medical Association 2004; 117: 1207.

41. Doyle TJ, Glynn MK, Groseclose SL. Completeness of notifiable infectious disease reporting in the United States: an analytical literature review. American Journal of Epidemiology 2002; 155: 866.

42. Rosenberg ML, Marr JS, Gangarosa EJ, Pollard RA, Wallace M, Brolnitsky O. *Shigella* surveillance in the United States, 1975. Journal of Infectious Diseases 1977; 136: 458.

43. For *capture–recapture software*, see Appendix C.

44. McCarty DJ, Tull ES, Moy CS, Twoh CK, LaPorte RE. Ascertainment corrected rates: applications of capture-recapture methods. International Journal of Epidemiology 1993; 22: 559.

45. Frischer M, Bloor M, Finlay A *et al.* A new method of estimating prevalence of injecting drug use in an urban population: results from a Scottish city. International Journal of Epidemiology 1991; 20: 997.

46. Stanton B, Clemens J, Aziz KMA, Khatun K, Ahmed S, Khatun J. Comparability of results obtained by 2-week home maintained diarrhoeal calendar with 2-week diarrhoeal recall. International Journal of Epidemiology 1987; 16: 595.

47. Verbrugge LM. Health diaries – problems and solutions in study design. In: Cannell CF, Groves RM (eds), Health survey research methods. DHHS publication no. PHS 84-3346. Rockville, MD: National Center for Health Services Research; 1984. pp. 171–192.

48. Heady P, Smith S, Avery V. 1991 census validation survey: coverage report. London: HMSO, 1994.

49. Thatcher AR. Trends in numbers and mortality at high ages in England and Wales. Population Studies 1992; 46: 411.

50. National Center for Health Statistics. Comparability of marital status, race, nativity, and country of origin on the death certificate and matching census record, United States, May–August, 1960. Vital and Health Statistics, series 2, no 34. Wshington, DC: Government Printing Office; 1969.

51. Garton MJ, Abdalla MI, Reid DM, Russell IT. Estimating the point accuracy of population registers using capture-recapture methods in Scotland. Journal of Epidemiology and Community Health 1996; 50: 99.

52. Finagle's three laws on information state: '(1) The information you have is not what you want. (2) The information you want is not what you need. (3) The information you need is not what you can obtain'. Cited by Murnaghan JH (Health indicators and information systems for the year 2000. New England Journal of Medicine 1974; 290: 603).

53. Neutel CI, Johansen HL, Walop W. 'New data from old': epidemiology and record linkage. Progress in Food and Nutrition Science 1991; 15: 85. See Gill L, Goldacre M, Simmons H, Bettley G, Griffith M (Computerized linking of medical records: methodological guidelines. Journal of Epidemiology and Community Health 1993; 47: 316) and Baldwin JA, Acheson ED, Graham WJ (Textbook of medical record linkage. New York, NY: Oxford University Press; 1987).

22

Planning the Records

Records cannot be properly planned until the study plan is almost complete. The planning of records requires prior decisions as to what variables will be studied, what scales of measurement will be used, and how the information will be collected and processed.

Apart from the forms used for recording the primary data collected in the study (the main topic of this chapter), a variety of other records may be required to ensure smooth working. These may include lists of people to be examined or interviewed, lists of potential controls from which some are to be chosen by matching or random selection, 'appointment book'-type records showing when examinations or re-examinations are scheduled, and so on. In a study in which various procedures are applied to the same subjects on different occasions or in different places (interview, physical examination, glucose tolerance test, chest X-ray, etc.), it is often helpful to maintain a 'record of procedures' for each individual, showing what has been performed (and if not, why not). In a large study, the organization of an efficient filing system may not be simple. Use may be made of card indexes in which the cards of people awaiting different procedures can be kept in separate sections or marked with variously coloured tags, or of 'virtual' card indexes created by a computer program.[1]

Record Forms

The most important forms are those used for recording the primary data of the study. These forms, or 'data sheets', may take the shape of questionnaires, examination schedules, forms for laboratory or other test results, extraction forms on to which data are copied from clinical or other records, etc., or they may be multipurpose forms with different sections to meet these various purposes.

The form may be printed on paper or cards, or may be designed for display on a computer screen.[2] It is usually advisable to use different forms for data (concerning a single individual) collected in different places, from different sources, by different observers or interviewers, or at different times. It may also be necessary to use different forms for different categories of subjects, e.g. when there are substantial differences in the questionnaires for men and women, or for living subjects and the surviving relatives of dead ones. If several paper forms are used, then it may be helpful to use different colours.

Specimens of special-purpose clinical questionnaires can be viewed on the Internet:[3] some, like the SF-36 health survey, for self-administration; others, like the Glasgow Coma Scale, presumably not.

Research Methods in Community Medicine: Surveys, Epidemiological Research, Programme Evaluation, Clinical Trials   J. H. Abramson and Z. H. Abramson   Copyright © 2008, John Wiley & Sons Ltd

The record forms should, if possible, meet four requirements:

1. Only one individual per form.
2. All the required information should be specified.
3. The form should be easy to use.
4. The form should be geared to the needs of data processing.

Most requirements are easily met if the form is designed by a data-entry program.[2]

Only one individual per form

It is advisable to use a separate form for each individual studied ('individual' here means the individual unit of the study – this may be a collective unit, such as a family or school). This usually greatly facilitates the subsequent handling of the data. Lists showing many individuals, with columns for different pieces of information (the 'ledger', 'register', or 'exercise book' method), have limited value; if hand tallying (p. 234) is used, errors are likely if more than two or three variables are recorded in such a list. Swaroop tells of a director of public health who analysed several thousand registers of cholera patients to determine how many had died, then repeated the process to obtain the same information for each sex, and when he found that he was unable to reach the same total 'threw up his hands and exclaimed, "Now I *really* wish those people had not died"'.[4]

Identification data are usually required on the form, although not necessarily for use in the analysis. In addition to the person's name, use may be made of his or her sex, age, address, hospital number, personal identity number, etc. In a long-term follow-up study, it is often helpful to add the name and address of a close friend or relative, to help in finding the person after a change of address; an e-mail address may also be helpful. Each record should also have space for a number that distinctively identifies the individual to whom it refers. This identifying number is usually a serial number or 'study number' arbitrarily allocated for the specific purpose of the study. The same identifying number should appear on all records pertaining to the individual. In an investigation where anonymity is guaranteed, this number will be the only identification on the record.

In studies where computers are used, a *check digit*[5] may be added to the serial number. This is a digit that is derived from the digits in the number, using a predetermined rule, and that is placed after it to make a new serial number that has a logical consistency. An error made in transcribing or in computer entry is likely to produce an 'illogical' number, which the computer can detect. A simple method is to choose a digit that will provide zero or a multiple of 10 when alternate digits are added and subtracted. If the original number is 1568, the check digit is 6, since $(+1 - 5 + 6 - 8 + 6) = 0$, and the new serial number is 15686. If this is accidentally rendered as 16586, the error can be detected, since $(+1 - 6 + 5 - 8 + 6) = -2$.

All the required information should be specified

Physical examination schedules are frequently unsatisfactory, in that they do not specify all the variables about which the investigator wishes to obtain information. If we wish to know about swelling of the legs, for instance, there is little point in using a form that merely has a heading 'Lower extremities', with a blank space beneath it. If the space remains blank after the examination, or if some other abnormality is noted, we will not know whether the examiner looked for oedema. At the least, then, the heading 'oedema of legs' should be printed.

Furthermore (and this applies to questionnaires as well as to examination schedules), all the alternative categories of measurement should appear on the form. If the heading 'oedema' has only a space beneath it, which the examiner leaves empty, we will still be uncertain that this sign was sought. The words 'present' and 'absent' should be printed, for the examiner to mark whichever is applicable; the findings are then clear and unequivocal. This item in the schedule might have the following format:

Oedema:	Right	Left
Absent	☐	☐
Present	☐	☐

As an extra precaution, the examiner may be asked to write 'not examined' (and state the reason) if any part of the examination is omitted, or to enter a prearranged number, say 9, in the appropriate box.

The same principle applies to questionnaires, in which (except in the case of open-ended questions) all the possible responses to each question should be printed, including (if necessary) a category of 'other' – or, more usefully, 'other (specify) …'. One exception to this rule is that some investigators prefer not to include a 'don't know' or 'unknown' category, in order to reduce the frequency of such answers, which (if given to an interviewer) can be written in. To avoid the possibility of ambiguous 'blank' responses when a question requests a numerical answer ('On how many days of a week do you eat meat?'), the instruction 'If not at all, write 0' should be stated.

The form should be easy to use

The easier the form is to use, the fewer errors there will be. The items should follow the sequence in which the data are to be collected. This requirement may present especial difficulties in the planning of a schedule for a clinical examination, and flaws in the schedule may not be detected until the form is submitted to a pretest.

As far as possible, the need for writing or entering text should be avoided, both to simplify the task of the observer, interviewer or extractor, and to reduce the need to decipher unintelligible scrawls. Wherever possible, the relevant findings or responses should be indicated with a check mark (a tick or cross), or circling or underlining, or (if on a computer screen) by a mouse click.

The form should, as far as possible, be self-explanatory. The main instructions should be clearly stated in the form itself, even if a more detailed manual has been prepared for examiners or interviewers. Although written instructions cannot always replace oral explanations, they serve as a constant guide and reminder. Instructions are particularly important when, as often happens, certain items are applicable only to some individuals. In a paper questionnaire, the instructions should be spelled out in detail, e.g. by saying 'If male and 18 years or older, ask:' or 'If "no", proceed to question 17. If "yes", ask next question'. Such instructions are best printed in a different font or shown in parentheses. Arrows may be helpful, as in the examples below. In a 'skip' instruction in a self-administered questionnaire, a page number ('go to page 3') may be better than a question number ('go to question 17'). When designing a computer questionnaire, automatic 'skip' patterns can be built in.

Other self-explanatory conventions may be used (not in self-administered questionnaires). For example, it is useful to divide a questionnaire into sections by horizontal lines, and instruct the interviewers that whenever the response they receive is one that is marked by double underlining, they should go on to the next section (see the second of the following two boxes).

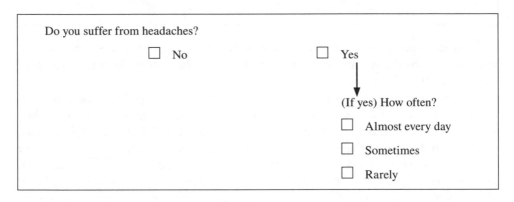

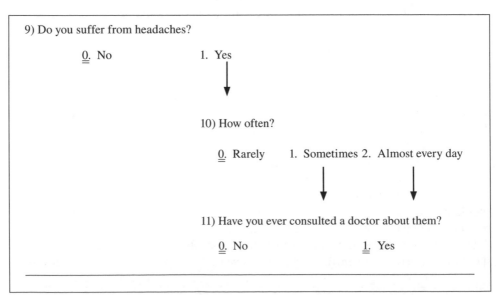

Clear and simple instructions are particularly important in self-administered question-naires. The method of marking responses should be clearly explained. In a study to be carried out in Trinidad, for example, the introduction (after explaining who is performing the study and why, and inviting the respondent's co-operation) might state:

Most of the questions can be answered by putting an 'X' in the box next to the answer that fits you best. For example:

Do you live in Trinidad?   ☒ Yes   ☐ No

The layout of the form should make for its easy use. The items should not be crowded, and the places for answers should be clearly shown.

The form should be geared to the needs of data processing.

If responses to a paper questionnaire are to be coded manually, then boxes should be printed for the codes; this will facilitate computer entry.

The use of a precoded form permits coding to be done at the time the data are collected. The code digits are printed on the form, and are either marked by circling or by checking an appropriately numbered box, or are written in a box provided for the purpose. Graphic rating scales (see p. 194) may also be used. A different approach is employed in each of the pot-pourri of items in the form below. (In practice, the use of such a medley of methods in a single form would be confusing.) The figures on the right

---

24. Pulse rate. (If under 100, put a zero in front of the number.

If pulse rate is 72, write 072)   ☐☐☐   42–44

25. Systolic pulmonic murmur. (Circle the appropriate number)

    1. Absent

    2. Present   45

26. Character of murmur. (Write the appropriate number in the box.)

    1. Blowing

    2. Musical

    3. Harsh

              ☐   46

27. Diastolic murmurs. (Circle the appropriate numbers.)

	Absent	Present Grade of intensity					
Apical	0	1	2	3	4	5	47
Mid-precordial	0	1	2	3	4	5	48
Pulmonic	0	1	2	3	4	5	49
Aortic	0	1	2	3	4	5	50

are the numbers of the columns in which the data will be stored in the computer record,[6] and are not needed if a data-entry program is to be used.

An alternative approach, preferred by some investigators, is to provide an interviewer with only a single questionnaire form, on which the coded alternatives to each question are stated, and to have a separate 'answer sheet' filled in for each respondent. This sheet need contain only the subject's name, etc., and the numbers of the questions, with either a box or a row of the alternative code numbers (for circling) next to each question number. This makes the form more compact, but there may be more errors when it is filled in.

A method that is likely to increase in popularity is the use of machine-readable forms, marks on which are read by an optical scanner and transferred to a computer record.

Precoding is best avoided in self-administered questionnaires, since it may confuse the respondent. It may, however, be used if the code numbers are kept small and inconspicuous.

Decisions about Coding

To facilitate computer processing and analysis, codes must be assigned to the categories of variables that have nominal, ordinal or dichotomous scales. Numbers are generally used for this purpose. Coding is not needed for simple numerical data, unless it is decided to group the data into prespecified classes (a job better left to a computer), and for data that will not be analysed (e.g. subjects' names).

The codes should be decided in advance where possible, particularly if precoded records are to be used. For questionnaires or other record forms to be displayed by a computer, decisions on coding are an integral part of the programming process.

Coding requires the preparation of a *coding key* that shows the codes used for each variable, and their meanings. If coding is complicated, then detailed coding instructions may be needed. These should be clear and unambiguous, in order to ensure coding reliability. Voluminous instructions may be needed if the responses to open-ended questions or statements made in relatively unstructured interviews have to be coded, particularly with respect to attitudes, motivation, etc. (content analysis).

Standardized conventions should be used wherever possible, so as to simplify both the coding process and the analysis. If there are 'yes–no' questions, for example, 1 might be allocated to all 'yes' answers and 0 to all 'no' answers. It is particularly important to use standard codes for 'unknown' and 'not applicable' – for example, 'unknown' might be entered as 9, 99, or 999 (choosing a number that is outside the range of possible data), and 'not applicable' as 8, 88, etc. This is advisable for numerical as well as categorical data, to reduce errors during data entry or analysis. Distinctive codes are sometimes used for 'unknown' values of different kinds, especially those resulting from refusal or failure to answer a question, explicit 'don't know' responses, and errors in the recording or handling of data.

A specimen portion of an imaginary coding key, incorporating coding instructions, is shown in Table 22.1. When coding is complicated, as for relative weight in this example,

Table 22.1   Coding key

Variable	Code	Coding instructions
Sex	1 Male 2 Female 9 Unknown	Precoded (question 1). If missing, look at subject's name, and see whether questions 3–5 (for females only) have been asked. If sex is still uncertain, code 9.
Marital status	1 Single 2 Married 3 Widowed 4 Divorced 9 Unknown	Precoded (question 2). If missing, code 9.
Social class	1 SC I 2 SC II 3 SC III 4 SC IV 5 SC V 8 Unclassifiable 9 No data on occupation	Code the occupation stated in the answer to question 6, using the attached instructions. If occupation not stated, code 9.
Height	999 Unknown	Centimetres (ignore fractions or decimals). If missing, code 999.
Relative weight	888 Unclassified 999 Unknown	Consult appended weight-for-height tables to find standard weight for a person of the subject's sex and height. Divide subject's weight by the standard weight, multiply by 100, round off downwards, and enter. Code 888 if height falls outside range shown in tables. Code 999 if sex, height or weight is unknown.

it is best done by a computer; the coding key might then include the relevant computer instructions (algorithm).

A more ambitious *codebook* may be prepared, including additional information such as operational definitions (see Table 10.1, p. 105) and other relevant explanations (to what subgroups of study subjects the variable is applicable, how the data have been edited or manipulated, ranges of values regarded as acceptable, the variables' positions in the electronic record, etc.).

New *derived variables* are often created by manipulating the original data; this may be done during data entry (with appropriate software and programming) or afterwards. If their creation is planned in advance, then they can be included in the coding key or codebook from the outset; otherwise, they should be added later. Their method of creation should be explained. A *recoded variable* is created by altering the variable's coding – age in years might be recoded by 5-year age groups, or data on the number of cigarettes smoked might be used to categorize subjects as nonsmokers or light, moderate or heavy smokers. The new variable may also be based on numeric transformation of the original value, e.g. using its square or logarithm, or adding or subtracting a constant. A *constructed variable* is derived from two or more other variables, like the relative weight shown in Table 22.1; diagnostic criteria may be brought together so as to categorize subjects in terms of the presence or absence of a disease.

Coding is less important if the data are to be processed by hand. But even then, it may be convenient to make use of symbols or standard abbreviations such as + (present), − (absent), ? (unknown), M (male) and F (female).

Coding errors are not infrequent. In one study in which coding was done by the interviewers, half of all the mistakes made by interviewers (detected by comparing replicate interview records) were coding errors.[7] Coding by the examiner or interviewer at the time that data are collected is obviously a cheap and fast method, and it does not impose a burden if the coding is simple. But coding errors can then be detected and rectified only if the record forms make provision for the full data as well as the codes.

Notes and References

1. For examples of computer programs that can create virtual card indexes, see Appendix C.
2. For software, see Appendix C. A tutorial on questionnaire design, as part of a tutorial on the conduct of a community survey using **Epi Info**, is available at http://www.cdc.gov/epiinfo/communityhealth.htm.
3. A number of questionnaires used for special purposes in clinical medicine are available at http://_www.medalreg.com/qhc/.
4. Swaroop S. Statistical methods in malaria eradication. Geneva: WHO; 1966. p. 20.
5. Acheson ED. Record linkage in medicine. Edinburgh: Livingstone; 1968. pp. 181–183.
6. See note 8, Chapter 23.
7. Horwitz RI, Yu EC. Assessing the reliability of epidemiologic data obtained from medical records. International Journal of Epidemiology 1985; 463: 14.

23

Planning the Handling of Data

Before data collection starts, decisions must be made about the method of processing, the preparation of a data set, and data checking and cleaning. These decisions are interrelated.

Decisions about Data Processing

Data processing may be done by a personal computer or a mainframe computer (usually accessed through a personal computer), or (if the study is a small one) the data may be processed manually. Personal computer software is generally more 'user friendly' (providing on-screen explanations, warnings and instructions) than mainframe computer programs, and it may offer more possibilities of interaction (permitting decisions to be made in an ongoing way during the course of a statistical analysis session).

There are, today, few studies that do not use computers. But a few words of caution about computer use are not out of place. First, some people still believe that 'the computer is never wrong'. The computer is no mental giant, but a moron that slavishly follows instructions. It cannot be accurate if the humans who operate it make errors, and to err is human. Data may be inaccurate or entered inaccurately ('garbage in, garbage out'), errors may be made in giving instructions, or the programs may have unknown bugs. 'Because of the faith that is placed in computers, the possibility of undetected human error may be greater when computers are used'.[1] Second, analysis by computer is so easy that there may be a temptation to examine trivial hypotheses, or hypotheses based on 'data snooping' (i.e. constructed only after examining the findings) – which may lead to unwarranted conclusions (see p. 259). Third, complex statistical procedures have become so readily available that they are often used even if they are inappropriate for the data or for answering the questions that the study asks. One statistician laments that 'in the past we have had misgivings about "cook book" statistics, and now what has evolved would have to be termed the "TV dinner" … Previously, we could believe that the user would at least have to read the recipe!'[2] Others observe that 'it is not hard to do a bad analysis … All that is needed is a canned computer program … and a lack of competence in biostatistics. These resources are widely available'.[3] 'Output from commercial computer programs, with their beautifully formatted tables, graphs, and matrices, can make garbage look like roses'.[4]

Research Methods in Community Medicine: Surveys, Epidemiological Research, Programme Evaluation, Clinical Trials   J. H. Abramson and Z. H. Abramson   Copyright © 2008, John Wiley & Sons Ltd

However processing is to be done, during the planning stage the investigator should decide, at least in broad outline, how the data will be analysed in order to meet the specific objectives of the study. It is often helpful to draw up a number of specimen skeleton tables, with column and row headings but containing no figures, and to consider how different kinds of result will be interpreted. This process of 'thinking forward' to the analysis often reveals gaps in the data (variables omitted, no information on the denominator population, etc.), defects in scales of measurement, or the superfluity of certain data. It provides a further opportunity for second thoughts as to whether the study, as planned, is likely to meet its objectives.

Thought should be given not only to the format of the tables, but to the statistical techniques to be used in the analysis (see Chap. 26), the general lines of which should always be decided in advance. Sometimes a detailed plan can be prepared (this may be obligatory if an application is made for research funds), but options should be left open, since the findings, as they emerge, may call for new or different analyses.

A statistician's help is often needed, although it is a consoling thought that the analysis of a well-planned study sometimes requires only the simplest of statistical techniques. It is foolhardy to decide to use complex procedures without adequate statistical knowledge or expert guidance. If a statistician is to be consulted, then this should be done during the planning phase, when the design of the investigation can still be influenced, and not after the data have been collected, when they may be found unsuitable for analysis. 'To call in the statistician after the experiment is done may be no more than asking him to perform a postmortem examination: he may be able to say what the experiment died of'.[5] When consulting a statistician, it must be remembered that a silly question gets a silly answer. Unless the investigator can explain very precisely and specifically what is hoped to be learned from the study, the advice received, however erudite and well meaning, may be inadequate and even misleading.

Manual data-processing methods

Manual data-processing methods (hand tallying and hand sorting) are appropriate for small-scale studies only, and may be tedious, but are favoured by some investigators on the grounds that they keep them 'close to their data'. 'The figures that we are analyzing represent the patients, animals, things or processes that we are studying, and the more familiar we become with them, the more likely we are to know about their interrelationships, oddities and defects; and the more likely we are to catch hints of explanations and clues for further research.'[6]

Hand tallying is the most primitive method. A tally sheet is prepared in the form of a skeleton table, and a tally mark is made in the requisite cell for each individual. The usual method is to make a vertical mark for each individual. Every fifth individual in a cell is indicated by a diagonal line drawn through the preceding four. This facilitates subsequent counting.

An alternative method is to make dots (arranged in a square) for the first four, then to draw a line (joining two dots) for each of the next four, making a square, which means a count of 8. A diagonal is then drawn for each of the next two, so that a complete set of 10 looks like a little flag with a St Patrick's Cross.

When a tabulation is done directly from lists (containing information on different individuals on the same page) or from unwieldy records (e.g. voluminous clinical files), hand tallying may be a convenient method. Its disadvantages are that it is laborious and time-consuming, and errors are prone to creep in, especially if a complicated cross-tabulation is being used. If an error is detected (e.g. if it is found that the total number shown in the table is one less than the actual number of individuals), this requires the repetition of the entire process, unless differently coloured inks have been used for different batches of records to help in the localization of errors.

Hand sorting is usually preferable to hand tallying. This requires a separate and easily handled record for each individual. The records are sorted and physically separated into piles conforming with the cells in the skeleton table, and the numbers in each pile are then counted, recounted, and entered. If an error is detected, it is usually necessary to repeat only part of the procedure. To prepare a cross-classification, the records are usually sorted 'hierarchically'; that is, they are sorted into piles according to one variable, then each pile is sorted according to a second variable, and so on until the cross-classification is complete. Each pile is then counted. Sorting is relatively easy if small cards are used, information on each variable is written in a standard position, and heavy lines or different colours are used to facilitate the visual identification of data.

Preparing the Data Set

Decisions must be made about the preparation of the *data set* (or *database*) that will be used in the analysis phase. 'Getting from a questionnaire or an interview to an actual data record', it has been said, 'is a perilous journey with many potential accidents waiting to happen'.[7]

If the data are collected by a computer-assisted process, then they go into the database automatically. Results of chemical, electrocardiographic and other instrumental examinations can also be put straight into the electronic record, as can data read by optical scanning. Usually, however, data are coded manually (if not precoded) and then entered manually, using a computer keyboard.

Accurate manual coding may not be easy to achieve, even with detailed written instructions (see p. 230). Careful training and monitoring may be needed. As a check on coding reliability, double coding (by the same or different coders) may be done for all records, a sample of records, or selected hard-to-code variables. The codes may be written or marked on the original data sheets, or may be copied to code sheets. Unnecessary transcription should be avoided, to avoid errors; if the codes are copied, then this process too may need checking. The process is simplified if coding is done at the time the data are collected, by the person who collects the data. But later checks and corrections are then possible only if the original data are recorded, as well as the codes. Manual coding and data entry should be separated, to permit concentration on one task at a time.

Before data are entered, the structure[8] and content of the data set must be decided – what variables will be entered, and in what order, whether entries will be treated as numbers or as strings of text ('alphanumerical'), with how many decimal places, and so on. The data for each individual are entered into a separate *record* (or series of records), with the variables in a preset sequence and each variable in a separate *field* (which can accommodate one or more numbers, letters or other characters) in the record. Use may be made of a *free field format*, in which the variables are recorded in fields without preset lengths but separated by blank spaces, commas, carriage returns, or other delimiters, or a *fixed format*, in which the length of the fields (and hence their locations in the record) are decided in advance.

The coded data are best entered with data-entry software,[9] which can check for errors by finding wild codes and out-of-range values and performing consistency checks (see p. 237) and may also be able to incorporate *skip patterns* (conditional jumps that bypass irrelevant variables), insert 'missing data' codes and 'not applicable' codes consistent with the skip patterns, create derived variables (see p. 231), and offer a *verification* procedure whereby the data can be re-entered ('double keying') and discrepancies identified. It is usually easy to get the program to provide a screen image of the record form, so that during data entry the items appear on the screen in the same order and with the same spatial arrangement as on the record form. Spreadsheet programs can also be used for data entry, and some can conduct checks and create new variables. Text editors (see Appendix C) or word-processing programs, too, can be used, by simply typing strings of digits or other characters, with or without delimiters to separate the variables; but they cannot perform checks.

One trial of methods of data entry showed that use of a word processor to produce a data file was more than adequate for short record forms. For longer forms, a simple program using a screen image of the form was fastest and most liked. A more sophisticated program, with inbuilt logical checks and skip patterns, did not realize its theoretical advantages. It was slower and identified only 10% of errors. Most errors caused by incorrect key-punching (at least 1% of all digits entered can be expected to be wrong)[10] are not detected by these checks. The recommended method was the simple one using a screen image of the record form, followed by re-entry for verification.[11]

The more elaborate statistical programs have their own data-entry mechanisms and their own data sets, although not always with the same checking capabilities as data-entry programs.

Although most investigators can themselves run statistical analysis programs, the creation, maintenance and management of the data set in large studies are often left to experts. This is best done by giving detailed explanations of the objectives and study plan to an expert early in the planning phase, in order to obtain the best possible aid and advice with regard not only to data processing, but also to the planning of forms and record systems.

Decisions about Data Checks and Data Cleaning

Data should be checked during the data collection process, as well as afterwards. Early planning is especially important if data are to be transferred to an electronic medium as an intrinsic part of the data collection process, as in computer-assisted interviewing.

In all studies, data should be checked for completeness and obvious errors as it is collected – preferably by checking every record form, but at least by checking a sample. This requires planning: what will be checked, by whom, when, and how will corrections be made? (See 'Quality control' in Chapter 25). The sooner an error is found, the easier it may be to correct it.

With appropriate data-entry software and programming, checks can be done on the fly – the computer can display a warning or refuse to accept the entry if an impermissible entry is made or if a record is re-entered. For a coded categorical variable, a *wild code* not included in the coding key would be illegal. For an interval-scale or ratio-scale entry, a range of acceptable values can be defined in advance so that *out-of-range values* can be identified. With suitable programming the computer can also perform *consistency checks* (*logical checks, machine edits*), comparing entries for different variables and providing warnings when obvious errors are found, e.g. a man who immigrated before his date of birth, a woman who was married before she was born, or who has given up smoking but smokes a pack a day, a person aged 342 years, or a man who is still menstruating. These checks can be done either during data entry (*interactive checking*) or after data entry (*batch checking*). Typing errors can also be checked by double data entry, preferably by different persons, followed by a search for differences (*validation* of the entries).

If quality control procedures are used during the collection of data (see p. 237), and especially if data-entry software is used to prepare the data set, the data set should not present big surprises when it is used. But one should never forget to perform a simple count; data forms – and electronic records – have a nasty habit of going astray.

Errors, which may have been made when the data were collected or may have occurred during coding or data entry, can be corrected if possible. Otherwise, the unacceptable values may be changed to 'unknown' and the individuals concerned may be excluded from specific analyses or from the analysis as a whole. Erroneous and missing values may also sometimes be changed to *imputed*[12] ones.

It is arguable that, since some data errors are probably inevitable, *data cleaning* is no less important than sound study design and sound study conduct. A systematic approach has been suggested,[13] comprising screening, diagnosing, and editing processes, carried out at three stages: when the record forms are collected, when the data are entered in the database, and when the data set is ready for analysis. Screening, based mainly on descriptive analyses (some of which can be automated 'logical checks'), would look for absence of data, excess of data (e.g. due to repeated entry of the same results), outliers, strange patterns in joint distributions, and other unexpected results. In the diagnostic phase, an effort is made to explain the worrisome findings; this may involve checks against previous records, repetition of measurements, or the collection of additional information. In the editing phase, the options are correcting the data (by imputation if necessary), deletion, or leaving the data unchanged. It may be decided to use *robust measures*,[14] such as *trimmed means*, which are relatively uninfluenced by outliers. Whatever the decisions, they should be documented and (it has been suggested) described in the study report:

We recommend that medical scientific reports include data cleaning methods. These methods should include error types and rates, at least for the primary outcome variables, with the associated deletion and correction rate, justification for imputations, and differences in outcome with and without remaining outliers.[7]

Data-set management tasks may persist throughout the process of analysis: new needs may arise for derived variables, or for work files confined to a subgroup of the sample or selected variables, or for new files appropriate for use with specific statistical software. It is important to have a backup copy of the data set, kept elsewhere for safety.

Notes and References

1. Blum ML, Foos PW. Data gathering: experimental methods plus. New York, NY: Harper & Row; 1986. p. 80.
2. Schucany WR. Comment. Journal of the American Statistical Association 1978; 73: 92.
3. Bross IDJ. Scientific strategies to save your life: a statistical approach to primary prevention. New York, NY: Marcel Dekker; 1981. pp. 42–43.
4. Tabachnick BG, Fidell LS. (Using multivariate statistics, 5th edn. Allyn & Bacon; 2006) try throughout their book 'to suggest clues for when the true message in the output more closely resembles the fertilizer than the flowers'.
5. Fisher RA. At an Indian Statistical Congress in Sankhya; 1938.
6. Mainland D. Elementary medical statistics. Philadelphia, PA: Saunders; 1964. p. 168.
7. Inter-university Consortium for Political and Social Research. ICPSR guide to social science data preparation and archiving; 1997. Available at http://www.icpsr.umich.edu/ICPSR/access/dataprep.pdf.
8. *Structure of the data set.* The data set may contain one or more data files, stored on disk, tape, or other medium. A data file is a collection of data records, which may be of any length, but are sometimes 'card-images' each containing 80 'columns' (i.e. accommodating 80 characters, like the old IBM punch card). Each record stores a predecided sequence of fields; the fields may have a predecided size (fixed format) or be separated by predecided characters (free field format). In the former instance, the data file is *rectangular* (the records are of the same length).

    The guide cited in note 7 provides useful advice on file formats and file structure, codes and codebooks, and other aspects of data-set preparation, and contains a useful glossary of technical terms.
9. **EpiData**, **Epi Info**, and **EpiSurveyor** are free programs (see Appendix C) that streamline data entry. All you need do is type the questionnaire or data entry form, using certain conventions for numeric, yes/no and other fields. This is subsequently shown on the screen so that each subject's data can be entered and stored. The program allocates variable names, field lengths, etc., using information derived from the form. Data entry constraints (acceptable ranges, etc.) and skip patterns can be built in. The program can convert the data to formats appropriate for various statistical programs. The questionnaires can be used in computer-assisted interviews.
10. Martin JNT, Morton J, Ottley P. Experiments on copying digit strings. Ergonomics 1977; 20: 409.
11. Crombie IK, Irving JM. An investigation of data entry methods with a personal computer. Computers and Biomedical Research 1986; 19: 543.
12. Erroneous and missing values are sometimes replaced by *imputed* ones, especially if exclusion of the subjects from the analysis is likely to cause bias. The imputed value may be derived from the values of other characteristics and the distribution of the variable. Simple methods of

imputation may lead to bias or overestimation of the precision of associations. Better results are obtained by *multiple imputation*, which makes use of values imputed in different ways, and then uses a complicated statistical procedure that brings together the results obtained by using different imputed values (Donders ART, van der Heijden GJMG, Stijnen T, Moons KGM. Review: a gentle introduction to imputation of missing values. Journal of Clinical Epidemiology 2006; 59: 1087).

Imputation is particularly problematic if the probability of being missing depends on the value itself (e.g. if better-off respondents tend to withhold information about their income) or reasons connected to the purpose of the study (*nonignorable*, or *missing not at random*, as opposed to *missing at random*). 'When addressing problems of missing data the issues of why the data are missing can be more important than how to cope with the resulting imbalance' (Armitage P, Berry G, Matthews JNS. Statistical methods in medical research, 4th edn. Blackwell Science; 2002. p. 246).

The pros and cons of different methods of imputation are discussed by Acock AC (Working with missing values. Journal of Marriage and Family 2005; 67: 1012). Basic information about the methods is available at http://www.stat.psu.edu/~jls/mifaq.html. For software, see Appendix C.

Whatever method is used, it may be wise to do the analysis without the 'guessed' values as well as with them, so that the effect of their inclusion can be observed and (if necessary) taken into account.

13. The *data cleaning* process described in the text is based on Van den Broeck J, Cunningham SA, Eeckels R, Herbst K (Data cleaning: detecting, diagnosing, and editing data abnormalities. PloS Medicine 2005; 2(10): e267).

14. *Robust measures and tests* are those that are little affected by failure to meet the assumptions on which they are based. *Trimmed means* are computed after omitting extreme observations.

24

Pretests and Other Preparations

Before the collection of data can be started, it is usually necessary to test the methods, and practical preparations must be made. If the planning phase was the gestation period, then this is the stage of parturition. It may not be free of pain; and if there are practical problems that cannot be overcome, then the study may yet be stillborn.

Pretests

Pretests, or prior tests of methods, vary in their scope. A pretest may consist of a single visit to a clinic to see whether patients' weights or other items of information are routinely recorded on their cards, or may take the form of a large and well-planned methodological study or a full-scale *pilot study*, a dress rehearsal of the main investigation. Pretests may be required in order to examine the practicability, reliability or validity of methods of study, and their planning varies according to their purposes. A pretest may be a well-constructed study aimed at yielding definitive results, or it may be designed to provide only a 'feel' of the suitability of a method. Pretests of examination schedules and questionnaires are usually of the latter type. If a data-entry program is to be used, it is wise to pretest it on a number of cases; this may reveal unexpected difficulties.

In a typical small-scale pretest of a questionnaire, 10–30 subjects are interviewed.[1] These may be chosen haphazardly, but should not be potential members of the study sample, since participation in the pretest interview may reduce willingness to be interviewed in the study proper, or may affect the responses given in the study proper. Subjects are usually chosen who are similar in their characteristics to the members of the study population. Sometimes, in order to highlight possible flaws in the questionnaire, 'difficult customers', e.g. people with an especially low or high educational level, are purposely chosen. The interviewer may be asked to record not only the responses for which the questionnaire makes provision, but also maybe the respondent's reactions (boredom, irritation, impatience, antagonism – or even interest!), to make verbatim notes of the respondent's comments, to record the time taken by the interview, and to make criticisms and suggestions concerning the questions, their sequence, and skip patterns ('If "No", go to…'). The interviewer (or another interviewer, in a special call-back visit) may be requested to discuss the questions with the respondent after they have been answered, asking whether they seemed clear, what the answers meant, why a 'Don't

Research Methods in Community Medicine: Surveys, Epidemiological Research, Programme Evaluation, Clinical Trials   J. H. Abramson and Z. H. Abramson   Copyright © 2008, John Wiley & Sons Ltd

know' response was made, etc. This may be done informally, or a formal procedure may be used – after explaining that this is a test of some of the questions, the interviewer reads out each question with its response and requests an explanation of exactly how the answer was arrived at; this is followed by preplanned questions designed to find out how particular terms were understood by the respondent.[2]

The best strategy is often to begin with a small-scale pretest that includes detailed questioning of the respondents about their reactions (a *participating pretest*[1]). This may require hand-picked respondents: 'investigators may find themselves relying on that familiar source of forced labor – colleagues, friends and family'.[1]

On the basis of all this information, it is often possible to identify 'difficult' questions – those that are offensive, hard to understand, or do not seem to elicit the information they are intended to get – and awkward sequences of items. If a question elicits many 'Don't know' answers, then it is probably unsatisfactory. If it produces many qualifying comments, then the response categories are probably not suitable. Inconsistencies between the answers to related questions, or uniform answers by all respondents ('all-or-none' responses), may also point to flaws. If questions were omitted, or asked when they should not have been, then the questionnaire's arrangement or provision of instructions is probably defective.

The pretest usually points to a need for changes in the questionnaire and the interviewing instructions. These changes are made, and a new version is available for pretesting.

Participation in pretesting can be a valuable component of the training of interviewers, and can also help to give interviewers a feeling of identification with the study.

The Internet can be used for easy and rapid pretests of questionnaires,[3] especially to see which questions often remain unanswered, presumably because they are not good ones. But the results may be of limited applicability, since the sample (motivated Internet users) may not resemble the study population in which the questionnaire is to be used, and the problems that are revealed may differ from those that are likely to arise when the questionnaire is used in a different way.

Enlisting Cooperation

It is particularly important to enlist the good will of people who will be involved in the study (subjects who will be examined or interviewed, administrators and others who can provide access to records or various facilities and services, etc.) and those (such as some colleagues) who think they are involved in the study or feel they should have been involved in the study. In clinical studies or studies using clinical material, the treating physicians should consent or at least be informed.

In a community study, cooperation can be enhanced by suitable public relations and preparatory educational work in the community. The best results are provided by contacts with key individuals and organizations in the community, but use may also be made of mass media, such as local television channels, radio talks, newspaper articles, pamphlets and posters. In such contacts, people should be told what they can expect to 'get out of' the study, but no false promises should be made. In medical surveys, 'the two most generally effective motivations are the desire to contribute to the community effort to benefit health through science, and the subject's own interest in a free medical examination'.[4] Many investigators dislike the idea of offering financial incentives (cash, vouchers, lottery tickets or gifts), but randomized trials of their use have usually shown improved compliance.[5] It may be decided to send out letters telling prospective respondents about the study and the impending visit or phone call by an interviewer (it is usually unwise to make the initial contact by telephone – this invites refusals). It may also be decided to prepare 'reminder' and 'thank you' letters. In studies in which access to confidential medical records is necessary, people may be required to give their approval in writing, and consent forms should be printed for this purpose.

Other Practical Preparations

A budget may have to be prepared and funds found (a process that probably commenced as soon as the study objectives and methods took shape, or maybe sooner), and arrangements made for administering them. Some few lucky people are experts in grantsmanship. Others should seek help from such an expert or from the numerous Internet sources that provide lists of funding opportunities and hints on the writing of grant applications.[6]

There may be many other practical preparations to be made before data can be collected. Approval may have to be obtained from an ethical committee. Accommodation, equipment and its maintenance, supplies, transportation, and access to laboratory, data processing, or other facilities may have to be arranged. Personnel may have to be found or trained. Record forms must be printed. Maps may have to be found or prepared, or a census of the study population may have to be performed. Sampling frames may have to be prepared, cases of a disease identified, and samples or controls selected. In a blind or double-blind experiment, complicated practical preparations may be needed to ensure secrecy (dummy medicinal preparations, containers identified by symbols, etc.). In a study involving a sequence of procedures performed by different examiners, logistic problems may require solution. An inspired researcher is not necessarily a good administrator (and vice versa, as the activities of many public health departments, hospitals and other medical services eloquently testify), and in a large investigation it is often wise to appoint a study coordinator or field-work director with a bent for practical matters.

If observational methods of data collection are to be used (by persons other than the investigator who has planned them), then they should be carefully explained and demonstrated, and 'running-in' exercises should be arranged. An examiner's manual may be required, both for training purposes and for subsequent consultation. If necessary, reference standards should be made available, such as standard photographs of skin abnormalities or (for laboratory tests) solutions of known chemical composition.

If interviewers have to be found, then they should be carefully selected, the main requirements being that they should be capable, personable, honest, interested, able to establish rapport, and good listeners. Interviewers who are new to the job should be given a general training[7] in interview methods (see p. 186), and all interviewers should receive an explanation of the objectives and methods of the study, should be told or shown, unhurriedly and in detail, what they are expected to do, and should conduct trial interviews before starting work on the study proper.[8] An interviewer's manual should be prepared if it is thought this will be helpful.

If documentary sources are to be used, then steps should be taken to ensure that there is access to them – confidentiality and poor systems of record storage and retrieval often pose problems – and that they contain the desired types of information. The people who are to extract the data should receive detailed instructions. Whatever methods are to be used, arrangements should now be made for quality control during the stage of data collection (see Chapter 25).

If the data are to be coded, then practical preparations for coding should be made, although these may sometimes be delayed until a later stage. Coding keys and coding instructions should be prepared, coders trained, and arrangements made for the testing and control of coding reliability.

Finally, a word of advice from Cochran *et al.*:[9] when the study plan is near completion, find a 'devil's advocate' – a colleague who is willing to examine the plan and find its methodological weaknesses (not recommended for sensitive souls).

Notes and References

1. Converse JM, Presser S. (Survey questions: handcrafting the standardized questionnaire, 2nd edn. Beverly Hills, CA: Sage Publications; 1986.) who provide detailed advice on pretests of questionnaires, write: 'The Magic N for a pretest is of course as many as you can get. We see 25–75 as a valuable pretest range'.
2. Belson WA. The design and understanding of survey questions. Aldershot: Gower; 1981.
3. Suchard MA, Adamson S, Kennedy S. Netpoints: piloting patient attitudinal surveys on the web. British Medical Journal 1997; 315: 529.

    A message sent to an Internet discussion group for epidemiologists read 'I am composing a short questionnaire for a project about SCUBA divers … I need to validate the questionnaire. I am looking for anyone who is a recreational SCUBA diver that will be willing to fill out the questionnaire twice (Test–Retest approach)…'. This pretest would presumably lead to the development of a superb questionnaire for a study of cooperative scuba divers who use the Internet and are epidemiologists.
4. Rose GA, Blackburn H. Cardiovascular survey methods. Geneva: WHO; 1968. p. 58.
5. According to meta-analyses of trials, incentives generally improve response rates in mail, face-to-face and telephone surveys (Edwards P, Cooper R, Roberts I, Frost C. Meta-analysis of randomised trial of monetary incentives and response to mailed questionnaires. Journal of Epidemiology and Community Health 2005; 59: 987. Singer E, van Hoewyk J, Gebler N, Raghunathan T, McGonable K. The effect of incentives on response rates in interviewer-mediated surveys. Journal of Official Statistics 1999; 15: 217).

    If a prize is to be raffled among participants, it should probably be big. In a controlled trial in England, small prizes had no effect on response rates (Mortagy AK, Howell JBL, Waters WE. A useless raffle. Journal of Epidemiology and Community Health 1985; 39: 183).

    Financial incentives may deter well-off people from participating (Campanelli P. Minimising non-response before it happens: what can be done. Survey Methods Bulletin 1995; 37: 35).

6. A great deal of advice on obtaining research funds is available on the Internet. To find it, google for "(grant-writing OR grantsmanship)".

    Simple tips – the first of which, and possibly the most useful, is 'Ask a successfully funded researcher to critique your grant proposal before you submit it' – are provided by Hopkin K (How to wow a study section: a grantsmanship lesson. The Scientist 1998; 12(5): 110). See Kraicer J (The art of grantsmanship. 1997. Available at http://www.utoronto.ca/cip/sa_ArtGt.pdf).

    Information on sources of research funds can also be found on the Internet at, for example, http://rdfunding.org.uk/.funds.

7. For fuller advice on the training of interviewers, see Bowling A (Research methods in health: investigating health and health services, 2nd edn. Buckingham: Open University Press; 2002 Chapter 13).

8. Preparations for a household survey in a disadvantaged community in South Africa, including the selection and training of community members as interviewers, are described by Hildebrandt E (Survey data collection: operationalizing the research design. Public Health Nursing 1996; 13: 135). She points out that 'surveys are conceived and designed in offices at desks by people who are concerned about validity, reliability, randomization, sample size and research rigor. These same surveys are carried out by people who have agreed to walk miles of city streets or dusty roads, knock on door after door, develop trusting relationships with absolute strangers, and subsequently probe these strangers' lives. It is a vulnerability of survey research that it is difficult to control the data-collection process in this "living test tube"'.

9. Cochran WG, Moses LE, Mosteller F (eds). Planning and analysis of observational studies. New York, NY: Wiley; 1983. p. 71.

25

Collecting the Data

After the intellectual stimulation of the planning phase, the investigator now comes to a rather dull period when data are collected in a routine and predetermined manner. The greater the forethought and effort that were put into the planning and preparation, the more uneventful this new phase is likely to be.

However, the best-laid plans of good and bad researchers gang aft agley.[1] All kinds of unexpected contingencies may arise, and the investigator must be prepared to make running repairs as they become necessary.

Apart from this kind of troubleshooting, the investigator should take positive steps to test whether the collection of the data is in fact proceeding as it should. This may be done by instituting 'spot checks' (in Carl Becker's words, 'we need, from time to time, to take a look at the things that go without saying to see if they are still going') or, preferably, by regular periodic or ongoing surveillance and monitoring.

This has two main aspects. *Quality control* measures should be instituted[2] and *records of performance* should be maintained in an ongoing way, both for each subject and for the subjects as a whole (How many people have been examined? How many have refused to be interviewed? etc.).

Each questionnaire or examination record should be checked for errors and omissions, as soon after its completion as possible; coding (if required) can be done at the same time. Sometimes, omissions and errors can be corrected on the spot by editing; at other times, it may be necessary to refer to the person who completed the record, or even, if the omission or error is an important one, to repeat part of the examination or interview. If it is not possible to check all records, then a sample should be scrutinized. Regular meetings with examiners or interviewers are advisable, to discuss problems and maintain interest. If appropriate software is used, then quality control can also be built into the data-entry procedure (see p. 237). Quality control is an inbuilt feature of computer-assisted questionnaire programs (see p. 181). Additional checking and cleaning will usually be necessary after the preparation of the data set, and only when this has been done can data collection be regarded as complete.

Checks on reliability (see p. 155) form an important part of quality control. It is not often possible to conduct repeated examinations or interviews of the same persons, but sometimes the reliability of examinations is tested by having the same subjects examined on the same occasion by two examiners. Sometimes, limited analyses of

Research Methods in Community Medicine: Surveys, Epidemiological Research, Programme Evaluation, Clinical Trials J. H. Abramson and Z. H. Abramson Copyright © 2008, John Wiley & Sons Ltd

the findings are performed, to permit comparisons of the data obtained (for different individuals) by different examiners or interviewers, or at different times by the same examiners or interviewers. If, for example, one examiner finds a far higher rate of varicose veins than others, then it is worth exploring the possibility that this is due to a difference not in the subjects, but in the methods of diagnosing varicose veins. Similarly, if the hypertension rate springs up in a specific month, then this may be due to a defect in the instrument used. All measuring equipment should be checked periodically. If laboratory procedures are used, then reliability should be checked by periodic comparisons with standards and by the examination of replicate specimens ('blinded duplicates' with different labels). In addition, systematic differences between laboratories, or in the same laboratory at different times, may sometimes be detected by comparing the results of determinations (of different batches), in terms of their average values or the proportions of determinations falling above or below predetermined cutting points.

If these tests lead to substantive mid-study changes in methods or operational definitions then it is important to ensure that the subjects affected by the changes can subsequently be identified, or to use the new method in parallel with the old, so that the effect of the change can be appraised.

Throughout this stage, detailed records should be kept of people who are omitted from the study – subjects who are replaced, nonrespondents, persons who drop out or are excluded because of side-effects, etc. – so as to permit possible selection bias to be taken into account in the analysis (see p. 261). A record should be kept of their demographic characteristics and any other relevant information that can be easily obtained. Sometimes it is feasible to concentrate resources upon an attempt to obtain fuller information about a sample of nonrespondents.

Identifying the subjects, finding them and persuading them to cooperate may require hard work, patience and ingenuity. In a case-control study, the identification of cases may involve tedious searches through clinical records, disease registers, diagnostic indexes of hospitals, or other sources. The selection of controls, too, may be far from easy, especially if they are to be matched. If the subjects were identified from old or incorrect records, then it may be difficult to locate them. Names change – especially those of nubile females – and are often wrongly spelt. Recorded addresses may be incomplete, incorrect, or out of date. People who have moved may be difficult to trace, especially those who were living alone or as lodgers, and the divorced and widowed.[3] With luck, the present residents at the previous address may know where the subjects went, or a letter may be forwarded by the post office. In other cases, intensive detective work may be needed, including contacts with ex-neighbours, known relatives and friends, local shopkeepers, the postman, the local doctor or public health nurse, and so on.

Finding the subjects may be a real problem in a longitudinal study. Tracking them is facilitated if detailed information (e.g. nicknames, place of employment, whereabouts of family members, and home addresses of migrant workers) was recorded, if the time gap between contacts is short, if respondents are made to feel part of the study, and if interviewers are well trained and motivated.[4]

Even in a simple household survey, it may not be easy to make contact, especially if the family is childless or all its members go out to work. The only solution, of course, is to try, try, try again, sometimes in the morning, sometimes in the late afternoon or evening, sometimes at weekends. Once contact has been made, obtaining cooperation usually presents little difficulty in an interview survey. More nonresponse is to be expected if medical examinations or blood samples are needed. The examination process should be made as painless as possible – flexible schedules, no waiting around, and above all a pleasant atmosphere – but broken appointments and frank refusals can be expected, however convenient the arrangements. Here, too, perseverance is needed. Response rates can be boosted by establishing rapport, by repeated contacts and patient persuasion, by a judicious unreadiness to take 'no' for an answer (at least the first or second time it is said) – and, often, by a readiness to call for the help of a more irresistible member of the study team.

The longer these efforts go on, the more subjects will be traced, and the more nonrespondents will turn into respondents. But a line has to be drawn, and it is important to know where to draw it. A time comes when the added benefits fall far short of keeping pace with the added investment of effort, and the investigator should not hesitate to cry halt. This law of diminishing returns has been rephrased as the Ninety-Ninety Rule: 'The first 90 per cent of the task takes 90 per cent of the time, and the last 10 per cent takes the other 90 per cent'.[5]

Notes and References

1. Some readers have complained that this phrase is Greek to them. It is not, it is Scottish – 'gang aft agley' means 'often go wrong'.

   The following Will Rogers quotation may be substituted: 'There ain't but one place that a plan is any good and that's on paper. But the minute you get it off the sheet of paper and get it out in the air, it blows away, that's all' (Sterling BR, Sterling FN. Will Rogers speaks. New York, NY: Evans, 1996. p. 221).

   In an account of the day-to-day working of a cohort study in a family practice, a nurse and two doctors describe little things that can go wrong. When patients are asked to sign a consent form before blood-taking 'a few are illiterate, others arrive without their reading glasses ...'. The date of starting prophylactic aspirin therapy 'might be dated from a hospital summary provided the patient had not neglected to bring it ... [or] from an entry by the regular physician ... or by the nurse ... Sometimes all three sources are available but do not agree ... the information may be tucked away in a thick file containing tens of pages ... the energy with which the abstracter pursues the search is also a factor in determining what figure will ultimately be entered ... banal mistakes such as neglecting to rotate a test tube containing anticoagulants or a misplaced sticker ... A worm's-eye view has afforded us some sobering insights into what can go wrong with a project after issues of method have been decided' (Naveh P, Yaphe J, Herman J. Research in primary care: a worm's-eye view. Journal of Clinical Epidemiology 1996; 49: 1323).

2. For a detailed account of the *quality control measures* used in a large-scale health examination survey, see National Center for Health Statistics (Quality control in a national health examination survey. Vital and Health Statistics, series 2, no 44. Washington, DC: Public Health Service; 1972).

3. For descriptions of methods used to trace *hard-to-find subjects*, see Skeels HM, Skodak M (Techniques of a high-yield follow-up study in the field. Public Health Reports 1965; 80: 249), Modan B (Some methodological aspects of a retrospective follow-up study. American Journal of Epidemiology 1966; 82: 297) and Bright M (A follow-up study of the Commission on Chronic Illness Morbidity survey in Baltimore: I. Tracing a large population sample over time. Journal of Chronic Diseases 1967; 20: 707; A follow-up study of the Commission on Chronic Illness Morbidity survey in Baltimore: III. Residential mobility and prospective studies. Journal of Chronic Diseases 1969; 21: 749).

4. Hill Z. Reducing attrition in panel studies in developing countries. International Journal of Epidemiology 2004; 33: 493.

5. Wallechinsky D, Wallace I, Wallace A. The book of lists. London: Cassell; 1977. p. 300.

26

Statistical Analysis

When the data have been collected, entered, checked and cleaned, we can at last start on the analysis, and begin to reap the fruit of our labours. 'O frabjous day, callooh, callay' we can chortle in our joy. (Unless we have come to 'regard ... statistical tools more as instruments of torture than as diagnostic aids in the art and science of data analysis'.)[1]

But this book has no pretensions to being a statistics textbook. We will deal with general strategy only, and will not try to suggest statistical procedures or explain them or their rationale. There are many statistics textbooks,[2] a number of statistics primers on the Internet,[3] and a much larger number of statisticians who can provide advice and help. Nor will we suggest what statistical software should be used, apart from remarking that many good free programs are available on the Internet; some of these are listed in Appendix C, which also indicates which of them provide simple descriptive statistics, bivariate analyses, stratified analyses, and other specific statistical procedures.

The choice of statistical methods, particularly when more elaborate analyses are contemplated, requires a degree of statistical knowledge – knowing, for example, what procedures are appropriate for ordinal or other types of variable, and whether nonparametric procedures (which make no assumptions about the frequency distributions of the variables) are indicated. Recourse can be had to the decision trees and guides to the choice of tests and other procedures that are provided in many textbooks and on the Internet,[4] which are based mainly on the type and number of the variables. But 'no algorithm can address the most important aspect of selection: the judgement needed to know what you want to learn from the data'.[5]

The detailed analysis plan must obviously depend on the nature and objectives of the study. We have previously stressed the importance of having clearly formulated study objectives, expressed in measurable terms (Chapter 4). The investigator should have a clear idea of what kinds of results will meet these objectives, and this should determine the choice of methods. Skeleton tables (p. 128) may help to crystallize ideas about the analysis, and can serve as a basis for the instructions to be given to the computer. On the increasingly rare occasions when data are processed manually, these tables can be used as work sheets.

Whatever statistical software is used, and whether the investigator is personally involved in running it or not, he or she should have, or should acquire, a sufficient understanding of what the program does and the options it provides (RTFM!)[6] to be able to read the output.

Research Methods in Community Medicine: Surveys, Epidemiological Research, Programme Evaluation, Clinical Trials   J. H. Abramson and Z. H. Abramson   Copyright © 2008, John Wiley & Sons Ltd

Every set of results should be checked. Are the totals and marginal totals[7] correct? Are missing values handled correctly? Are there blatant errors – results that just 'don't make sense' (the interocular traumatic test)?[8]

The more elaborate statistical programs can use any data set; some have their own data-entry mechanisms and their own data sets, and some can import data sets from other programs. Some programs can use data pasted from a spreadsheet or a text file. And still others require keyboard entry of data – sometimes the raw data, and sometimes counts or summary figures that have been prepared previously, either manually or by using a program that processes primary data.

Adequate documentation of the analysis is important. Tables and other results should be fully labelled and listed, and records should be kept of the categories of individuals who were included or excluded, how missing values were handled, and how variables and their categories have been defined. All this information may come ready printed in computer outputs, but the investigator should make sure they can decode it.

We discuss statistical analysis in this chapter, and the interpretation of results in the next. But analysis and interpretation are interdependent, and should be seen as activities that go hand in hand, rather than as separate stages. Except in the simplest of investigations, the investigator produces or obtains a set of analytic results, then carefully considers them, sees what inferences may be drawn from them and what further questions they open up, decides what further facts are needed in order to test the inferences or answer the questions, produces or obtains the new tabulations or calculations that are required, thinks about the new facts, does more analyses if necessary, and so on. Each set of results influences decisions about the next analysis.

Sequence

No hard and fast rules can be laid down for the sequence of the analysis, but most investigators would agree that simple descriptive results should be produced first, enabling the investigator to 'get to know the data', and that more elaborate analyses, such as multivariate analyses that permit the simultaneous examination of relationships involving many variables, should come last.

---

1. Get to know the data.
2. Do simple analyses.
3. Do more elaborate analyses.

There may be a temptation to jump in at the deep end and start with a multivariate analysis (e.g. multiple logistic regression), knowing that this is what will provide the main results required to meet the study's objectives, but most experts would consider this unwise:

> We regard this approach as unsound, and instead recommend a more orderly application of analytic methods, beginning with simple descriptive statistical displays and summaries. Gaps, patterns and inconsistencies in the data can be discovered and further analyses suggested by this examination. Next, relationships between variables

can be explored by means of simple cross-tabulations, scatter plans, and measures of association ... Once again, patterns and inconsistencies are sought and, when found, lead to additional tabulations. Finally, multivariate methods may be applied to the data after a full exploration has been conducted using simpler techniques.[9]

A textbook on multivariate statistics devotes a whole chapter to 'Screening data prior to analysis'.[10]

Let us see how the above general strategy (getting to know the data, then simple analyses, then more elaborate analyses) might work out in practice. As an illustration, our scenario is a cross-sectional community study of haemoglobin levels, anaemia, and risk factors for anaemia. But the principles apply to any study.

It is usually advisable to start with *simple descriptive statistics*, examining the frequency distributions of all relevant variables. That is, a separate table is prepared for each variable, showing how many individuals fall into each category or at each value of the variable. It is best to use detailed scales of measurement at this stage (i.e. narrow categories, with little or no 'collapsing') so that the distributions can provide a basis for decisions about the categories to be used in subsequent stages.

The frequency distributions provide an opportunity to check the data (Are the totals correct? Are missing values handled correctly?) and to begin to get to know the data. They may influence decisions about subsequent steps in the analysis. Plans for a detailed study of relationships between social class and anaemia, for example, may have to be abandoned if the study population turns out to be very homogeneous in social class. ('Make sure your variables vary.')[11] If there are only three cases of anaemia, then there is little point in planning complicated tables on its epidemiology, unless we modify our definition of the disease. If there are an excessive number of individuals in an 'unknown' category, then it may be decided that the variable cannot be studied. Moreover, peculiarities in a distribution may throw doubt on the accuracy of the data (low face validity). Outliers may be found, i.e. values that differ very markedly from the others; these can have an unduly large effect on the results, and may necessitate special handling.[12]

Simple *indices that summarize frequency distributions*,[13] such as means, proportions, and rates, may be calculated at this time. They may, of course, come ready made from a computer together with the frequency distributions.

The next step is usually the performance of *bivariate*[14] analyses, i.e. the examination of pairs of variables. In most community medicine studies it is helpful if associations between relevant variables and selected 'universal' variables (see p. 103) are explored early in the analysis. This may be done by repeating the descriptive analysis in selected strata, by looking at the frequency distribution of relevant variables in (say) different age or sex or ethnic groups, or in different seasons of the year. Also, in epidemiological studies whose main thrust is the assessment of associations with risk factors or possible causes of a disease, and in clinical and programme trials, the relationships between the dependent variable and each of the independent variables are generally appraised. This may be called 'screening for associations', with the aim of determining which of the independent variables are strongly enough associated with the dependent variable to justify their inclusion in a multivariate analysis.

These bivariate relationships may be explored by obtaining *contingency tables* (cross-tabulations), as on page 270, or by scrutinizing the scattergrams (scatter-plots) produced by some computer programs, or by calculating *measures of the strength of the association*, such as the difference between mean values (e.g. mean haemoglobin values), or the difference between proportions or rates (e.g. of anaemia), or the ratio of proportions or of rates, or the odds ratio, or correlation or regression coefficients, or a variety of other measures.

In some studies, the above analyses will yield all the information needed to fulfil the study's objectives. In others, further exploration may be needed, and associations that are of interest will need to be investigated more intensively, along the lines discussed in Chapter 27. This will generally necessitate a *multivariate analysis* that involves more than two variables.

Age, sex and other 'universal' variables are among those most frequently introduced into the analysis, bivariate or multivariate. In addition, consideration is usually given to other variables known or suspected to be associated with the dependent variable. No set rules can be laid down. Decisions depend on the aims of the study, on feasibility, and above all on the imaginativeness and ingenuity of the investigator.

The simplest method of multivariate analysis is *stratification* (subclassification), i.e. the construction of multiple contingency tables that allow for simultaneous cross-classification by three or more variables; for a simple example, see Table 28.2 (p. 271). The analysis generally uses the Mantel–Haenszel procedure, or a similar one. These procedures aim to clarify the relationship between a dependent variable (e.g. anaemia) and an independent variable (say, pregnancy) by (a) seeing whether the relationship differs in different strata, which would indicate that the stratifying variable (say, educational level) has a *modifying effect* (see p. 271), (b) assessing the strength and statistical significance of the association when the effect of the stratify-ing measure is (mathematically) controlled, and (c) seeing whether controlling the effect of the stratifying variable alters the strength of the association, which might suggest *confounding* by the stratifying variable. A number of different procedures may be used for this purpose, depending on whether the variables are dichotomous, nominal, ordinal, or numerical, and whether the study is based on matched observa-tions, as in an individually matched case-control study. The stratification method is, of course, unwieldy if the data have to be stratified by many independent variables.

Alternatively, a *mathematical model* to express the effects of the independent vari-ables can be chosen and applied to the data, and the results (assuming that the model is an apt one) can be used to indicate how strong these effects are, and to point to effect modification and confounding effects. The available procedures, which use different models and are appropriate in different circumstances, include multiple linear regres-sion, multiple logistic regression, multiple Poisson regression, and Cox proportional hazards regression. (The analysis of multilevel studies requires particularly compli-cated models and methods.)[15] The vogue today is to use logistic regression or Cox regression. These techniques permit the simultaneous examination of relationships involving a number of variables, and permit controlling of confounding. Since the mathematical models on which they are based may or may not be appropriate in a specific situation ('all models are wrong but some are useful'),[17] their results should be used only if there is evidence suggesting a good fit between the facts and the model, e.g. by performing a goodness-of-fit test if logistic regression is used. (This proviso, it may be remarked, is usually ignored by investigators.)[18]

It is often helpful to do an analysis by stratification techniques first, so as to identify and get some understanding of important interrelationships.

It is, of course, not essential to follow the above sequence. Instead, other variables may be built into the analysis from the outset. This applies especially to 'universal' variables; tables are often broken down by age and sex[19] from a very early stage of the analysis. When there are two or more study populations, e.g. cases and controls, they are often analysed separately from the outset.

Notes and References

1. Cobb GW. Introductory textbooks: a framework for evaluation. Journal of the American Statistical Association 1987; 82: 321.
2. *Statistics textbooks* with special relevance to the analysis of health data include the following. The books are arranged by the number of their pages, as a rough guide to their simplicity or complexity.

   Harris M, Taylor G. Medical statistics made easy. Taylor & Francis; 2003. 120 pp.

   Stewart A. Basic statistics and epidemiology: a practical guide. Radcliffe Publishing; 2002. 144 pp.

   Campbell MJ. Statistics at square two. BMJ Books; 2006. 144 pp.

   Petrie A, Sabin C. Medical statistics at a glance, 2nd edn. Blackwell Publishing; 2005. 160 pp.

   Campbell MJ. Statistics at square one. BMJ Books; 2002. 160 pp.

   Campbell MJ. Medical statistics: a commonsense approach for health professionals. Wiley; 2007. 256 pp.

   McNeil D. Epidemiological research methods. New York, NY: Wiley; 1996. 305 pp.

   Peat J, Barton B. Medical statistics: a guide to data analysis and critical appraisal. BMJ Books; 2005. 336 pp.

   Jewell NP. Statistics for epidemiology. CRC Press; 2003. 352 pp.

   Dawson B, Trapp R. Basic and clinical biostatistics. McGraw-Hill; 2004. 416 pp.

   Bland JM. An introduction to medical statistics, 3rd edn. Oxford University Press; 2000. 422 pp.

   Selvin S. Statistical analysis of epidemiologic data, 3rd edn. Oxford University Press; 2004. 492 pp.

   Glantz SA. Primer biostatistics, 6th edn. Appleton and Lange; 2005. 500 pp.

   Gerstman BB. Basic biostatistics: statistics for public health practice. Boston, MA: Jones and Bartlett; 2007. 537 pp.

   Altman DG. Practical statistics for medical research. London: Chapman & Hall; 1991. 611 pp.

   Armitage P. Statistical methods in medical research, 4th edn. Oxford: Blackwell Science; 2002. 817 pp.

   Van Belle G, Fisher LD, Heagerty PJ, Lumley TS. Biostatistics: a methodology for the health sciences, 2nd edn. Wiley; 2004. 872 pp.

   Zar JH. Biostatistical analysis, 4th edn. Prentice Hall; 1998. 942 pp.

Daniel W W 2005 Biostatistics: a foundation for analysis in the health sciences. 8th edn. John Wiley & Sons. 944 pp.

3. A number of statistics primers are available on the Internet:

    Dallal GE. The little handbook of statistical practice; 2006. http://www.tufts.edu/~gdallal/LHSP.HTM.

    Gerstman BB. StatPrimer; 2003 http://www.sjsu.edu/faculty/gerstman/StatPrimer.

    Lane D. HyperStat online statistics textbook; 2006 http://davidmlane.com/hyperstat/index.html.

    Swinscow TDV. Statistics at square one, 9th edn. BMJ Books; 1997. http://www.bmj.com/collections/statsbk/index.dtl.

    StatSoft, Inc. Electronic statistics textbook; 2006. http://www.statsoft.com/textbook/stathome.html.

    Altman D, Bland M. Statistics notes; 1994–2006. (Published in the British Medical Journal.) http://www-users.york.ac.uk/~mb55/pubs/pbstnote.htm.

    Simple introductions to data analysis basics (among other topics) are available at http://www2.sph.unc.edu/nccphp/focus/issuelist.htm.

4. *Guides to the choice of statistical procedures*, based mainly on the number and type of the variables, are available at the following sites:

    http://bama.ua.edu/~jleeper/627/choosestat.htm

    http://www.socialresearchmethods.net/selstat/p5_3.htm

    http://www.graphpad.com/www/Book/Choose.htm.

5. Gerstman BB. How to know what to use; 2001. Available at http://www.sjsu.edu/faculty/gerstman/StatPrimer/HowTo_Know.PDF.

6. A computer-speak acronym for 'Read The Fact-filled Manual'.

7. In a table showing a cross-classification, the totals of the figures in each column and row are referred to as 'marginal totals'. These are the totals in each category of the variables shown, i.e. simple frequency distributions. When one inspects the frequency distributions of variables (see p. 253) one can impress the uninitiated by saying that one is looking at the marginals.

8. It hits you between the eyes.

9. Stolley PD, Schlesselman JJ. Planning and conducting a study. In: Schlesselman JJ (ed.), Case-control studies: design, conduct, analysis. New York, NY: Oxford University Press; 1982. pp. 69–104.

10. Tabachnick BG, Fidell LS. Using multivariate statistics, 5th edn. Allyn & Bacon; 2006. Chapter 4.

11. 'If the heart of research is to compare cases which fall in different categories, the research worker must have plenty of cases which differ in their classification. It is hard to argue with such a truism, but it is easy to forget it' (Davis JA. Elementary survey analysis. Englewood Cliff, NJ: Prentice Hall; 1971).

12. There is no simple solution to the problem of *outliers*. The least that should be done is to be aware of their presence, and it is generally worth seeing how their exclusion affects the findings. It may be decided to modify the scale of measurement (e.g. by collapsing categories) so that outliers are grouped together with less extreme values, or to exclude the outliers, or to change them to less extreme values. See Tabachnick and Fidell (1989; see note 10), pp. 66–70.

    Robust means, e.g. *trimmed means*, are calculated by ignoring extreme values at both ends of the distribution.

13. Indices that may be used to describe frequency distributions include measures of central tendency, measures of dispersion, and proportions.

    The commonest *measures of central tendency* are the arithmetic mean (used for interval or ratio scales) and the *median* or *50th percentile*, which is the value of the middle observation when all the observations are arranged in ascending order (for ordinal, interval or ratio scales).

The commonest *measure of dispersion* around the mean is the *standard deviation* (not to be confused with the standard error of the mean). *Quartiles* (the values below which fall one-quarter, one-half, and three-quarters respectively of all values) or the *interquartile range* between the upper and lower quartiles may be used to measure dispersion around a median. Use is frequently made of *percentiles* (the values below which fall 3%, 10%, etc. of the observations), especially to summarize anthropometric data.

The number of individuals in a category may be expressed as a *relative frequency*, i.e. as a *proportion* (e.g. a *percentage*) of the total. The data may be combined to show what proportions of individuals have values that lie above (or below) successive levels (*cumulative frequencies*). *Rates* are briefly discussed in note 3, Chapter 10.

14. In statistics, a *bivariate analysis* is an analysis involving two variables. But epidemiologists often refer to such analyses as *univariate*, thinking of only the independent variable, because they usually assess the association of each independent variable (in turn) with the dependent variable (a series of 'univariate' analyses) before putting them together into a multivariate analysis.

15. Methods of *multilevel analysis* (*hierarchical modelling*) are described, *inter alia*, by Diez-Roux AV (Multilevel analysis in public health research. Annual Review of Public Health 2000; 21: 171) and Teachman J, Crowder K (Multilevel models in family research: some conceptual and methodological issues. Journal of Marriage and Family 2002; 64: 280). For software, see Appendix C.

The use of logistic regression is discussed by Merlo J, Chaix B, Ohlsson H, Beckman AS, Johnell K, Hjerpe P, Rastam L, Larsen K (A brief conceptual tutorial of multilevel analysis in social epidemiology: using measures of clustering in multilevel logistic regression to investigate contextual phenomena. Journal of Epidemiology and Community Health 2006; 60: 290).

16. For succinct advice on the formulation of a model, see Kleinbaum DG (Epidemiologic methods: the 'art' in the state of the art. Journal of Clinical Epidemiology 2002; 55: 1196).

17. Box GEP. Robustness in the strategy of scientific model building. In: Launer L, Wilkinson GN (eds), Robustness in statistics. New York, NY: Academic Press; 1979.

18. Regrettably, the proviso that *the model's appropriateness* should be examined is honoured more in the breach than in the observance. In a meta-analysis of peer-reviewed studies of patients' interest in genetic testing for cancer susceptibility, using logistic regression, not a single study was found that reported tests of goodness of fit or other appraisals of the validity of a logistic model (Bagley SC, White H, Golomb BA. Logistic regression in the medical literature: standards for use and reporting, with particular attention to one medical domain. Journal of Clinical Epidemiology 2001; 54: 979).

A review of articles using logistic regression in two major epidemiological journals revealed that only 19% reported tests of goodness of fit (Ottenbacher KJ, Ottenbacher HR, Tooth L, Ostir GV. A review of two journals found that articles using multivariable logistic regression frequently did not report commonly recommended assumptions. Journal of Clinical Epidemiology 2004; 57: 1147).

This is not the only instance of disregard for statistical precepts. Logistic regression can use a conditional approach (suitable for matched data) and an unconditional one. A review of 917 articles using logistic regression for matched data (e.g. matched case-control studies) revealed that only 50% reported use of the conditional method; 5% used the unconditional method (which can seriously overestimate odds ratios), and 45% gave no indication of what approach was used (Rahman M, Sakamoto J, Fukui T. Conditional versus unconditional logistic regression in the medical literature. Journal of Clinical Epidemiology 2003; 56: 101).

19. Hopefully, unlike the investigator.

27

Interpreting the Findings

Now has come the time to *really* reap the fruits of the study, by considering its findings and using them to answer the questions that were specified as study objectives.

There may also be fringe benefits – interest is sometimes extended to finding answers to questions that were not posed at the outset. This exploration can be useful, provided that it is done with reservations – since the study was not designed to answer these other questions, the answers may be inadequate or misleading. The testing of hypotheses that the study was not designed to test, but that are suggested by the data, has been referred to as *data dredging*.[1] Any large set of variables is likely to show some associations that have occurred only by chance ('if you torture the data long enough, they will confess'),[1] and misleading conclusions may be reached if the possibility is ignored that some or all of the associations detected are due to chance. In Ontario, a study without prior hypotheses revealed 72 significant associations between the astrological signs under which residents were born and their causes of hospitalization, but when allowance was made for multiple testing, no associations were significant.[2] An association brought to the surface by data dredging is best treated not as evidence that the relationship exists – that is, that it is likely to be found in other data sets also – but only as a clue suggesting that it *may* exist. Other studies can then be designed to test this hypothesis. This problem may arise whenever multiple significance tests are applied to the same body of data.[3]

The interpretation of findings may be child's play,[4] or it may present formidable difficulties. Usually, the task is more exacting than it seems on the surface. In one investigator's words of warning:

> An eminent British biostatistician, Major Greenwood, remarked that once the proper questions are asked and the relevant facts collected, any sensible person can reach the correct conclusions. There are two limitations. The facts are never quite complete nor completely accurate, and, as Voltaire pointed out in his Dictionnaire Philosophique, 'Common sense is not so common'.[5]

When interpreting the findings, the first and main task is to 'make sense' of them, in the context of the population that was studied or sampled. Consideration should be given to the possible effects of random sampling variation and bias, both of which will be discussed in this chapter. What is the *internal validity* of the study, i.e. can it yield sound conclusions relating to the study population? Interpreting the findings is generally more

Research Methods in Community Medicine: Surveys, Epidemiological Research, Programme Evaluation, Clinical Trials   J. H. Abramson and Z. H. Abramson   Copyright © 2008, John Wiley & Sons Ltd

difficult in analytic studies, which investigate associations between variables, than in simple descriptive ones. (The appraisal of associations will be discussed in the next chapter.)

The second task is to draw inferences that go beyond the specific findings in the specific study population. This has two aspects, both of which are discussed in Chapter 29. First, is it possible to make generalizations to a broader population? That is, what is the *external validity* of the study (its capacity to yield sound generalizations going outside the study population)? Internal validity is a prerequisite for, but does not guarantee, external validity. Second, what are the practical implications of the results? Do the findings point to a need for changes in the provision of medical care, for public health action, for further studies, for the development of new investigative tools, etc.?

We have previously emphasized the interdependence of the statistical analysis and the interpretation of findings. Throughout the process of interpretation, a need may arise for new analyses, and sometimes for supplementary data.

Random Sampling Variation

Caution is required in drawing inferences from findings in samples, even if the samples are randomly selected, since chance differences may be expected between different samples drawn randomly from the same population. Differences may similarly arise by chance in a trial in which subjects are randomly assigned to experimental and control groups.

One of the advantages of random sampling and random assignment, however, is that it is easy to estimate the findings in the sampled population. Using formulae, tables, or a computer program, we can estimate, with a specified degree of certainty (usually 95 or 99% – this is the *confidence level*), within what range (*confidence interval*) the value in the sampled population probably lies.[6] The narrower this range, the greater the precision of the estimate. If a prevalence of 10% is detected in a simple random sample containing 200 individuals, then there is an exact 95% probability that the rate in the population is between 6.2 and 15.0% (the lower and upper confidence limits). If the sample contains only 30 individuals then the interval is much wider, from 2.1 to 26.5%. Confidence intervals can also be calculated for means and other measures of a distribution, and for rate ratios, odds ratios, and other measures of the strength of an association.

Bias

Bias is defined as 'any trend in the collection, analysis, interpretation, publication, or review of data that can lead to conclusions that are systematically [i.e. one-sidedly] different from the truth'.[7]

'Bias' is not used here as a synonym for 'prejudice'. The investigator's preconceived opinions and preferences are, of course, among the factors that may lead – as a result, it may be hoped, of unconscious processes only – to biased findings or to distortions in the interpretation and use of findings. A study of 106 review articles on passive smoking revealed that 74% of those written by authors with tobacco industry affiliations concluded that passive smoking was not harmful, as compared with 15% of those written by authors without such affiliations; publications about drugs used for allergies and lung diseases reported favourable results in almost all (98%) of the studies sponsored by pharmaceutical companies, but in only 32% of the nonsponsored studies; and a meta-analysis of scientific articles on the health effects of soft drinks, fruit juices, and milk showed a significant association with the funding source – no studies sponsored by the food industry reported results unfavourable to commercial interests.[8] A selective blindness to awkward facts, a failure to look for contrary evidence, and a too-easy acceptance of incomplete proof may lead to conclusions that happen to coincide with what the investigator wanted ('wish bias') or expected. This is part of the 'self-fulfilling prophecy' syndrome.[8] The investigator should seek insight into his or her motivations – how strong is the felt need to 'prove a case' or come up with a 'discovery'? An investigator aware of being prejudiced, or of a possible conflict of interests, should take special pains to interpret findings objectively and fairly, should use every opportunity to discuss the interpretation with colleagues, and should then not only hear but also listen to what they have to say.

Avoiding bias is an important element in the planning and performance of a study, as stressed in previous chapters, where many specific sources of bias were mentioned. At the present stage, before interpreting the findings, the investigator should systematically consider the possibility that they may be biased, as a result of shortcomings either in the study plan or (by the ineluctable operation of Murphy's Law)[9] in its execution. It may not be too hard, if the study's imperfections are not yet known, to find a colleague who will gladly point them out.

Biases may be classified in different ways.[7] We will here consider two kinds of bias: *selection bias* and *information bias*. Confounding, which may also be regarded as a kind of bias, will be discussed in Chapter 28 and biases that are specific to trials will be discussed in Chapter 32.

Selection bias

Selection bias is the distortion produced by the manner in which subjects are selected for study, or by the loss of subjects who have been selected. If the individuals for whom data are available are not representative of the study population, then this may obviously impair the study's validity with respect to whatever the investigator wants to know about the study population – the prevalence of a disease, the strength of an association with a disease, etc. – as well as the capacity to make valid generalizations. The bias may be caused by (*inter alia*) failure to choose or study an appropriate sample (*sample bias, noncoverage bias*) or by losses or exclusions of study subjects (e.g. *nonresponse* or *nonconsent bias*) or *missing data bias*.

In analytic studies in which groups are compared, selection bias may be caused by differences between the groups with respect to subject selection or subject losses, such that the associations found in the study are different from those that would have been found if these differences had not occurred. Common causes are *detection bias* (failure to include certain cases, e.g. those diagnosed outside hospitals) and *differential nonresponse*. In case-control studies, other common sources of bias are the drawing of cases and controls from different study bases, *incidence-prevalence bias* (*selective survival* or *Neyman bias*, resulting from the influence of a risk factor on mortality from the disease),[10] the selection of inappropriate controls, and selective factors in the identification of study subjects, e.g. when inclusion in a case register is influenced by exposure to a possible causal factor,[11] or when inclusion as a control is influenced by possession of a telephone. In cohort studies and trials, selective losses are a common cause of selection bias. In a cohort study or trial, there may be *follow-up or drop-out bias* if the risk of developing the outcome condition is different for subjects who are censored (i.e. withdrawn from the analysis because of loss of contact, refusal to continue, death, etc.) and for those who remain in the analysis. In a trial, selection bias may be caused by nonrandom allocation to treatment and control groups, and by the exclusion of subjects who stopped their treatment (see intention-to-treat analysis, p. 333).

The ability to generalize findings from the study population to a reference population may obviously be affected by the above sources of bias, which can hence impair both external as well as internal validity. There are also kinds of selection bias that may affect external validity without necessarily affecting internal validity, as a result of the choice of a study population that is not representative of the broader population to whom the investigator wishes to apply the results. A study of hospital patients, for example, may yield completely sound conclusions about factors associated with a given disease in the study population, but these may not be applicable in the population at large (*referral filter bias*, *Berksonian bias*, etc.). This kind of problem may arise in any study performed in a 'special' or 'different' study population. It may result from selective admission to the study population, as in a study of volunteers (*self-selection bias*) or of bus drivers, vegetarians, or other groups defined by their occupations or behaviour; examples are listed on pp. 64–66. It may also result from *selective migration* into or out of a population, or from *selective survival*. The 'special' nature of a study population, of course, does not lead to bias if interest is limited to this special population.

Selection bias can have a marked impact on a study's results.[12] While selectivity can seldom be completely avoided, its degree should always be appraised. To do this, the way in which the sample or samples were chosen should be critically reviewed. Special attention should be paid to substitutions (see p. 83), nonrespondents, nonparticipants, patients who were removed from a clinical trial because of side-effects, and drop-outs. How numerous were these, and what were the reasons? Bias is particularly likely if the selective factors were illness, death, or other reasons that might be connected with the variables under study. Unless the rates of substitutions, nonresponse and drop-outs were negligible, the individuals included in the study should be compared with those who were omitted, using any demographic and other relevant information available. In a study in which repeated efforts are made to enlist response, it may be helpful to compare early and late respondents to obtain insights into factors affecting response (although it cannot be assumed that nonrespondents necessarily resemble late respondents).[13] Even at this stage, it may not be too late to collect further data to make these comparisons possible. Any differences that are found, such as an underrepresentation of working mothers among the respondents, may be helpful in the interpretation of the findings. An absence of such differences increases the likelihood that there is no important selection bias; unfortunately, it can never guarantee this, especially if non-response or drop-out rates are high.

Sometimes it is possible to control selection bias by statistical manipulations during the analysis. If there was a low response or follow-up rate in some age groups, for example, then the findings can be weighted in accordance with the age composition of the total study population to obtain an estimate that compensates for this selectivity.[14] This method of adjustment becomes complicated if many variables (age, sex, social class, etc.) are taken into account, and is especially unwieldy if stratified sampling was used, so that different weights are needed in each stratum; multivariate procedures can simplify the computation. Alternatively, the findings in separate groups (age-specific rates, etc.) might suffice, without using the global finding in the total study population. A disadvantage is that these methods are based on the assumption that, within each defined category of the population, respondents and nonrespondents are similar, which is not necessarily true. Weighting may actually increase bias, if a greater weight happens to be given to a stratum where the respondents are especially unrepresentative.

Adjustments may also be based on assumed dissimilarities between the individuals for whom data are and are not available. In a study of causes of death, for example, the data were adjusted to compensate for the fact that (in different years) between 4 and 16% of deaths were not medically certified. Two alternative assumptions were made: (1) that the proportion of deaths from each cause (in a given age–sex stratum and in a given year) was twice as high among the uncertified cases as among the certified cases; and (2) that it was half as high. The two sets of alternative estimates yielded similar conclusions concerning trends of mortality from specific causes.[15] Even more extreme assumptions are sometimes made, e.g. that all or no nonresponders smoke, so as to obtain maximal and minimal estimates.

Probably the best way of handling nonresponse bias, although seldom a practicable one, is to invest intensive efforts in a drive to obtain full information about a sufficiently large and representative sample of the nonrespondents. These can then be compared with the respondents with respect to the characteristics the investigator wishes to study.

Information bias

Information bias is bias caused by shortcomings in the collecting, recording, coding or processing of data. Its origins include the people who collected information (*observer bias*, *interviewer bias*), the use of defective questionnaires or other instruments (*measurement procedure bias*, *insensitive measure bias*, *instrument bias*, etc.), the use of proxy variables (e.g. date of diagnosis instead of date of onset, or current diet to represent previous diet), and one-sided responses by the people studied (*recall bias*, *response bias*, *social undesirability bias*). It may arise because 'blind' procedures (see p. 146) were not used, or because of deviations in compliance with experimental or other study procedures. Biased information about categorical variables may be termed *misclassification bias*.

Information bias is particularly troublesome when its presence, degree or direction varies in different groups of subjects. Differential validity (see p. 163) of this kind may occur if (among other possibilities) the data for the various groups under comparison were not collected in a standard way – there may have been different observers or interviewers, or different operational definitions or criteria may have been used, or different instruments or techniques, or different follow-up periods. Differential misclassification can either exaggerate or downplay an effect.[16]

In a case-control or cross-sectional study of a supposed cause of a disease, bias may be produced by the fact that information about the supposed cause is collected after the occurrence of the disease; this may result in *exposure suspicion bias* (knowledge of the subject's disease status may influence the intensity of a search for exposure to the cause), *rumination bias* (a form of recall bias: cases may ruminate about causes for their illnesses and thus report different prior exposures than controls), or *obsequiousness bias* (subjects may alter their responses to fit what they think the investigator wants). Conversely, if there is a known history of exposure (in a cohort or cross-sectional study or a trial) then there may be a more energetic hunt for the disease (*diagnostic suspicion bias*, a form of detection bias).

When possible bias is suspected, evidence of its presence should be sought. In a study in which people with and without cancer were interviewed, for example, the presence of interviewer bias caused by awareness that respondents had cancer was tested by looking separately at the data for patients whose cancer diagnoses were subsequently disproved.[17]

When possible, the direction and magnitude of the bias should be appraised so that allowances can be made when inferences are drawn. The effects of the bias can sometimes be controlled or corrected. If, for example, there is a constant bias in laboratory results, due to a mistake in the preparation of a standard solution, then it may be rectified by applying a correction factor to the results. Special analyses may be required, as in a case-control study of a form of cancer, where there was a suspicion that the differences observed between patients and controls might be partly due to the fact that proxy informants had been far more often used for patients (many of whom had died) than for controls. Therefore, special analyses were conducted, restricted to data with high face validity. When parity was investigated, attention was confined to cases and controls who themselves reported their parity. When the subjects' home circumstances in their childhood were investigated, use was made of information provided by subjects or their parents or siblings, but not by other informants.[18] Computations may be used to assess the effects of misclassification.[19]

Notes and References

1. Finding an association by *data dredging* and then using the same data to test its significance may lead to unwarranted conclusions; data dredging 'should be considered as useful, if at

all, only for generating hypotheses for examination in further studies' (Altman DG. Practical statistics for medical research. London: Chapman & Hall; 1991).

On the other hand, there are proponents of data dredging who stress 'the important danger of not studying an association when it actually exists', which they call a 'type zero error' (Michels KB, Rosner BA. Data trawling: to fish or not to fish. Lancet 1996; 348: 1152). The noteworthiness of an association (or its absence) depends on whether it provides new knowledge and on the quality of the data, not on its statistical significance or whether the hypothesis was formulated *a priori*, says Marshall JR (Data dredging and noteworthiness. Epidemiology 1990; 1: 5).

A British Medical Journal editorialist points out that data dredging is a major source of the 'health scare of the week' that appears each Friday and is controverted by subsequent studies, and suggests that findings with a P value more than 0.001 should be ignored (Smith GD. Data dredging, bias, or confounding: they can all get you into the BMJ and the Friday papers. British Medical Journal 2002; 325: 1437). He cites a solution proposed by medical journalist James Le Fanu: 'The simple expedient of closing down most university departments of epidemiology could ... extinguish this endlessly fertile source of anxiety mongering'.

The aphorism 'If you torture the data long enough, they will confess' is attributed to the economist Ronald Coase.

2. In a study of a randomly selected half of the population of Ontario, in which thousands of significance tests were done (without prior hypotheses) to detect associations between 223 causes for hospitalization and the signs of the zodiac, 72 significant associations were found. But when the 24 strongest of these were tested in the other half of the population, only two remained significant – residents born under Sagittarius were especially likely to be hospitalized because of fractures of the humerus, and Leos because of gastrointestinal haemorrhages. When the significance level was adjusted to account for multiple comparisons (see note 3), there were no significant associations in either half of the population (Austin PC, Mamdani MM, Jourlink DN, Hux JE. Testing multiple statistical hypotheses resulted in spurious associations: a study of astrological signs and health. Journal of Clinical Epidemiology 2006; 59: 964).

    Misleading conclusions are possible if an association is tested separately (without prior hypotheses) in a number of subgroups, e.g. age–sex groups, 'in the hope that "something will turn up" that has a P value lower than 0.05. This approach to analysis is similar to the sharpshooter who fires at a barn and then paints a target around the bullet hole. A target shows how accurate the shot was only if it was in place before the shooting' (Fletcher J. Subgroup analyses: how to avoid being misled. British Medical Journal 2007; 335: 96).

3. *Multiple comparison* or simultaneous inference procedures, which adjust P values by taking account of the performance of multiple tests, reduce the danger that associations will be reported as significant when they are flukes (Bland JM, Altman DG. Multiple significance tests: the Bonferroni method. British Medical Journal 1995; 310: 170). Software is available for a number of such procedures (see Appendix C).

    Opinions on their use vary. 'It is to be hoped that they will become as much a part of accepted statistical practice as unadjusted P values are now,' says Wright PS (Adjusted P-values for simultaneous inference. Biometrics 1992; 48: 1005). Others consider them unnecessary, misleading, or inefficient (Rothman KJ, Greenland S. Modern epidemiology, 2nd edn. Philadelphia, PA: Lippincott-Raven; 1998. pp. 227–228). Bender and Lange say that 'different persons may have different but nevertheless reasonable opinions', but they 'prefer that data of exploratory studies be analyzed without multiplicity adjustment. "Significant" results ... should clearly be labeled as exploratory results. To confirm these results the corresponding hypotheses have to be tested in further confirmatory studies' (Bender R, Lange S. Adjusting for multiple testing – when and how? Journal of Clinical Epidemiology 2001; 54: 343).

Perneger concludes that these procedures make sense in only a few situations. These include 'when searching for significant associations without pre-established hypotheses' (Perneger TV. What's wrong with Bonferroni adjustments. British Medical Journal 1998; 316: 123).

In clinical trials in which *multiple outcome measures* are used, suggested solutions (instead of adjusting the P values) are selection of a single primary outcome measure or creation of a global assessment measure (Feise DJ. Do multiple outcome measures require p-value adjustment? BMC Medical Research Methodology 2002; 2: 8).

4. See our companion book: Abramson JH, Abramson ZH. Making sense of data: a self-instruction manual on the interpretation of epidemiological data, 3rd edn. New York, NY: Oxford University Press; 2001.

5. Mann GV. Diet–heart: end of an era. New England Journal of Medicine 1977; 297: 644.

6. More strictly, the 95% confidence interval for a value is the interval calculated from a random sample by a procedure which, if applied to an infinite number of random samples of the same size, would, in 95% of instances, contain the true value in the population. To unravel this, see a statistics textbook. Recommended: Altman DG, Machin D, Bryant TN, Gardner MJ (eds). Statistics with confidence: confidence intervals and statistical guidelines, 2nd edn. BMJ Books; 2000.

A guide to the use of confidence intervals is available at http://www.doh.wa.gov/Data/ Guidelines/ConfIntguide.htm.

It would seem pointless to estimate a confidence interval if the whole of the study population was studied, but the study population can be visualized as a sample of an imaginary larger population (see note 10, Chapter 28).

7. Definition of *bias* from Last JM (ed.) (A dictionary of epidemiology, 4th edn. New York, NY: Oxford University Press; 2001).

Catalogues of biases are provided by Sackett DL (Bias in analytic research. Journal of Chronic Diseases 1979; 32: 51), who includes 'hot stuff bias', 'looking for the pony bias', and 'tidying-up bias', Choi BCK, Pak AWP (Bias, overview. In: Armitage P, Colton T (eds), Encyclopedia of biostatistics. Chichester: Wiley; 1998. pp. 331–338), who include 'faking bad bias', 'faking good bias', and 'obsequiousness bias', and Delgado-Rodriguez M, Llorca J (Glossary: bias. Journal of Epidemiology and Community Health 2006; 58: 635), who include 'mimicry bias', 'sick quitter bias', and the 'Will Rogers phenomenon'.

8. The study of review articles on passive smoking is reported by Barnes DE, Bero LA (Why review articles on the health effects of passive smoking reach different conclusions. Journal of the American Medical Association 1998; 279: 1566), who found that (controlling for article quality, peer review status and other factors) the odds ratio expressing the association between reported nonharmfulness and tobacco industry affiliations was 88. The study pointing to bias in the publication of studies sponsored by pharmaceutical companies is by Liss H (Publication bias in the pulmonary/allergy literature: effect of pharmaceutical company sponsorship. Israel Medical Association Journal 2006; 8: 451). In the study of nutrition articles, the odds ratio against an unfavourable conclusion was 6.2 (Lesser LI, Ebbeling CB, Goozner M, Wypij D, Ludwig DS. Relationship between funding source and conclusion among nutrition-related scientific articles. PloS Medicine 2007; 4(1): e5).

The *self-fulfilling prophecy syndrome* refers to 'the bias a researcher is inclined to project into his methodology and treatment that subtly shapes the data in the direction of his foregone conclusions'. (Isaac S, Michael WB. Handbook in research and evaluation for education and the behavioral sciences. San Diego, CA: EdITS; 1977. p. 58). Maier's Law is relevant here: 'If the facts do not conform to the theory, they must be disposed of'. If the investigator's prejudice is a reflection of a conventional or fashionable belief, then the findings may tend to confirm this belief. This is the *self-perpetuating myth syndrome*; see Fleiss JL, Levin B, Paik MC (Statistical methods for rates and proportions, 3rd edn. Wiley; 2003. p. 576).

9. Murphy's Law: 'If anything can go wrong, it will'. Murphy's corollary: 'If nothing can go wrong, it will anyway'. O'Toole's commentary: 'Murphy was an optimist'.

10. For an example of Neyman's bias, see Hill G, Connelly J, Hebert R, Lindsay J, Millar W (Neyman's bias revisited. Journal of Clinical Epidemiology 2003; 56: 293).

11. As an example of selective factors in the identification of study subjects, men with prostatic cancer are far more likely to be detected if they undergo screening, leading to possible bias in the appraisal of associations with variables related to screening, such as social class. As another example, patients with aplastic anaemia were especially likely to be reported to the American Registry of Blood Dyscrasias if they had taken chloramphenicol (which had been reported to be associated with the disease), and this led to an overestimation of the association with the disease (Shapiro S, Rosenberg L. Bias in case-control studies. In: Gail MH, Benichou J (eds), Encyclopedia of epidemiologic methods. Wiley; 2000. pp. 83–92).

12. Examples showing how selection bias can lead to misleading or entirely incorrect results are presented by Ellenberg JH (Selection bias in observational and experimental studies. Statistics in Medicine 1994; 13: 557), who would like studies with selection bias to be considered 'scientifically "politically incorrect"', so that the scientific community will 'just say no' to them.

13. Sheikh H. Late response vs. non-response to mail questionnaire. Annals of Epidemiology 1998; 8: 75.

14. For a numerical example of this method of *adjusting for nonresponse bias*, see Moser CA, Kalton G (Survey methods in social investigation, 2nd edn. London: Heinemann; 1972. pp. 181–184).

This book also describes the Politz–Simmons technique for dealing with the *not-at-home* problem in household interview surveys (pp. 178–181). The results are weighted in accordance with the proportion of days the respondent is ordinarily at home at the time of the interview. Most weight is given to respondents who are seldom at home, who represent a group with a high nonresponse rate.

15. Abramson JH, Gofin R. Mortality and its causes among Moslems, Druze and Christians in Israel. Israel Journal of Medical Sciences 1979; 15: 965.

16. In a study of the association between an exposure and a disease, *differential misclassification* of exposure or the disease can either exaggerate or underestimate the strength of the association.

Nondifferential misclassification may be expected to reduce the strength of the association (or, in extreme instances, to reverse its direction), unless there are more than two categories of exposure and the misclassification is between two of these. This is the expected effect on the average estimate; but random variation could result in a spuriously increased strength in a particular study (Jurek AM, Greenland S, Maldonaldo G, Church TR. Proper interpretation of non-differential misclassification effects: expectation vs observations. International Journal of Epidemiology 2005; 34: 680. Fosgate GT. Non-differential measurement error does not always bias diagnostic likelihood ratios towards the null. Emerging Themes in Epidemiology 2006; 3: 7).

Nondifferential misclassification of a confounder is a serious problem, since it can cause a bias in either direction, and is difficult to control. See Rothman KJ, Greenland S (Modern epidemiology, 2nd edn. Lippincott-Raven; 1998. pp. 125–133).

17. Lilienfeld AM, Lilienfeld DE. Foundations of epidemiology, 2nd edn. New York, NY: Oxford University Press; 1980 pp. 208–209.

18. Abramson JH, Pridan H, Sacks MI, Avitzour M, Peritz E. A case-control study of Hodgkin's disease. Journal of the National Cancer Institute 1978; 61: 307.

19. The *arithmetical control of misclassification errors* is explained by Greenland S (Basic methods for sensitivity analysis of biases. International Journal of Epidemiology 1996;

25: 1107), by Fleiss JL, Levin B, Paik MC (Statistical methods for rates and proportions, 3rd edn.Wiley; 2003. pp. 565–574) and by Kleinbaum DG, Kupper LL, Morgenstern H. (Epidemiologic research: principles and quantitative methods. Belmont, CA: Lifetime Learning Publications; 1982. Chapter 12). For software, see Appendix C.

Also see Greenland S, Gustafson P (Accounting for independent nondifferential misclassification does not increase certainty that an observed association is in the correct direction. American Journal of Epidemiology 2006; 164: 63).

28

Making Sense of Associations

The exploration of associations[1] between variables is usually the most challenging and rewarding part of the analysis. This is especially true in analytic epidemiological studies in which causal hypotheses are tested, and in clinical and programme trials, which aim at testing hypotheses about the effects of health care.

Associations may be detected in different ways, e.g. by examining simple or multiple contingency tables, by computing differences, ratios, or other measures, and by applying logistic regression and other models. The association may be *positive* – i.e. the *dependent variable* (generally a measure of health status, health behaviour, or health care) and the *independent variable* (see p. 101) may tend to 'go along with one another' – or *negative* (or *inverse*), when the variables tend to go in opposite directions – e.g. if the presence of one characteristic is associated with the absence of another, or if high values of one variable are associated with low values of another.

Whenever an association is found, there are six basic questions that may be asked.

Questions about an association

1. Actual or artefactual? (Influence of bias?)
2. How strong?
3. Consistent? (Influence of modifying factors?)
4. Nonfortuitous?
5. Influence of confounding factors?
6. Causal?

The first three are always applicable, and the other three are important if the investigator wants to explain the findings, and not only describe them.

As will be pointed out, some of these questions may also be asked about the *absence* of an association.

Artefacts

The first question, always worth asking, is whether the association actually exists or whether it may be an artefact, i.e. ask *whether* before asking *why* there is an association.

Research Methods in Community Medicine: Surveys, Epidemiological Research, Programme Evaluation, Clinical Trials J. H. Abramson and Z. H. Abramson Copyright © 2008, John Wiley & Sons Ltd

Artefactual (spurious)[2] associations may be produced by flaws in the design or execution of the study that result in selection bias or information bias (see Chapter 27). They may also be reflections of regression to the mean (see p. 74). The prevalence of anaemia may appear to be higher in one town or one group of patients than in another because of the use of different sources of data, different definitions of anaemia, different methods of measuring haemoglobin, etc. Artefactual associations may be caused by errors, often remediable ones, in the handling of data. Not uncommonly they result from mistakes in arithmetic or computer programming. Flawed methods may, of course, not only produce an artefactual association, they may also weaken, obscure, strengthen, or change the direction of an actual association. If marked bias is strongly suspected and there is no way of correcting or controlling its effects, then further examination of the association is usually pointless.

Strength

The strength of an association may be a measure of its importance. If anaemia is found among 30% of pregnant women and 1.5% of nonpregnant women (see Table 28.1), then this marked disparity indicates a strong relationship between anaemia and pregnancy. The strength of the association might be measured not only by the difference between the rates (28.5 per 100) but also by their ratio (20) or by an odds ratio[3] (28.1). How strong an association must be if it is to be regarded as important is a matter of judgement. A difference of 1.5 per 100 in anaemia rates would probably be considered trivial, but the same difference in infant mortality rates, i.e. 15 extra infant deaths per 1000 live births, would be more likely to be regarded as important.

Many measures of the strength of an association (measures of *effect*) are available. They include the *difference between rates or proportions, the ratio of rates or proportions*, the *odds ratio* (all three used in the above example) and measures based on them (e.g. the *relative risk reduction* and the *number needed to treat*),[4] the *difference between means* (e.g. of haemoglobin values), and *correlation and regression coefficients*,[5] and experts sometimes disagree about their utility.[3] Odds ratios have advantages for use in analyses, but clinicians may find them deceptive. The term *relative risk* is best avoided, since it is sometimes used as a synonym for a ratio of rates or proportions, sometimes for an odds ratio, and sometimes for the hazard risk ratio provided by some analyses.

Different measures may be appropriate for the analysis of causal processes and for direct application in clinical or public health practice. For example, absolute differences between rates are helpful if there is interest in the magnitude of a public health problem, as are measures of impact that are based on these differences, i.e. *attributable*

Table 28.1 Contingency table showing relationship between pregnancy and anaemia among 10,000 women (imaginary data)

	No anaemia	Anaemia	Total
Pregnant	*a*: 1400 (70%)	*b*: 600 (30%)	2000 (100%)
Not pregnant	*c*: 7880 (98.5%)	*d*: 120 (1.5%)	8000 (100%)

(aetiological), prevented and preventable fractions, which measure the impact of a harmful or protective factor on the health of people exposed to it, or on the total community. The *attributable fraction in the population*, for example, is the percentage of the disease in the population that can be attributed to a given cause.

Whatever measure is used, a confidence interval may be informative. This is the range within which we can assume the true value (in the population from which the study sample was drawn) to lie, with a specified degree of confidence.[6]

As will be seen below, conclusions about the strength of an association may sometimes be modified when additional variables are incorporated into the analysis. Therefore, an association should not be prematurely discarded as unimportant. This, it must be said, is not easy advice to follow; it is very tempting to restrict further analysis to associations that 'come through loud and clear' from the beginning.

Consistency of the Association

An association may vary in different parts of the population or in different circumstances. The simplest way of detecting this is to stratify the data in accordance with the categories of another variable, and then inspect the findings in each stratum separately. In Table 28.1, for example, we saw an association between pregnancy and anaemia. Table 28.2 additionally subclassifies the same data according to educational level, so that education can be 'held constant' in the analysis. (This could, of course, be done better by using more than two educational categories, so as to ensure greater homogeneity within each educational stratum.) This table shows a much stronger association between pregnancy and anaemia among the poorly educated (where the relative risk, i.e. the ratio of the proportions, is 50% ÷ 2%, i.e. 25) than among the better educated (relative risk = 10% ÷ 1%, i.e. 10). If odds ratios are used, the respective values are 49 and 11. If a significance test is used (see 'Nonfortuitousness' below), the difference between the two associations is statistically significant: $P = 0.00002$ (a test that compares the associations in two or more strata is called a *test of heterogeneity*).[7]

In such analyses, the additional variable (education) may be called a *modifier variable*,[7] since it 'modifies' the relationship between pregnancy and anaemia. In statistical parlance, there is *statistical interaction* between education and pregnancy.

Table 28.2 Multiple contingency table showing relationship between pregnancy and anaemia among 10,000 women, by educational level (imaginary data)

	No anaemia	Anaemia	Total
High educational level			
Pregnant	900 (90%)	100 (10%)	1000 (100%)
Not pregnant	3960 (99%)	40 (1%)	4000 (100%)
Low educational level			
Pregnant	500 (50%)	500 (50%)	1000 (100%)
Not pregnant	3920 (98%)	80 (2%)	4000 (100%)

This means that the association between pregnancy and anaemia differs when educational level varies, and also (check this in the table) that the association between poor education and anaemia is different in pregnant women (*relative risk*, or *risk ratio* = 50% ÷ 10%, i.e. 5) and nonpregnant women (relative risk = 2% ÷ 1%, i.e. 2).

Effect modification always refers to a specific measure of association. In the above calculations we used the ratio of the proportions with anaemia. We would also find evidence of interaction if we used the difference between the proportions, which is 50% minus 2%, i.e. 48%, among the poorly educated, and only 10% minus 1%, i.e. 9%, among the better educated. But a modifying variable may affect different measures differently. For example, if the proportions with anaemia were 40% and 20% in one stratum and 4% and 2% in another, then the ratio of proportions would be identical (2) in each stratum, but the differences between proportions would be 20% and 2% respectively.

If multiple regression analysis is used, then modifying effects can be appraised by including appropriate *interaction terms* in the model. They can afterwards be omitted if they are clearly not significant.

The findings in Table 28.2 can be usefully looked at in a different way, by comparing the prevalence of anaemia when both risk factors – pregnancy and low educational level – are present with the prevalence when only one is present, using the women with neither risk factor as a reference group when calculating ratios and differences (Table 28.3).

Using Table 28.3, we can now compare the joint effect of the risk factors with their combined separate effects. The two factors multiply the anaemia prevalence by 10 and 2 respectively, so that their expected combined effect is a 20-fold prevalence. But the observed joint effect is much stronger: a 50-fold prevalence. The 95% confidence interval for the joint effect is 37–68, a range that does not include 20. This is *positive interaction* on a multiplicative scale. We could instead look at the differences (and that is what is usually done): the two factors raise the anaemia prevalence by 9% and 1% respectively, so that their expected combined effect is a rise of 10%. But the observed joint effect is a rise of 49% – positive interaction on an additive scale. If a joint effect is smaller than any single effect, then this is *negative interaction*. Statistical interaction, positive or negative, may or may not point to biological interaction (causal interaction).

The different findings in different strata are often of interest in their own right. They may have important practical implications. It may be possible, for example, to identify vulnerable 'high-risk' population groups who may require special health care. The presence of positive interaction (on the additive or multiplicative scale) may point to particularly vulnerable groups. In an evaluative study, a care procedure or programme may be found to be more effective among some categories of patients or population groups than among others.

Table 28.3   Prevalence of anaemia, in relation to presence of two risk factors

	Anaemia prevalence (%)	Ratio	Difference (%)
No risk factors (reference group)	1	1	–
Pregnancy only	10	10	9
Low educational level only	2	2	1
Both risk factors (joint effect)	50	50	49

The detection of effect modification is also a fruitful source of clues for the investigator who wishes not only to describe associations, but also to explain them. It often suggests what directions the subsequent analysis (or a subsequent study) should take; for example, can an explanation be found for a finding of synergism or antagonism?

Consistency may sometimes be worth investigating even when no overall association has been found, since an association that occurs only in a relatively small stratum can be drowned by the findings in other strata, so that no association is observed in the data as a whole. An association may also (less commonly) be concealed if there are positive and negative associations in different strata, so that they cancel each other out.

Nonfortuitousness

Anything[8] may happen by chance. However strong the association that is observed between two variables, it may be fortuitous, unlikely though this may be. 'The "one chance in a million" will undoubtedly occur, with no less and no more than its appropriate frequency, however surprised we may be that it should occur to *us*'.[9] The absence of an association may also be a fortuitous occurrence. The question is not whether the association observed in the study may have occurred by chance – the answer to which is almost always 'yes' – but whether we are prepared to regard it as nonfortuitous. Occasionally, e.g. if there is a big difference between the rates observed in two groups, and the groups are large, just looking at the results may enable us to decide whether to regard the association as nonfortuitous. When this 'eye test' is not enough, a *test of statistical significance*[10] may be used to enable us to make this decision.

Significance tests should not be done when they are not needed. In some studies, especially in simple descriptive surveys and programme reviews in which probability sampling was not used, the issue of fortuitousness may have little importance. For practical purposes it may be enough to know that housebound patients are concentrated in certain neighbourhoods of a city or that the proportion of women given postnatal guidance on family planning is lower in one clinic than in others, without worrying about deciding whether these associations occurred by chance. There is little point in doing a significance test on an association that is likely to be an artefact or on one that is so weak that it would be of no consequence even if it were regarded as nonfortuitous.

An association is adjudged to be statistically significant if the test yields a *P value* that is less than an arbitrarily chosen significance level (*alpha*). Critical levels often selected are 5% (0.05) and 1% (0.01). Whatever level is chosen, it must be remembered that significance tests have 'built-in errors'. Using a significance level of 5%, purely random processes will produce a verdict of 'statistically significant' in about 5 of every 100 significance tests performed, even if no real associations exist ('making a fool of yourself five times out of every 100').[11] This is an important consideration if many tests are performed.[12] The probability of such errors may be reduced by lowering the critical level, but can never be eliminated.

If the association is statistically significant we may regard it as nonfortuitous, without forgetting that, because of the 'built-in errors', we have not proved beyond doubt that the difference is not due to chance. A 'statistically significant' result does not mean that the relationship is necessarily strong, and it tells us nothing about the importance of the relationship. If the prevalence of anaemia is 30% in one group of pregnant women and 32% in another, this difference might be considered negligible even if it were statistically significant, which it would be if each group contained 5000 women. If the result is 'not statistically significant', then this does not necessarily mean that the association is fortuitous (any more than a negative sputum test for the tubercle bacillus necessarily means that a patient does not have tuberculosis). The verdict is 'not proven'. If the samples are large, then such a result may, however, be taken to mean that there is unlikely to be a nonfortuitous association of any great strength.

Helpful though significance tests may be, they have limitations. Not only do their built-in errors make them open to misinterpretation, they tell us nothing about the strength of an association. They are based on arbitrary conventions, and when only two alternative outcomes are presented (i.e. either 'significant' or 'not significant') this 'is not helpful and encourages lazy thinking'.[13] It is generally more useful to know in what range the true value of a measure of association probably lies in the population, i.e. its confidence interval (see p. 266), than merely to know whether the difference is statistically significant. This was illustrated by a review of 71 randomized controlled clinical trials that yielded 'negative' results, i.e. there was no statistically significant difference between the outcomes in the experimental and control groups. When 90% confidence intervals were calculated, however, it was found that in half the studies the interval included a 50% reduction in mortality or whatever other outcome condition was used in the study, so that an appreciable favourable effect of the therapy could not be ruled out.[14]

Confidence intervals can be used to provide an indication of statistical significance. If, for example, the 95% confidence interval for a difference between two rates or means does not include zero, or if the 95% confidence interval for the rate ratio or odds ratio does not include one, then this means a significant difference (by most two-sided tests) at the 5% level.

Confounding Effects

All studies of samples of children will display a correlation between shoe size and vocabulary: children with larger feet tend to know more words. The possible explanations include an increased transmission of mitogenic impulses to the extremities when Broca's area (a language centre in the brain) is active, and the secretion by tarsal and metatarsal osteocytes of a central nervous system stimulant that selectively activates the grey cells. Or, of course, age differences may explain the association: older children, who have bigger feet, also know more words.

This is a simple example of confounding:[15] the distortion of an association between two variables by the influence of another variable. This is of obvious concern to an investigator who wants to understand the findings. As another example, a survey in Massachusetts revealed that the children of fathers who smoked tended to have lower birth weights than those of fathers who did not smoke. This apparently occurred because smokers tended to have wives who smoked, and women who smoked during pregnancy tended to have lighter babies.[16]

As another example:

> Consider the association between storks and babies (which, depending on time and place, is almost always small but positive). Few people believe that storks bring babies, and the small positive relation is undoubtedly due to rural areas having both a large number of storks and a higher birth rate than urban areas.[17]

People who give up cigarettes have a high death rate in the next year or two. This occurs not because smoking is good for you, but because decisions to give up smoking are often due to the onset of diseases that carry a high fatality. Women who have cosmetic breast implants have higher suicide rates.[18] But is this an effect of the implants? Statistics show that the larger the number of fire engines that come to deal with a fire, the greater the fire damage. But does this necessarily mean that it is the fire engines that cause the damage?

Similarly, elderly people who live alone use chiropody services more than those who do not live alone. But this is a distorted finding, caused by the fact that those who live alone are older and include more women. When age and sex are held constant in the analysis, i.e. when people of the same age and sex are compared, it is found that those who live alone receive much less chiropody care.[19]

In each of these instances the association that was originally observed was a *secondary* one, resulting from the fact that both variables were related to a *confounding*[15] variable (or, in the chiropody example, two confounding variables). This may be portrayed as $A - C \rightarrow B$, where A and B, the independent and dependent variables respectively, are both linked with C, the confounding factor. Variable A is a *passenger variable*[20] that C has carried into its association with B. It follows that the variables that should be investigated as possible confounders are those with known or suspected associations with both the dependent and independent variables.

As a numerical illustration, we can use the findings in the subgroup of 2000 pregnant women in our fictional sample. In these pregnant women there was an association (relative risk = 5) between anaemia and poor education (Table 28.2). These data are subclassified in Table 28.4 according to an additional variable, the presence of

Table 28.4 Multiple contingency table showing relationship between educational level and anaemia among 2000 pregnant women, by presence of hookworm infestation (imaginary data)

	No anaemia	Anaemia	Total
Hookworm infestation			
High educational level	36 (36%)	64 (64%)	100 (100%)
Low educational level	260 (35%)	490 (65%)	750 (100%)
No hookworm infestation			
High educational level	864 (96%)	36 (4%)	900 (100%)
Low educational level	240 (96%)	10 (4%)	250 (100%)
Total			
High educational level	900 (90%)	100 (10%)	1000 (100%)
Low educational level	500 (50%)	500 (50%)	1000 (100%)

hookworm infestation. When separate attention is paid to women with hookworm and those without, no association between anaemia and poor education is found in either stratum, although in the total sample of pregnant women the relative risk was 5. The association observed in the total sample is a distortion of the true situation – hookworm infestation is apparently a confounding variable. This effect arises from the strong relationships of hookworm both with poor education (750 of the 1000 poorly educated women in this sample had hookworm, compared with 100 of the 1000 better-educated women) and with anaemia – 554 of the 600 anaemic women (92%) had hookworm, compared with 296 of the 1400 nonanaemic women (21%), a risk ratio of 4.4. We can also look at the hookworm–anaemia relationship separately in the poorly educated and the better-educated women. In the poorly educated women, hookworm was found in 490 of the 500 who were anaemic (98%), but in only 260 of the 500 who were not anaemic (52%; risk ratio = 1.9). In the better-educated women, hookworm was found in 64 of the 100 who were anaemic (64%), but in only 36 of the 900 who were not anaemic (4%; risk ratio = 16). The latter relationships (holding educational level constant) are examples of *conditional associations*, which are usually more important than overall (unconditional) associations in the mechanism of confounding.

It must be stressed that if an association disappears or is altered when another variable is controlled, then this does not necessarily mean that there is a confounding effect. This could also happen if the pattern of associations was $A \rightarrow C \rightarrow B$, i.e. if A produces or affects C, and C produces or affects B. In this pattern, C is an *intermediate* or *intervening cause*, and not necessarily a confounder. A is then an *indirect cause* of B. In the present instance, the possibility must be considered that poor education, or some closely related factor for which poor education serves as a proxy, is a cause of hookworm infestation and hence, indirectly, of anaemia. To the extent that this is true, the relationship between education and anaemia may be causal. Even the association between fathers' smoking habits and their babies' birth weights may to an extent be causal, if men's smoking habits affect their wives' smoking habits. (The relationship between A and C may be complex, and C can be both a causal factor and, to an extent, a confounder.)

To confound an association between variables A and B, variable C must (1) influence or be a cause of B (or be a closely associated stand-in for a variable that influences or causes B), and it must (2) be associated with A in the study population, but (3) not simply because it is caused or influenced by A. Only if its associations with A and B are strong can C have a confounding effect of any importance. The associations with A and B do not mean that C is a confounder; they only make it a *potential confounder*. Note that the associations with A and B may not be readily visible to the naked eye – they may be conditional ones, apparent only when other variables are held constant.

The way that a confounding variable distorts an association depends on the strength and direction of its relationships with the other variables. Controlling a confounding variable may make an association disappear (as in the above example); it may weaken it, exaggerate it, or change its direction (from positive to negative or vice versa); and it may reveal an association not previously apparent.

Confounding effects can be detected and handled only if there was sufficient forethought in the planning stage of the study to ensure that possible confounders were selected as study variables (see p. 102), and hence measured. This requires prior knowledge or at least a prior suspicion that each such variable meets the above requirements for a potential confounder. An endeavour to cope with confounding can then be made when planning the study design, by *restricting* the study to a homogeneous group (see p. 62) or by using *matching* (Chapter 7) or *randomization* (Chapter 32). If the latter methods are used, their effectiveness should afterwards be tested by checking the similarity of the groups that are to be compared.

In multilevel studies, confounding may occur at any level, or across levels. Possible confounders at all levels should be included as study variables.

Potential confounders are sometimes detected during the course of the analysis, when the examination of associations reveals variables that could meet the above requirements.

To decide whether a potential confounder is an actual confounder, it is necessary to control its effect on the association under study, and compare the observed ('factual') strength of the association with its calculated ('counterfactual')[21] strength when the possible confounding effect is controlled. The magnitude of the difference between 'actual' and 'counterfactual', i.e. the degree of distortion, is then an indication of the strength of the confounding effect.

Once data have been collected, there are three main approaches to the assessment and control of confounding effects:

1. The variable suspected of being a confounding factor can be held constant by *stratification*. The study population is divided into strata in accordance with the categories of the suspected confounder, and the association between the dependent and independent variables is measured separately in each stratum and compared with the association found in the data as a whole. If, as in the above example, this comparison reveals a difference large enough to be considered meaningful by the investigator,[22] and if the suspected confounder is not an intermediate cause, then the difference is evidence of a confounding effect. The stratum-specific data provide estimates of the strength of the 'true' association when the confounding variable is controlled. As pointed out on p. 271, stratification also permits the inspection of modifier effects.

2. The confounder can be *neutralized*. The strength of the association is measured by a statistical technique, such as standardization, multiple linear or logistic regression, the Mantel–Haenszel procedure, etc., that 'holds constant' and thus nullifies the effect of the suspected confounder or confounders, and computes an *adjusted* (counterfactual) measure of the strength of the association. The difference between this adjusted measure and the corresponding *crude* measure (not controlling for confounding) is an indication of the degree of confounding. It should be remembered, though, that 'overadjustment' may have the same effects as overmatching (see p. 71) – the association that the investigation was designed to study may be masked, and unnecessary adjustment (for variables that are not confounders) may impair the precision with which this association can be measured.[23]

3. Unmeasured confounding factors can occasionally be *reasoned away*; that is, it may be possible to deduce that an observed association between A and B is unlikely to be a secondary one caused by their common association with C. The reasoning

is based on known and assumed facts about C's relationships with A and B, which must be very strong to produce an appreciable confounding effect (the effect is a relatively weak echo). This approach can be applied in calculations that appraise the possible effects of an unmeasured confounder.[24]

It is the *amount* of confounding that a variable produces that matters, i.e. the *degree* of distortion that it causes. Variables that have mild confounding effects can usually be ignored, and are usually omitted when a final selection of the confounders to be controlled in the analysis is made. This requires a decision on a cut-off point – a change of 10% or more[22] in the measure of effect, for example, might be regarded as important. Statistical significance is sometimes used as a criterion for the importance of confounders, but this is not recommended, unless a 0.20 or higher *alpha* level is used as the cut-point, not 0.05.[22]

Adjusted measures that control for confounding should be used with discretion. They may not be appropriate if the confounders have strong modifying effects. If, for example, a study in Guinea-Bissau shows that various risk factors have different associations with diarrhoea in older (weaned) and younger (breast-fed) children,[25] then these conditional associations may provide a basis for appropriate intervention of different kinds in children of different ages, but controlling for age to obtain adjusted (overall) measures may not be very helpful. If regression models are used, then they may provide misleading findings if they do not include interaction terms, or if there is a poor fit with the regression model. If the confounder is a strong effect modifier, standardization too can yield misleading results; in Britain, age-standardized mortality data show persistent differences between regions, but obscure the fact that the differences have become small at younger ages, although not at older ages.[26]

Causality

Finally, we come to the question of causality. How can we know whether the association between A and B (i.e. $A - B$) is a cause–effect one? Does A, or a factor of which A is a proxy measure, produce or affect B (i.e. $A \rightarrow B$)? (Or, of course, vice versa: $A \leftarrow B$.)

Let us pause to consider what we mean by causality.[27] For our purpose, a causal association may be defined as 'an association between two categories of events in which a change in the frequency or quality of one is observed to follow alteration in the other. In certain instances the possibility of alteration must be presumed and a presumptive classification of an association as causal may be justified'.[28] A cause may be defined, for example, as a factor that alters the probability of occurrence of a disease.[29]

Usually, we wish to obtain information that can be put to practical use, now or in the long run. We want to identify factors that, if altered, would lead to a reduction in something we consider undesirable – premature deaths, disease, etc. – or to an improvement in something we regard as desirable, such as health care. For us, these factors are causes, even if manipulating them is unfeasible or unacceptable. In a clinical or programme trial, we want to know what effects, desirable and undesirable, can be attributed to intervention.

Not only do we want to know whether *A* causes *B*, we may also want to know what the mechanism is: by what process is this influence exerted? In the chain of causation *A* → *X* → *Y* → *Z* → *B*, we may be interested not only in *A*, but also in the intervening causes *X*, *Y* and *Z*. Information about these intermediate links, while it is not essential, may make us more certain that the association is a causal one. In an evaluative study, we may be interested not only in the achievement of changes in health and other desirable outcomes, but also in the chain of activities and intermediate outcomes that led to these end results. A report that a Ministry of Health recommendation for folic acid supplementation in early pregnancy resulted in a reduction in the national rate of spina bifida in the newborn would be far from convincing if we were not told that the recommendation was followed by a measured increase in the proportion of pregnant women who took folic acid supplements.[30] A report of a randomized trial of training for nutritional counselling, which showed that babies who attended a facility whose staff had received this training grew faster, became more convincing when it was shown that there had been increases in the number of mothers counselled and improvements in mothers' feeding behaviours and in children's dietary intake.[31]

Having learned about *X*, *Y* and *Z*, we can endeavour to modify them as well as or instead of *A*, so as to modify *B*. What we may actually want (but can probably never attain) is a complete picture not only of all the links in the chain of causation, but also of the other variables that influence *A*, *X*, *Y*, *Z* and *B* or the processes by which they affect each other (Figure 28.1).

In fact, we may want to know the total nexus, the 'web of causation',[28] incorporating not only the *A* → *B* chain and its intervening causes and modifying factors, as shown in Figure 28.1, but also any other chains of causation that culminate in *B*, as well as the interactions between chains. From our immediate pragmatic viewpoint all these variables – *A*, *X*, *Y*, *Z*, and the other variables shown in the diagram – the various *O*s, *C* (which may also be a confounder), and *M* (which is a modifier) – can be regarded as causes of *B*. All of the following, and more, are causes of deaths from gastroenteritis: various microorganisms, dirty feeding bottles, early weaning, poverty, malnutrition, respiratory infections, treatment by traditional practitioners, a lack of clinics.

The web will include causes that operate at different levels (molecular, cellular, personal, familial, community, societal, etc.). Some few causes may be *sufficient* to produce or influence *B* without the participation of other causes (beheading is enough to produce

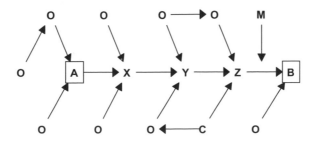

Figure 28.1   The web of causation.

death), but even they will have antecedent causes. Some causes may be *necessary* ones, without which *B* cannot occur or be modified, but on their own they will seldom be sufficient – exposure to HIV is a necessary cause of AIDS, but not everyone who is exposed develops the disease. Clearly, causes are always multiple[32] and effects are always the *joint effects* of multiple causes.

A *sufficient* cause can be defined as a set of minimal conditions and events that inevitably produces a given disease (or other effect) when an individual is exposed to them, 'minimal' meaning that there are no superfluous factors in the set.[33] Many alternative constellations of causes (known or unknown) may be involved in the aetiological process in different individuals, and no single constellation is therefore a necessary cause. But in each constellation, every component is a necessary element, i.e. the effect will not occur without the interaction between the components. Following this line of thinking, the importance of any cause in a given population will depend on the prevalence of the other components of the constellations in which it features.

The better we understand the causal processes, the better the prospect of finding an effective way of prevention; but this does not mean that a complete picture is essential for this purpose – many effective preventive procedures have been based on data connecting a cause and effect[34] without knowledge of the contents of the mysterious 'black box' concealing the intermediate mechanism (the web and constellations are now in a box!). What we need is to identify causes that are always or frequently necessary, i.e. that feature in all constellations of causes or in many of the frequently operating constellations that lead to the effect. If we can remove or minify (or block the action of) even a single such cause then we have a 'preventive broom'[35] that can sweep away the causal web or a good part of it, whether it is in a black box or not (or, stating this less ambitiously, we can break 'selected strands of this causal web'[36]). Immunization, for example, aims to control an always necessary cause (low level of immunity), and wearing of seat belts or the manufacture of vehicles with a low centre of gravity and a wide base may prevent many severe road accident injuries. If we extend the model to include causes at different levels, ranging from the molecular to the societal, then we may find preventive actions that operate at different levels; this replaces the black box with a nest of 'Chinese boxes, each containing a succession of smaller ones … we envisage successive levels of organization, each of which encompasses the next and simpler level, all with intimate links between them'.[37]

Trials versus observational studies

The accepted wisdom is that the best evidence for a causal relationship comes from a randomized controlled trial, especially if the findings are replicated in other randomized controlled trials. Proponents of evidence-based medicine and public health have used a hierarchical ranking of research designs, using internal validity as their criterion, with most credence being given to randomized controlled trials, followed by well-designed trials without randomization, then well-designed cohort or case-control studies, and then time-series studies.[38] Well-designed cohort studies are, in general, deemed more convincing than case-control studies, which are particularly subject to bias, or to cross-sectional studies, which do not indicate temporal relationships.

But comparisons of the results of experimental and nonexperimental studies – controlled cohort studies and case-control studies – suggest that what really matters may be the quality of the study and the characteristics and circumstances of its subjects, rather than the type of study. One comparison of meta-analyses of trials and meta-analyses of nonexperimental studies of five treatments or interventions (e.g. BCG vaccination and screening mammography) revealed remarkably similar average results. Another comparison found that treatment effects were similar for 17 of the 19 treatments studied, and another (a study of 22 treatments) led to the conclusion that 'results of randomized controlled trials and other studies do not inevitably differ'; it highlighted the effects of differences in the characteristics of the subjects, and advised caution in extrapolation from the samples included in trials – 'a well-designed non-randomised study is preferable to a small, poorly designed and exclusive RCT'. Meta-analyses of topics related to digestive surgery showed discrepancies in the primary outcome in 4 of 16 topics; the observational studies displayed more between-study heterogeneity than the trials.[39]

Studies of the effects of postmenopausal hormone therapy[40] have shown a major discrepancy (which has put many women and health professionals in a quandary) between observational studies and the large Women's Health Initiative trial with respect to the risk of coronary disease – a discrepancy which, it has been suggested, may be due to an age difference, since most of the subjects in the observational studies started treatment at the time of their menopausal symptoms, whereas most participants in the trial began at the age of 60 or more.

Differences between the results of trials and observational studies, such as the markedly greater effectiveness of statins in reducing mortality in observational studies than in trials,[41] may of course be attributable, in part, both to the restrictiveness of trials and to selection bias in the observational study. Suggested explanations for the fact that statins seem to protect against hip fractures in observational studies but not in trials may be that people who use statins are more health conscious and, therefore, are more active or eat healthier diets, or that physicians choose not to prescribe statins to patients they perceive as frail. These conjectures underline the need to measure and report on the characteristics of the subjects, as well as possible confounders.

It must of course be remembered that randomized controlled trials of some interventions are precluded by ethical or practical difficulties, and there is then no alternative to the use of observational studies. In a seminal meta-analysis of randomized controlled trials of parachute use to prevent death and major trauma related to gravitational challenge, for example, an extensive literature search revealed not a single trial, leading to the conclusion that 'individuals who insist that all interventions need to be validated by a randomized controlled trial need to come down to earth with a bump'.[42]

The value of evidence from a nonexperimental study depends on how well the study was designed and conducted – how close was it to a good experiment, with respect to the avoidance or control of selection and information bias and confounding? This is not easy to achieve, and it is not unusual for nonexperimental studies to yield conflicting results.[43]

The Cochrane Collaboration, an international organization that produces and disseminates systematic reviews of health-care interventions, is cautious in its recommendations:

> Randomised controlled trials (RCTs) are considered by many the *sine qua non* when addressing questions regarding therapeutic efficacy, whereas other study designs are appropriate for addressing other types of questions. For example, questions relating to aetiology or risk factors may be addressed by case-control and cohort studies... Well designed observational studies have provided useful data regarding the effects of interventions such as mandatory use of helmets by motorcyclists, screening for cervical cancer, dissemination of clinical practice guidelines to change professional practice and rare adverse effects of medication... The major difference between randomized trials and observational studies has to do with selection bias and the need to identify and account for potential confounders in observational studies... A great deal of judgement is necessary in assessing the validity of observational studies. Judgement is also needed when the validity of randomized trials is assessed, but the nature of observational studies makes them even more difficult to critically appraise ... Caution is needed.[44]

Sizing up causality

Whatever kind of study the evidence comes from, four conditions must be met before we can seriously entertain the possibility that *A* may be a cause of *B*. First, *A* and *B* must be associated. Second, we must be sure that *A* preceded *B*, or at least that *A* *may* have come before *B*. This is essential, although a time sequence cannot by itself prove causation: 'if winter comes, can spring be far behind?', but does winter cause spring? Third, we must satisfy ourselves that there is little likelihood that the association is an artefact (see p. 269) caused by shortcomings in the study methods. And fourth, we must decide that the association is probably not wholly attributable to confounding (see p. 274). We can, of course, never be quite sure that there are no confounding factors that were not taken into account in the design or analysis of the study and that were not measured, and that we may not even suspect. The fact that a study of married men aged 45–59 showed that those who had sexual intercourse at least twice a week had a relatively low mortality in a 10-year follow-up, and that this association held up when a set of possible confounders (age, blood pressure, cholesterol level, social class, smoking, and the presence of coronary heart disease at the outset) were controlled,[45] does not necessarily mean that sexual activity protects against death. There may well be other confounders, notably a good marital relationship and its other benefits. Confounders may be factors that we do not even know of – a simulation study has shown that the well-known association between birth weight and neonatal mortality could theoretically be explained by a strong confounding effect of some rare unknown factor or factors.[46]

We can never really 'prove' a causal relationship. What we want, however, is 'reasonable proof', strong enough to be used as a basis for decision and action. To this end, we should review the way that possible confounders were handled in the study. Can we think of any important factors that were not measured,[47] in themselves or by proxy, or that were measured unsatisfactorily? How well were possible confounding influences explored and controlled in the analysis? Do the size of the sample and the nature and complexity of the findings permit a thoroughgoing analysis of these influences? If not, to what extent can confounding influences be 'reasoned away' (see p. 278)?

If these conditions are met, then we can consider other evidence. Basically, we see how well the facts fit in with what we might expect to find if the association were causal. This is not quite the same thing as 'proving' a causal association, but it is the best we can do. For this purpose, use may be made of the following additional criteria,[48] which (taken together) may strengthen or weaken the case for causality, although none of them is essential or conclusive:

1. *Statistical significance.* This supports the case for a causal association. Its absence weakens the case, but only if the test is sufficiently powerful[9] (this usually means 'if the sample is large enough'). But note that less conventional statisticians, supporters of a *Bayesian* approach to statistical inference,[49] regard the usual statistical tests as maybe misleading.
2. *Strength of the association.* The stronger it is, the more likely that it is causal, and not produced by bias or confounding. But a weak association may also be (weakly) causal.
3. *Dose–response relationship.* The case for causality is supported if there is a correlation between the amount, intensity or duration of exposure to the 'cause' and the amount or severity of the 'effect'. But a dose–response relationship does not 'prove' causality – the significant association found (in at least one study)[50] between the severity of heartburn in pregnancy and the offspring's hairiness is not proof that heartburn promotes hair growth. There may also be a correlation between an 'effect' and the dose of a placebo.[51] Nor does the absence of dose–response effect disprove causation; there may be an 'all-or-none' response that appears only when the causative factor reaches a threshold level, or a relationship between cause and effect that is U- or J-shaped (or inverted U- or J-shaped) rather than linear.
4. *Time–response relationship.* If the incidence of the 'effect' (e.g. the rate of new cases of a disease) rises to a peak some time after a brief exposure to the 'cause' and then decreases, this supports the case.
5. *Predictive performance.* If surveys or experiments provide new knowledge supporting an *a priori* causal hypothesis, this supports the case; a failed prediction weakens the case.[52]
6. *Specificity.* The finding that the 'effect' is related to only one 'cause', or that the 'cause' is related to only one 'effect', may be regarded as supporting the case. But a lack of specificity in no way negates a causal relationship.
7. *Consistency* (in different populations or circumstances, and in studies by different investigators or methods). If the same association is found repeatedly, this strongly

supports the case. If results are inconsistent, and the variation cannot be attributed to modifying factors or differences in study methods, this weakens the case.

8. *Coherence* with current theory and knowledge – in particular, the availability of a satisfactory explanation of the mechanism by which *A* may affect *B* – supports the case. But the investigator who cannot think up some plausible explanation for a finding must indeed be a rare bird.[53] If no plausible explanation can be suggested, then a cause–effect relationship may be difficult to accept, but should probably not be ruled out. Incompatibility with known facts weakens the case.

These 'rules of evidence'[4] are not clear-cut, and the appraisal of causality is a matter of judgement. Experts often differ in their conclusions. Critics emphasize this heavy reliance on judgement, stating that 'epidemiological attribution of causation is not a science but an activity more akin to the arguing of a case in law: based on evidence but not dictated by the evidence' – epidemiology cannot produce predictions as reliable as those produced by some other disciplines, and 'cannot be regarded as a scientific discipline because it aims at concrete usefulness rather than abstract truthfulness'.[54]

There is no disagreement, however, about the usefulness of these judgements as a basis for decisions about health care in situations where (as almost always) there is no completely valid answer.

There is usually interest in knowing not only *whether A* is a cause of *B*, but also *how* it interrelates with other causes in producing *B*. We have seen how even simple techniques of analysis can point to the role of an intervening cause (p. 276) and demonstrate modifying effects (p. 271), which often supply clues to the intricacies of causal processes.[55] Multivariate analysis can streamline the production of information about the inte-relationships among a series of factors. It does not, unfortunately, eliminate the need for causal interpretation of the findings.

The temporal characteristics of causes may be of interest. A cause of an infectious disease may influence the probability of infection, of subsequent pathogenesis, or of progression or recovery; and a cause of accidental injuries may influence the probability of accidents or the probability and severity of injury during the event, or it may affect the subsequent course. A distinction may be made between a *predisposing cause* or *precondition*, a *precipitating cause* or *initiator*, and a *promoter* (a later-acting cause in carcinogenesis); *concomitant causes* act simultaneously.

Conceptual models used in *life course epidemiology*[56] – the study of the effects of exposures before conception, during fetal or infant life, or in other phases of the life course on later health or disease risk) – include the *critical period model*, according to which an exposure during a specific period has lasting effects, sometimes modified by later experience, and the *accumulation of risk model*, according to which health or disease risk is affected by a set of earlier exposures, which may be independent of each other and have independent uncorrelated effects, or which may be clustered, or which may form a chain and have additive effects, or which may form a chain whose last link has a *trigger effect*.

Before leaving the subject of causality, it must be stressed that things may be more complicated than they seem, since not only may one cause have many effects and one effect many causes, but variables may simultaneously have more than one kind of association with each other. For example, there may be a reciprocal causal relationship, where A affects B, and B affects A ($A \leftrightarrow B$). Poverty may be a cause of chronic illness, for example, and chronic illness may lead to poverty. At the same time, there may be a secondary association between poverty and chronic illness, due to a common association with an identifiable factor such as ethnic group ($A \leftarrow C \rightarrow B$), or with unknown, possibly remote, common causes ($A \leftarrow ? \leftarrow ? \rightarrow ? \rightarrow B$). The association between A and B may thus be partly causal and partly noncausal. A third variable may be both a confounding factor and an intervening cause; or it may have both confounding and modifying effects, and so on. 'O, what a tangled web we perceive'. Even Sir Isaac Newton observed that 'to myself I seem to have been only like a boy playing on the sea-shore, and diverting myself in now and then finding a smoother pebble, or a prettier shell than ordinary, whilst the great ocean of truth lay all undiscovered before me'.[57] But let us take heart – we don't have to find all the answers (not all at once, anyway), only some useful answers, and this we can do.

Notes and References

1. *Associations* may be referred to nonspecifically *as relationships* or *concomitant variation* or by a variety of other terms. *Statistical dependence* is a nonspecific statistical term synonymous with 'association.

   The variables that are associated are usually designated as *dependent* (generally a measure of health status, health behaviour, or health care) and *independent* (see p. 101). The terms *criterion variable* and *response variable* refer to a dependent variable, and independent variables may be called *predictor, explanatory, stimulus* or *exposure* variables.

   The appraisal of associations (*epidemiologic inference*) and the pros and cons of different measures are discussed in most epidemiology textbooks. They are treated in depth in many writings, including Rothman KJ, Greenland S (Modern epidemiology, 2nd edn. Philadelphia, PA: Lippincott-Raven; 1998), Kleinbaum DG, Kupper LL, Morgenstern H (Epidemiologic research: principles and quantitative methods. Belmont, CA: Lifetime Learning Publications; 1982) and Greenland S (Concepts of validity in epidemiological research. In: Detels R, McEwen J, Beaglehole R, Tanaka H (eds), Oxford textbook of public health, 4th edn, vol 2. The methods of public health. New York, NY: Oxford University Press; 2002. pp. 621–639).

   For exercises in the appraisal of associations, see Abramson JH, Abramson ZH (Making sense of data: a self-instruction manual on the interpretation of epidemiological data, 3rd edn. New York, NY: Oxford University Press; 2001).

   Readers who are unsure of what an association is will find the following explanation, written over a century ago, unhelpful (Doolittle MH. Association ratios. Bulletin of the Philosophical Society of Washington 1888; 10: 83, 94). 'Having given the number of instances respectively in which things are both thus and so, in which they are thus and not so, in which they are so but not thus, and in which they are neither thus nor so, it is required to eliminate the general quantitative relativity inhering in the mere thingness of the things, and to determine the special quantitative relativity subsisting between the thusness and the soness of the things'.

2. Authors writing about associations between variables vary in their terminology and often use the same terms with different connotations. *Spurious* for example, is variously used to refer to *artefactual* associations, *fortuitous* ones, *secondary* ones, and *noncausal* associations as a whole. The terms used in the text of this chapter were chosen because they are relatively clear and unambiguous. Alternative terms may be mentioned in footnotes.

3. Using the symbols shown in Table 28.1, the simplest formula for the *odds ratio* (also called the *cross-ratio* or *cross-product ratio*) is *bc/ad*, which is the ratio of the odds *b/a* to the odds *d/c* (or the ratio of the odds *b/d* to the odds *a/c*). For the data in the table, this gives a value of 28.1 (the fact that this is also the number of the table can fairly safely be assumed to be a coincidence). Alternatively, 0.5 may first be added to *a*, *b*, *c*, and *d*. This, which carries certain advantages, gives a value of 28.0. The numerator and denominator in the formula may be transposed (*ad/bc*), giving a value of 1/28.1 instead of 28.1. These findings may be interpreted as meaning that, in this sample, the odds in favour of having anaemia are 28.1 times higher among pregnant than among nonpregnant women, or alternatively that the odds in favour of being pregnant are 28.1 times higher among anaemic than among nonanaemic women.

Odds ratios, unlike differences between proportions or rates, or the ratios of proportions or rates, can be computed in case-control studies as well as in cross-sectional and cohort studies (facilitating comparisons of results), and have useful statistical properties that make them particularly helpful in analytic studies that aim to investigate associations. However, they are easily misunderstood. An odds ratio may be very different in magnitude from a relative risk (risk ratio, ratio of proportions). Suppose that a ship struck an iceberg and sank, and that 709 male passengers died and 142 survived (risk of death = 83%), whereas 154 female passengers died and 308 survived (risk of death = 33%). As alternative measures of male supremacy in drownability (or of men's chivalry?), the odds ratio based on these figures would be (709 × 308) ÷ (142 × 154), i.e. 10, whereas the relative risk would be only 83% ÷ 33%, i.e. 2.5 (Simon SD. Understanding the odds ratio and the relative risk. Journal of Andrology 2001; 22: 533).

In Table 28.1, the odds ratio of 28.1 may be wrongly taken to mean that anaemia is 28.1 times more common in pregnant women, whereas the proportion with anaemia is 20 times higher (30% divided by 1.5%). After a survey of treatment decisions made by physicians presented with feigned patients with identical clinical pictures revealed that the odds ratio for referral for cardiac catheterization was 0.6 for Blacks, in comparison with Whites (Schulman KA, Berlin JA, Harness W, Kerner, JF, Sistrunk S, Gersh BJ, Dube R, Taleghani CK, Burke JE, Williams S, Eisenberg, JM, Escarce JJ. The effect of race and sex on physicians' recommendations for cardiac catheterization. New England Journal of Medicine 1999; 340: 618), this was widely reported in the media in such terms as 'Doctors are only 60% as likely to order cardiac catheterization for Blacks as for Whites'. The referral rates were 84.7% and 90.6% respectively, and the rate ratio corresponding to the odds ratio of 0.6 was 0.93 (Schwartz LM, Woloshin S, Welch HG. Misunderstandings about the effects of race and sex on physicians' referrals for cardiac catheterization. New England Journal of Medicine 1999; 341: 279).

If the disease (or other condition under study) is rare, then the odds ratio can be used as a substitute for the ratio of proportions. A rule of thumb is that the error in estimating the ratio of proportions will not exceed $100X$ per cent if X is the highest odds in any subgroup (Greenland S. Interpretation and choice of effect measures in epidemiologic analysis. American Journal of Epidemiology 1987; 125: 761). Under certain conditions, the odds ratio can also be used as a proxy for the ratio of person-time incidence rates.

The main shortcoming of odds ratios is their lack of what has been called 'plugability' (Hilden J. Effect measures in biostatistics. Journal of Clinical Epidemiology 2003; 56: 391), i.e. the ability to be plugged in directly as input to clinical decision analyses, health-economic evaluations, hospital planning, etc.

Another disadvantage is that, unlike risk ratios, they can behave paradoxically when applied to conditional probabilities. As shown by Newcombe RG (A deficiency of the odds ratio as a measure of effect size. Statistics in Medicine 2006; 25: 4235), in an example where a comparison of two groups of schoolboys yields a risk ratio of 3.11 expressing their responses to 'Have you ever had sex?' and a risk ratio of 1.47 expressing their nonuse of a condom the last time they had sex, the product of these two ratios, i.e. 4.57, coincides with the observed risk ratio expressing the overall probability of unprotected sex. But the product of the corresponding odds ratios (6.97 and 1.93), which is 13.45, is very different from the observed odds ratio expressing the overall probability of unprotected sex (6.26).

For discussions of odds ratios and other measures of effect, see Greenland (1987; see above), Walter SD (Choice of effect measure for epidemiological data. Journal of Clinical Epidemiology 2000; 53: 931) and the subsequent correspondence (Journal of Clinical Epidemiology 2002; 55: 424), and Abramson JH. (Cross-sectional studies. In: Detels R, McEwen J, Beaglehole R, Tanaka H (eds), Oxford textbook of public health, 4th edn, vol 2. The methods of public health. New York, NY: Oxford University Press; 2002. pp. 509–528).

4. If P^1 is the risk of an outcome among people who are treated and P^0 is the risk among those not treated, the *relative risk reduction* is $(P^1 - P^0)/P^1$.

The *number needed to treat* (NNT) in order to prevent one event is $1/(P^1 - P^0)$ if P^1 is more than P^0, and the *number needed to treat to produce one episode of harm* (NNTH) is $1/(P^0 - P^1)$ if P^0 is more than P^1.

NNT is an easily understood yardstick for the value of a treatment; but its use to compare treatments may be misleading if the treatments were applied to dissimilar patients or if the outcomes occur during different time periods (Wu LA, Kottke TE. Number needed to treat: *caveat emptor.* Journal of Clinical Epidemiology 2001; 54: 111). Patients who are told how many must be treated in order to prevent one case may understand this to mean that 'the treatment is like a lottery in which a few win the prize' (Kristiansen IS, Gyrd-Hansen D, Nexoe J, Nielsen JB. Number needed to treat: easily understood and intuitively meaningful? Theoretical considerations and a randomized trial. Journal of Clinical Epidemiology 2002; 55: 888). Because of misuses and misunderstandings of NNT, its supplementation by additional measures (basal NNT, interventional NNT) has been proposed (Curiel R, Rodriguez-Plaza L. Basal NNT and interventional NNT. Journal of Clinical Epidemiology 2005; 58: 1074), leading to the observation that NNT 'may become known as the "number needed to traumatize (the reader)"' (Walter SD. Is NNT now the number needed to traumatize? Journal of Clinical Epidemiology 2005; 58: 1075).

5. A *correlation coefficient* indicates the degree to which two variables have a linear relationship, but does not indicate how much each variable changes when the other changes; this requires a regression coefficient. A *logistic regression coefficient* is the log of an odds ratio, a *Poisson regression coefficient* is the log of a rate ratio, and a *Cox regression coefficient* is the log of a hazard ratio.

6. See note 6, Chapter 27. The 95% *confidence interval* for the difference between rates (28.5%) shown in Table 28.1 is from 26 to 31%. If the same rates had been found in a study of only 500 women, then the confidence interval would have been from 19 to 38%.

7. A *modifier variable* may also be termed an *effect-modifier* or a *moderator* or *qualifier variable*. It may also be called a *specifier* or *conditional* variable, since it specifies the conditions for examination of the association. The method of analysis shown in Table 28.2 (*subclassification* or *stratification*) may also be termed *specification*.

The associations observed in the separate strata of analysis are *conditional* relationships. If these differ in their strength or direction, then there is *statistical interaction* between the independent and modifier variables.

Tests of heterogeneity have a low power, i.e. they are not very good at determining that the difference is 'true'. 'A high P value ... does not show that the measure is uniform, it only means that heterogeneity ... was not detected by the test' (Rothman and Greenland, 1998 *op. cit.*; see note 1). To be on the safe side, a P value of over 0.1, over 0.2, or even more is generally demanded as reasonable evidence that there is no modifying effect of any importance.

Instead of relying on a significance test, *measures of heterogeneity* can be used (Higgins JPT, Thompson SG. Quantifying heterogeneity in a meta-analysis. Statistics in Medicine 2002; 21: 1539).

8. Well, almost anything.
9. Fisher RA. The design of experiments, 8th edn. Edinburgh: Oliver & Boyd; 1966. p. 13.
10. *Significance tests* are usually concerned *with random sampling variation* (see p. 260). At the risk of oversimplification, most tests can be said to measure the probability P that an association that is as strong as or stronger than that actually observed will occur in a random sample drawn from a wider population in which this association does not exist (i.e. in which the *null hypothesis* that there is no association holds true). That is, if a large number of random samples were drawn from this population, all of the same size as the sample actually studied, in what proportion of them could such an association be expected?

    When these tests are used in nonrandom samples or total populations they are generally based on the notion that the study sample or population is drawn from 'a hypothetical population which would be generated if an indefinitely large number of observations showing the same sort of random variation as those at our disposal could be made' (Armitage P, Berry G, Matthews JNS. Statistical methods in medical research, 4th edn. Oxford: Blackwell Scientific; 2002. p. 84). Many statisticians reject this use of what Feinstein AR (Clinical biostatistics. St Louis, MO: CV Mosby; 1977. p. 311) has called 'a great imaginary parent population out there somewhere in the sky', and they limit the use of the tests to situations where there is random sampling variation or another 'chance' process, such as random intrapersonal variation, random measurement error, and random permutation of the observations.

    Two-sided or *two-tailed* significance tests test the null hypothesis – that there is no difference between, say, the rates of anaemia in two groups – against the alternative that there *is* a difference, no matter in what direction. For a *one-sided* test, the alternative to the null hypothesis (the 'study hypothesis') is that there is a difference in a prespecified direction (e.g. that there is a higher rate in group 1) and the null hypothesis is that there is not a difference in this direction. It is easier to obtain significance with a one-sided test. Such a test should be used if, and only if, the null hypothesis and its alternative, stated before the analysis, are such as to warrant its use.

    The P value is the probability of rejecting the null hypothesis when in fact it is true, i.e. of concluding that there is a real association when actually there is none. This is a *type I error*. A *type II error* is the erroneous missing of a true association. The *power of a test* is its capacity to avoid type II errors.
11. Hamilton M. Lectures on the methodology of clinical research. Edinburgh: Churchill Livingstone; 1974. p. 43.
12. See note 3, Chapter 27 on multiple significance tests.
13. 'The confidence interval ... provides a range of possibilities for the population value, rather than an arbitrary dichotomy based solely on statistical significance. It conveys more useful information at the expense of precision of the P value. However, the actual P value is helpful in addition to the confidence interval, and preferably both should be presented. If one has to be excluded, however, it should be the P value' (Gardner MJ, Altman DG. Confidence intervals rather than P values. In: Altman DG, Machin D, Bryant TN, Gardner MJ (eds), Statistics with confidence, 2nd edn. BMJ Books; 2000).
14. Freiman JA, Chalmers TC, Smith H Jr, Kuebler RR. The importance of *beta*, the type II error and sample size in the design and interpretation of the randomized control trial: survey of 71 'negative' trials. New England Journal of Medicine 1978; 299: 690.
15. *Confounding* has diverse definitions. The working definition used here is that the measure of association has different values when the confounder is ignored and when its effects are held constant (by stratification, standardization or other methods). The presence and degree of confounding may vary, depending on what measure of association is used.

    For a fuller simple description of confounding, see Rothman and Greenland (1998, pp. 59–62, 120–126; see note 1).

A confounder may also be referred to as a *disturbing* or *nuisance* variable. The term 'intervening variable' is best avoided, as it may be misinterpreted as meaning an intervening cause (see note 32).

An association produced by confounding is sometimes called a *secondary association*, an *indirect association* (which may be misconstrued as an indirect causal association – see note 32), or a *spurious association*, a term which has several other connotations (see note 2).

16. MacMahon B, Alpert M, Salbert EJ. Infant weight and parental smoking habits. American Journal of Epidemiology 1966; 82: 247.
17. Labovitz S, Hagedorn S. Introduction to social research. New York, NY: McGraw-Hill; 1971. pp. 80–81.
18. Villeneuve PJ, Holowaty EJ, Brisson J, Xie L, Ugnat A-M, Latulippe L, Mao Y. Mortality among Canadian women with cosmetic breast implants. American Journal of Epidemiology 2006; 164: 334.
19. Harvey I, Frankel S, Marks R, Shalom D, Morgan M. Foot morbidity and exposure to chiropody: population based study. British Medical Journal 1997; 315: 1054.
20. A term suggested by Susser M (Causal thinking in the health sciences. New York, NY: Oxford University Press; 1973).
21. *Counterfactual*. Pertaining to, or expressing, what has not in fact happened, but might, could, or would, in different conditions (Oxford English Dictionary).
22. 'The exact cutoff for importance [of a confounder] is somewhat arbitrary but limited in range by the subject matter. For example, a 5% change in the risk ratio would be considered ignorable in most contexts, but rarely if ever would a 50% change... The most important point is that one should report the criterion used to select confounders for adjustment. [If significance tests are used] they must have high enough power to detect any important confounder effects. One way to insure adequate power is to raise the *alpha* level for rejecting the null (of no confounding) to 0.20 or even more' (Rothman and Greenland, 1998, *op. cit.*; see note 1).
23. Overadjustment: see Day NE, Byar DP, Green SB (Overadjustment in case-control studies. American Journal of Epidemiology 1980; 112: 696), and subsequent correspondence in the American Journal of Epidemiology (1982; 115: 797, 799).
24. A sensitivity analysis can show how an observed association would be affected by controlling for a hypothetical unmeasured confounder, based on different assumptions about the confounder's strength and prevalence (Lin DY, Psaty BM, Kronmal RA Assessing the sensitivity of regression results to unmeasured confounders in observational studies. Biometrics 1998; 54: 948). Inferences can then be made about the probable importance of the hypothetical confounding effect, in the light of the plausibility or implausibility of these assumptions. For software, see Appendix C.
25. Molbak K, Jensen H, Ingholt L, Aaby P. Risk factors for diarrhoeal disease- incidence in early childhood: a community cohort study from Guinea-Bissau. American Journal of Epidemiology 1997; 146: 273.
26. Illsley R, Le Grand J. Regional inequalities in mortality. Journal of Epidemiology and Community Health 1993; 47: 444.
27. *Causality*: See Rothman KJ, Greenland S (Causation and causal inference. In: Detels R, McEwen J, Beaglehole R, Tanaka H, eds. Oxford textbook of public health, 4th edn, vol 2. The methods of public health. New York, NY: Oxford University Press; 2002. pp. 641–665); also in Rothman KJ, Greenland S (Modern epidemiology, 2nd edn. Philadelphia, PA: Lippincott-Raven; 1998. pp. 7–28).

    Also, see Susser M (1973; see note 20), Charlton BG (Attribution of causation in epidemiology: chain or mosaic? Annals of Epidemiology 1996; 49: 105), Weed DL (On the use of causal criteria. International Journal of Epidemiology 1997; 26: 1137), and collections assembled by Greenland S (ed.) (Evolution of epidemiologic ideas: annotated readings on concepts and methods. Chestnut

Hill, MA: Epidemiologic Resources; 1987) and Rothman KJ (ed.) (Causal inference. Chestnut Hill, MA: Epidemiologic Resources; 1988).

For papers stressing social and ecological processes, see note 13, Chapter 2.

There is a growing body of literature about *counterfactual analysis* (see note 21) in the appraisal of causal effects. 'The theory of counterfactuals (1) provides a general framework for designing and analysing aetiologic studies; (2) shows that we must always depend on a substitution step when estimating effects, and therefore the validity of our estimate will always depend on the validity of the substitution; (3) leads to precise definitions of effect measure, confounding, confounder, and effect-measure modification; and (4) shows why effect measures should be expected to vary across populations whenever the distribution of causal factors varies across the populations' (Maldonado G, Greenland S. Estimating causal effects. International Journal of Epidemiology 2002; 31: 422). For commentaries and the authors' response, see International Journal of Epidemiology 2002; 31: 431–438. See also Greenland S, Brumback B (An overview of relations among causal modelling methods. International Journal of Epidemiology 2002; 31: 1030), Phillips C, Goodman KJ (Causal criteria and counterfactuals; nothing more (or less) than scientific common sense. Emerging Themes in Epidemiology 2006; 3: 5), and Herman MA (A definition of causal effect for epidemiological research. Journal of Epidemiology and Community Health 2006; 58: 265).

28. MacMahon B, Pugh TF. Epidemiology: principles and methods. Boston, MA: Little, Brown; 1970. pp. 17–27.

29. 'A *causal relationship* would be recognized to exist whenever evidence indicates that the factors form part of a complex of circumstances that increases the probability of occurrence of a disease and that a diminution of one or more of these factors decreases the frequency of that disease' (Lilienfeld AM, Lilienfeld DE. Foundations of epidemiology, 2nd edn. New York, NY: Oxford University Press; 1980. p. 295); '... the idea of cause has become meaningless other than as a convenient designation for the point in the chain of event sequences at which intervention is most practical' (Helman C. Culture, health and illness. Bristol: Wright; 1984). See Susser M (Causal thinking in the health sciences: concepts and strategies in epidemiology. New York: Oxford University Press; 1973, Rothman KJ (ed.) (Causal inference. Chestnut Hill, MA: Epidemiology Resources; 1988) and Rothman KJ (Modern epidemiology. Lippencott-Raven; 1998. Chapter 2: Causation and causal inference).

It has been argued that statements about causal relationships should be avoided because of confusion about the meaning of causation – 'when we say for lung cancer that smoking increases risk by ten times compared with those who do not smoke, the causal language is "increases risk by…" What is the purpose then of adding "and this is likely to be a causal relationship"?' (Lipton R, Odegaard T. Causal thinking and causal language in epidemiology: it's in the details. Epidemiologic Perspectives and Innovations 2005; 2: 8). To which one response has been a vignette of an epidemiologist who, when asked whether smoking causes lung cancer, instead of saying 'Yes', replies: 'I can tell you with 95 percent certainty that smoking two packs a day for N years increases your risk of lung cancer by between A and B times, assuming that there is no systematic error in my observations…I have tried to correct for biases C, D and E using…' – by which time 'the enquirer will probably have regretted asking the question in the first place and, while puffing away at their cigarette, poured themselves a stiff whisky too' (Tam CC. Causal thinking and causal language in epidemiology: a cause by any other name is still a cause: response to Lipton and Odegaard. Epidemiologic Perspectives and Innovations 2006; 3: 7).

30. Zlotogora J, Amitai Y, Leventhal A. Surveillance of neural tube defects in Israel: the effect of the recommendation for periconceptional folic acid. Israel Medical Association Journal 2006; 8: 601.

31. Santos IS, Victora CG, Martinez JC, Martines J, Goncalves H, Gigante DP, Valle NJ, Pelto G. Nutrition counseling increases with gain among Brazilian children. Journal of Nutrition 2001;

131: 2866. Victora CG, Habicht JP, Bryce J. Evidence-based public health: moving beyond randomized trials. American Journal of Public Health 2004; 94: 400.

32. We can never speak of *A* as *the* cause of *B*. *A* always has its own determinants, and these are also causes of *B*. Moreover, as we learn more about the mechanism by which *A* affects *B*, we can usually interpose *intervening (mediating) causes*, thereby changing *A* from a direct cause ($A \rightarrow B$) to an indirect one ($A \rightarrow X \rightarrow Y \rightarrow Z \rightarrow B$). A cause is seldom *sufficient* to produce an effect without the participation of other causes – the outcome of exposure to pathogenic germs, for example, depends upon the susceptibility of the persons exposed. Sometimes *A* can be defined as a *necessary* cause of *B*, without which *B* cannot occur. But this need not mean that there are no other causes of importance; only a small fraction of people infected with the tubercle bacillus become ill with tuberculosis, indicating that factors other than the bacillus (the necessary cause) play a crucial role.

  According to the 'constellations of causes' concept explained in the text, causes are components of various alternative constellations, each of which is sufficient to cause the effect in an individual, and all causes are necessary (in the specific constellations in which they feature).

33. Rothman KJ. Causes. American Journal of Epidemiology 1976; 104: 587.

34. There is an extreme view, which most epidemiologists do not share, that epidemiological evidence alone, without laboratory and clinical studies that support and explain a cause–effect relationship, can never be conclusive enough to warrant a preventive programme (Charlton BG. A critique of Geoffrey Rose's 'population strategy' for preventive medicine. Journal of the Royal Society of Medicine 1995; 88: 607). In this view, a preventive strategy at the population level is justified only if the 'black box' concealing the mysteries of causal mechanisms has been opened (Skrabanek P. The emptiness of the black box. Epidemiology 1994; 5: 553).

  Examples that refute this view include: the link between a dearth of fresh fruit and scurvy, demonstrated in 1753, long before vitamins were thought of; between exposure to soot and scrotal cancer, in 1775, when the carcinogenic role of polycyclic aromatic hydrocarbons was undreamt of; between polluted water and cholera, in 1855, before bacteria had been discovered; between a poor diet and pellagra at the beginning of the 20th century, when this was thought to be a communicable disease; between smoking and lung cancer and other diseases before the pathogenetic mechanisms were understood; and, more recently, between putting babies to sleep on their tummies and the sudden infant death syndrome.

35. Robertson LS. Causal webs, preventive brooms, and housekeepers. Social Science and Medicine 1998; 46: 53.

36. Krieger N. Epidemiology and the web of causation: has anyone seen the spider? Social Science and Medicine 1994; 39: 887.

37. The 'Chinese box' metaphor was suggested by Susser M, Susser E (Choosing a future for epidemiology: II. From black box to Chinese boxes and eco-epidemiology. American Journal of Public Health 1996; 86: 674).

  Metaphors suggested by Krieger (1994; see note 36) are a web spun by two spiders (one social and one biologic) or, preferably, a fractal structure – a 'branching bush' pattern repeated indefinitely at every level, societal to subcellular.

38. Preventive Services Task Force. Guide to clinical preventive services: report of the U.S. Preventive Services Task Force, 2nd edn. Baltimore, MD: Williams & Wilkins; 1996.

39. Smeeth L, Douglas I, Hubbard R. Commentary: we still need observational studies of drugs – they just need to be better. International Journal of Epidemiology 2006; 35: 1310.

40. *Comparison of the results of observational studies and controlled trials.* The references cited in the text are: Concato J, Shah N, Horwitz RI (Randomized, controlled trials, observational studies, and the hierarchy of research designs. New England Journal of Medicine 2000; 342: 1887); Benson K, Hartz AJ (A comparison of observational studies and randomized, controlled trials. New England Journal of 2000; 342: 1878); Britton A, McPherson K, McKee M,

Sanderson C, Black N, Bain C (Choosing between randomized and non-randomised studies: a systematic review. Health Technology Assessment 2: no. 13; 1998); Shikata S, Nakayama T, Noguchi Y, Taji Y, Yamagishi H (Comparison of effects in randomized controlled trials with observational studies in digestive surgery. Annals of Surgery 2006; 244: 668).

Meta-analyses based on observational studies generally yield similar conclusions to those based on randomized controlled trials, and there are advantages in including both, according to Shrier I, Bolvin J-F, Steele RJ, Platt RW, Furlan A, Kakuma R, Brophy J, Rossignol M (Should meta-analyses of interventions include observational studies in addition to randomized controlled trials? A critical examination of underlying principles. American Journal of Epidemiology. Advance Access published 21 August 2007. DOI: 10.1093/aje/kwm189).

The possibility that the difference with respect to the effect of postmenopausal hormone therapy on the risk of coronary heart disease is due to an age difference is propounded by Grodstein F, Clarkson TB, Manson JE (Understanding the divergent data on postmenopausal hormone therapy. New England Journal of Medicine 2003; 48: 645) and Stampfer M (Commentary: hormones and heart disease: do trials and observational studies address different questions? International Journal of Epidemiology 2004; 33: 454).

Too few reports of observational studies provide enough information about details of treatment, methods of assessment, and the subjects' characteristics and other possible confounders to permit a meaningful comparison with randomized controlled trials, according to a review of meta-analyses by Hartz A, Bentler S, Charlton M, Landka D, Butani Y, Soomro GM, Bendon K (Assessing observational studies of medical treatments. Emerging Themes in Epidemiology 2005; 2: 8). 'Patient-oriented researchers should emulate the sense of purpose demonstrated by laboratory-based researchers in the Human Genome Project, with a corresponding focus on studying and understanding clinical, social, and behavioural factors – in what could be called a human phenotype and habits project (The goal might be to conquer confounding by 2015)' (Concato J, Horwitz RI. Lancet 2004; 363: 1660).

41. Bavry AA, Bhatt DL (Interpreting observational studies – look before you leap. Journal of Clinical Epidemiology 2006; 59: 763) comment on the discrepant results concerning the effect of statins on mortality, despite control of known confounders, and urge caution in the implementation of results based on observational findings.

42. Smith GCS, Pell JP. Parachute use to prevent death and major trauma related to gravitational challenge: systematic review of randomised controlled trials. British Medical Journal 2003; 327: 1459.

43. For papers on *the use of experimental principles in non-experimental studies*, see Horwitz RI, Feinstein AR (The application of therapeutic-trial principles to improve the design of epidemiologic research: a case-control study suggesting that anticoagulants reduce mortality in patients with myocardial infarction. Journal of Chronic Diseases 1981; 34: 575) and Esdaile JM, Horwitz RI (Observational studies of cause–effect relationships: an analysis of methodologic problems as illustrated by the conflicting data for the role of oral contraceptives in the etiology of rheumatoid arthritis. Journal of Chronic Diseases 1986; 39: 841).

Contradictory results from case-control studies are listed by Mayes LC, Horwitz RO, Feinstein AR (A collection of 56 topics with contradictory results in case-control research. International Journal of Epidemiology 1988; 17: 680).

In a prospective survey in which precautions were taken to control bias and confounding, Gray-Donald K, Kramer MS (Causality inference in observational vs. experimental studies: an empirical comparison. American Journal of Epidemiology 1988; 127: 885) found a clear association between formula supplementation of newborn babies in hospital and a low breastfeeding rate at 9 weeks; but a controlled trial conducted in the same hospital demonstrated no association at all. This discrepancy was probably mainly attributable to confounders that were controlled in the trial but not measured (and, therefore, not controllable) in the survey (mothers' motivation to breast-feed and the occurrence of sore nipples or other indications for formula feeding).

44. Higgins JPT, Green S (eds) Cochrane handbook for systematic reviews of interventions 4.2.6 [updated September 2006]. In: The Cochrane Library, issue 4, 2004. Chichester: Wiley; 2006. Available at http://www.cochrane.org/resources/handbook/hbook.htm.

45. This study was conducted in Wales. The authors say 'Sexual activity seems to have a protective effect on men's health', but add that 'confounding may well account for our findings' because of the effects of imprecisely measured confounders or unmeasured or unknown ones, and that further investigation is indicated, and point out that 'the likely absence of randomised controlled trial data will make the matter difficult to resolve'. However, they say 'Intervention programs could ... be considered, perhaps based on the exciting "At least five a day" campaign aimed at increasing fruit and vegetable consumption – although the numerical imperative may have to be adjusted. The disappointing results observed in health promotion programmes in other domains may not be seen when potentially pleasurable activities are promoted'. (Smith GD, Frankel S, Yarnell J. Sex and death: are they related? Findings from the Caerphilly cohort study. British Medical Journal 1997; 315: 1641); Ebrahim S, May M, Ben Shlomo Y, McCarran P, Frankel S, Yarnell J, Smith GD. Sexual intercourse and risk of ischaemic stroke and coronary heart disease: the Caerphilly study. Journal of Epidemiology and Community Health 2007; 56: 99).

Interestingly, a 20-year follow-up (from which men with beards were excluded) revealed that men who shaved at least once a day also had a lower mortality. But, except for a relationship with stroke, this could be explained by confounding by smoking and social factors (Ebrahim S, Smith GD, May M, Yarnell J. 2003 Shaving, coronary heart disease, and stroke: the Caerphilly Study. American Journal of Epidemiology 157: 234).

46. The study showing that the association between birth weight and neonatal mortality could be explained by a rare unknown factor or factors (Basso O, Wilcox AJ, Weinberg CR. Birth weight and mortality: causality or confounding. American Journal of Epidemiology 2006; 164: 303) 'suggests a search for the proverbial needle in the haystack ... if there is a needle in the haystack, we would have to accidentally sit on it to find it' (Schisterman EF, Hernandez-Diaz S. Invited commentary: simple models for a complicated reality. American Journal of Epidemiology 2006; 164: 312).

47. *Unmeasured confounders* present a major problem. Efforts to deal with them include advanced statistical techniques such as *propensity score* calibration, which is too complicated to explain fully here. The subjects' propensity (predicted probability) for exposure to the postulated cause under study, based on their measured characteristics, is held constant in the analysis; e.g. see Stuermer T, Joshi M, Glynn RJ, Avorn J, Rothman KJ, Schneeweiss S (A review of the application of propensity score methods yielded increasing use, advantages in specific settings, but not substantially different estimates compared with conventional multivariable methods. Journal of Clinical Epidemiology 2006; 59: 437).

A simple and creative solution is to make assumptions about the strength of the associations between a hypothetical unmeasured confounder and the independent and dependent variables, and then see how (for different assumed prevalences of the confounder) controlling its effect would influence the findings. In a study of elderly people, this approach showed that in the most extreme scenario tested (a confounder that halves the likelihood of vaccination and triples the risk of death, and has a prevalence of 60%), influenza vaccination reduced the death rate by 33%, compared with 48% when the confounder was ignored (Nichol KL, Nordin JD, Nelson DB, Mullooly JP, Hak E. Effectiveness of influenza vaccine in the community-dwelling elderly. New England Journal of Medicine 2007; 357: 1373). See note 24 and (for software) Appendix C.

48. These *criteria for the appraisal of causality*, or similar ones, are explained in all epidemiology textbooks. Their resemblance to the *Rules by which to judge of causes and effects* written by the

philosopher Hume in 1740 has been pointed out by Morabia A (On the origins of Hill's causal criteria. Epidemiology 1991; 2: 367).

The list in the text is based in part on Susser M (The logic of Sir Karl Popper and the practice of epidemiology. American Journal of Epidemiology 1986; 124: 711). See also Hill AB (The environment and disease: association or causation? Proceedings of the Royal Society of Medicine 1965; 58: 296), Surgeon-General's Advisory Committee on Smoking and Health (Smoking and health. Public Health Service Publication no. 1103. Rockville, MD: Department of Health, Education and Welfare; 1964), Susser M (1973); and the other references cited in note 27.

For an illustration of how judgements using the same criteria may differ, see a debate by Burch PRJ and Lilienfeld AM (Journal of Chronic Diseases 1983; 36: 821, 837 and 1984; 37: 148) on the evidence concerning smoking and lung cancer.

49. Some statisticians regard the usual significance tests (which are based on a *frequentist* approach to statistical inference) as misleading, because they do not take account of what the known or assumed probability was before the study was conducted, as does the *Bayesian* approach. For a full explanation see (for example) Gurrin L, Kutinczuk JJ, Burton PR (Bayesian statistics in medical research: an intuitive alternative to conventional data analysis. Journal of Evaluation in Clinical Practice 2000; 6: 193), Blume JD (Tutorial in biostatistics: likelihood methods for measuring statistical evidence. Statistics in Medicine 2002; 21: 2563), and Nayarri MJ, Berger JO (The interplay of Bayesian and frequentist analysis. Statistical Science 2004; 19: 58). For software, see Appendix C.

A Bayesian approach leads to the conclusion that in a well-conducted clinical trial starting with a 50% chance that the treatment is effective, a statistically significant result (using a test with a power of 80%) will be 'true' only about 85% of the time (Ioannidis JPA. Why most published research findings are false. PLoS Medicine 2005; 2(8): e124). But if the significant finding is replicated in other studies, then Bayesian calculations show that (unless the same biases operate in all the studies), this enhances the 'truth' of the findings (Moonesinghe R, Khoury MJ, Janssens CJW. Most published research findings are false – but a little replication goes a long way. PLoS Medicine 2007; 4(2): e28).

50. In a study of 64 pregnant women, a significant linear relationship ($P < 0.001$) was found between the severity of heartburn, reported at 36 weeks' gestation, and the amount of hair afterwards seen in photographs of the neonate, as rated by 'blind' judges. The authors suggest that this confirmation of an old wives' tale linking heartburn with hairy babies may reflect dual consequences of rising levels of sex steroids (Costigan KA, Heather HL, DiPietro JA. Pregnancy folklore revisited: the case of heartburn and hair. Birth 2006; 33: 311).

51. Coronary Drug Project Research Group. Influence of adherence to treatment and response of cholesterol to mortality in the Coronary Drug Project. New England Journal of Medicine 1980; 303: 1038.

52. Susser M. Falsification, verification, and causal inference in epidemiology: reconsiderations in the light of Sir Karl Popper's philosophy. In: Susser M (ed.), Epidemiology, health, and society. New York, NY: Oxford University Press; 1987. pp. 82–93. Also in: Rothman KJ (ed.) (1988, pp. 33–57; see note 27).

53. The story (possibly true) is told of a trial comparing two treatments. When the statistician announced that one drug was superior, the researchers explained why this result could have been predicted, on the basis of prior knowledge about absorption, metabolism, tolerance, etc. When the statistician announced that he had confused the drugs, and it was the other that was superior, there was a short silence, and then a discussion that explained why the new result was consistent with expectations (Park CB. Attributable risk for recurrent events: an extension of Levin's measure. American Journal of Epidemiology 1981; 113: 491).

A paper on the 'biological plausibility' criterion points out that associations between smoking and subsequent suicide and between smoking and subsequent murder, detected in a large US risk factor study, are unlikely to be causal because they are biologically implausible (although they are strong, show clear dose–response relationships, and remain apparent when obvious confounders are controlled). 'It is likely that many more such associations ... are equally spurious, but are protected by their lack of obvious implausibility' (Smith GD, Phillips AN, Neaton JD. Smoking as 'independent" risk factor for suicide: illustration of an artifact from observational epidemiology? Lancet 1992; 340: 709).

When a study of Kenyan prostitutes showed that oral contraceptive use was positively related to risk of future HIV infection, several hypothetical mechanisms were forthcoming (Plummer FA, Simonsen JN, Cameron DW *et al.* Cofactors in male-female sexual transmission of human immunodeficiency virus type 1. Journal of Infectious Diseases 1991; 163: 233). But when a later study in Italians found that oral contraceptive use apparently protected against HIV infection, a plausible biological explanation was again available (Lazzarin A, Saracco A, Musicco M, Nicolosi A. Man-to-woman sexual transmission of the human immunodeficiency virus. Risk factors related to sexual behavior, man's infectiousness, and woman's susceptibility. Archives of Internal Medicine 1991; 151: 2411).

54. Charlton BG (1996; see note 27).

55. *Effect modification.* All effect modifiers are causes. Causes that have the same effect (i.e. that act on a common intermediate factor or process) may complement each other and manifest synergism. Causes that operate along the same pathway (one cause setting the stage for another) may have a multiplicative joint effect. Causes that operate in different pathways can have an almost additive joint effect. In each of these instances the effects may be less marked if other pathways are involved. If a cause–effect association is positive in some strata and negative in others, then the cause is both a risk factor and a preventive factor, with a varying balance between these actions.

Statistical interaction, positive or negative, may or may not point to biological interaction, i.e. to *biological synergism* or *antagonism* (see Ahlbom A, Alfredsson L. Interaction: a word with two meanings creates confusion. European Journal of Epidemiology 2005; 20: 563). This may be a difficult notion to swallow, but although positive statistical interaction between two causes means that the effect of each is enhanced when the other is present, it does not necessarily mean that their joint effect is stronger than a combination of their separate effects. The minimum requirement generally demanded before considering biological synergism is that the joint effect must be stronger than the *sum* of the separate effects. A joint effect that is stronger than the *product* of the separate effects (interaction on a multiplicative scale) is an excessive requirement. It is difficult to draw causal inferences from statistical measures of synergism because there is usually insufficient information to disentangle the relations between variables while controlling the confounding effects of other variables.

Statistical interaction and its measures are described by Rothman KJ (Modern epidemiology. Little Brown; 1986. pp. 310–326), Greenland S, Rothman KJ (Concepts of interaction. In: Rothman S, Greenland S (eds), Modern epidemiology, 2nd edn. Lippincott-Raven; 1998. pp. 329–342), and Kalilani L, Atashili J (Measuring additive interaction using odds ratios. Epidemiologic Perspectives and Innovations 2006; 3: 5). For software, see Appendix C.

56. *Life course epidemiology* is concerned with the effects of exposures before conception (including trans-generational influences), during fetal or infant life, or in other phases of the life course on later health or disease risk and other biological characteristics.

Terms and concepts used in life course epidemiology are explained by Kuh D, Ben-Shlomo Y, Lynch J, Hallqvist J, Power C (Glossary: life course epidemiology. Journal of Environmental and Community Health 2006; 57: 778), Ben-Shlomo Y, Kuh D (A life course approach to chronic disease epidemiology: conceptual models, empirical challenges and interdisciplinary challenges. International Journal of Epidemiology 2002; 31: 285), and Hall AJ, Yee LY, Thomas SL (Life course epidemiology and infectious diseases. International Journal of Epidemiology 2002; 31: 300).

A term that is becoming fashionable in epidemiological research is *embodiment* – the internalization, or incorporation into the body, of the material and social environment; see Krieger N (Embodiment: a conceptual glossary for epidemiology. Journal of Epidemiology and Community Health 2006; 59: 350).

Statistical issues are described by De Stavols BL, Nitsch D, Silva Id-S, McCormack V, Hardy R, Mann V, Cole TJ, Morton S, Leon DA. Statistical issues in life course epidemiology. American Journal of Epidemiology 2005; 163: 84.

57. Brewster D. Memoirs of the life, writings, and discoveries of Sir Isaac Newton, vol 2. Edinburgh: Thomas Constable; 1885. Chapter 27.

29

Application of the Study Findings

As part of the process of interpreting the study findings, thought should be given to the ways in which they can be applied. This chapter deals with two aspects: generalizations to a broader or different population, and the practical implications of the results.

Generalization from the Findings

We will often want to generalize from our findings. We may in fact have chosen the population we studied or sampled because we believed it was typical of a broader 'reference population' or 'external population' to which we wished to generalize the findings. Even if the study population was not chosen on these grounds, every population may be regarded as a part of a wider population, and we are often tempted to make generalizations. Having studied varicose veins in a single study neighbourhood, we may want to draw conclusions about their prevalence in the population at large, or to arrive at generalities that go beyond the population that was studied, about the strength of the association of varicose veins with fatness or leanness, the importance of occupation or tight garments as causal factors, and so on.

Consideration must, therefore, be given to the study's *generalizability* (its *external validity* or 'representativeness'), except in instances where interest is limited to the specific population studied. The study may be of solely local interest if it was performed in a practice setting as an aid in the planning, monitoring or evaluation of a specific health-care programme – in, for example, community-oriented primary health care (see Chap. 34), health care in a school or workplace, or district health care. Even in such instances, possible applications of the findings in other contexts may be contemplated.

Generalization from a sample to the study population requires, first, allowance for random sampling variation, by reporting confidence intervals (see p. 260). Confidence intervals are sometimes computed even when generalizations are made to a reference population from which the sample was *not* randomly chosen (e.g. to 'patients with peptic ulcer' or 'Canadian men'); this use of confidence intervals is open to debate (see note 6, Chapter 27).

But the main issue is not random variation, but whether the external population is sufficiently similar to the study population to warrant extrapolation of the findings.

Research Methods in Community Medicine: Surveys, Epidemiological Research, Programme Evaluation, Clinical Trials   J. H. Abramson and Z. H. Abramson   Copyright © 2008, John Wiley & Sons Ltd

Are the people similar, and are their circumstances (including health care) similar? Can the findings in one neighbourhood be applied to another? Can they be applied to the general population? Are the results of a study in one sex applicable to the other? Are the results applicable to other ethnic or age groups? Such questions may be difficult to answer. Populations and population groups differ in their health status, in the occurrence of risk and protective factors, and in their health care and other circumstances and exposures that may affect their health or the effectiveness of inter-ventions. Causal processes that are important in one population may be unimportant in another – not only may the prevalence of anaemia differ in a slum and a well-off neighbourhood, but different causes may operate in the two areas, or the modifying factors affecting their operation may vary – so that the risk associated with dietary iron deficiency may differ, as may the effectiveness of routine administration of iron or other supplements to pregnant women.

Clearly, the characteristics and circumstances of the study sample should be consid-ered and reported, if generalization is to be possible. Yet a recent review of epidemio-logical studies published in prestigious journals revealed that 59% did not even provide such elementary information as participation rates,[1] although consenters may clearly differ from nonconsenters.[2]

All this may seem obvious, yet how often do we read a statement like 'Conflicting findings are reported in the literature; A and B found something or other, C and D found something quite different, and E found something else again, which was not confirmed by F et al.', without any designation or description of the populations stud-ied by these investigators, let alone any effort to explain the discrepancies?

Although wide use was made of the results of the well-known Framingham Heart Study concerning risk factors for heart disease, for many years there was uncertainty about the generalizability of the results; the study started with a set of volunteers, who were then supplemented by a random sample of the town's population – with a response rate of 69%. Only in 1987, almost 40 years after the inception of the study, was it possible to compare the findings with those of a cohort study of a national prob-ability sample and confirm that the Framingham risk model predicted coronary deaths in the national sample 'remarkably well'.[3]

A decision to beware of generalization may, of course, be easy if there is sufficient selection bias to impair a study's internal validity (see p. 259), since this will obvi-ously also impair its external validity. Also, if the study was done in a very 'special' population (see p. 64) application of the findings to the general population may clearly be problematic; some study populations are representative of nothing but themselves.

Usually there is no simple foolproof way of deciding on generalizability. What is often done is to compare the demographic and other known characteristics of the study and ref-erence populations, or of the people included and excluded, so as to see whether there are obvious differences that may affect comparability. It may then be possible to try to com-pensate for these differences by making adjustments like those described on page 263.

Three questions that may not be obvious but are often worth asking are:

1. *Why was this study population chosen?* The reasons for the choice may be reflected in the findings: was the population chosen because of a high prevalence of a disease

or drug addiction or broken homes, or because of its ethnic heterogeneity or residential stability, or a local community's special interest in a health problem, etc.? In an evaluative study, reasons with a possible bearing on health care are of particular importance. The study population may have been 'chosen' simply because it was accessible, or because the staff of a particular clinic or health centre were motivated to perform or join in a study. Might this interest in research be a symptom of a high general standard of care? Was there special enthusiasm about the treatment or programme that was evaluated, and may this have influenced effectiveness? Was the study population chosen because there were especially good clinical records, or because special facilities were available? Was it chosen because a high level of cooperation or compliance was expected? Or was a captive population selected, whose diet or medical treatment could be manipulated with ease? If the population was selected because it was exposed to a novel health programme, why was this programme provided in this particular setting?

2. *May the study itself have produced an effect?* One distinctive feature of every study population is that a study was performed in it. Sometimes the performance of the study may in itself affect the results. Interviews and examinations, and especially the 'feedback' of examination findings to subjects, may lead to changes in health practices and health care. This possibility should be considered in longitudinal studies, particularly if investigations were repeated frequently. Weekly weighing of infants, or weekly interviews about their diet, may modify the growth pattern. The effect of the study itself is especially important in evaluative studies, where the subjects may be affected by their awareness that they are participating in an experiment, as well as by the experimental situation as a whole (see p. 73).

3. *Do operational definitions or other features of the study limit its applicability?* A study of the prognosis of diabetes may have limited relevance to diabetics diagnosed by other criteria, and the results of an evaluation of a diagnostic or surgical procedure performed by experts may not be applicable if the procedure is performed by people less skilled.

An obvious concern is the *generalizability of the results of clinical trials.* Not only do trials usually have strict eligibility and exclusion criteria, but informed consent is required; and, moreover, they are often performed in university hospitals or other institutions that have special facilities and highly trained staff. They are sometimes criticized as not being sufficiently relevant to the real world of clinical practice in the community. The precautions taken to ensure the trial's internal validity impair its external validity. The proportion of patients who are eligible for inclusion in a trial can be as low as 9% or 17%,[4] clearly raising doubts about the general clinical relevance of the results. Even in a trial conducted in family practices in England[5] that aimed to involve 'typical' patients with chronic heart failure and had very limited exclusion criteria, and where patients were invited to participate by a letter from their family doctor, with a subsequent reminder by telephone, only 36% agreed to participate. There were significant differences between those who consented and those who did not, with respect to sex, age, and the medicinal treatment they were receiving.

The distinction between trials that appraise efficacy (the effects under ideal conditions) and effectivity (the effects in real-life situations) has obvious relevance to the applicability of their findings in health care. The following criteria have been proposed as indications that a trial appraises effectiveness rather than efficacy (six of the seven criteria are required):[6]

- Subjects selected from a primary-care setting
- Non-stringent eligibility criteria
- The outcomes measured are changes in health
- Modalities (diagnostic methods, dosages, duration of follow-up) similar to those used in practice
- Assessment of adverse effects
- Adequate sample size
- Intention-to-treat analysis.

Practical Implications

It is arguable that just as every one of Aesop's fables has its moral ('Be content with your lot', 'Do not count your chickens before they are hatched', etc.), so should every study's findings be complemented by a statement of practical implications – what (if anything) ought to be done, and what are the expected consequences of doing or not doing it. Remember Will Rogers' salutary epigram 'The more we find out about anything the less we ever do about it'.

A clear-cut message concerning practical implications may reduce the likelihood that the findings will be ignored or misapplied. Decision makers, health workers and the public at large often exhibit two opposing tendencies: on the one hand, to disregard research findings or unnecessarily delay their application; and, on the other, to be unduly credulous and rush into injudicious action. The latter – and probably more regrettable – propensity generally results from undue reliance on a single study, ignoring the fact that different studies of the same topic often produce different results,[7,8] as a result of chance variation, differences in methods or circumstances, or differences between study populations. There is insufficient realization that 'what medical journals publish is not received wisdom, but rather working papers … Each study becomes a piece of a puzzle that, when assembled, will help either to confirm or to refute a hypothesis'.[7] Also, associations are too readily taken to mean causation, methodological shortcomings are too readily overlooked, and the specific circumstances in which the results may be applicable, as well as contraindications, may be ignored.

For the investigator, the minimal requirement is to specify whatever reservations there may be about the validity of the findings, to say whether there is a need to confirm conclusions by replicating the study or conducting other research, and (if relevant) to present the findings in a manner that facilitates decisions concerning possible changes in the provision of medical care, public health action, health behaviour, or other spheres.

But many feel that this is not enough and that the investigator should always go further and make recommendations on whether and how the study's results should be used, not just 'light the touch paper and then stand back'.[9] Whether this kind of advocacy is an ethical obligation is open to discussion.[10] If recommendations are made, then they should be based on an unbiased consideration of all the available objective evidence, and should be presented only as opinions. A reasonable role is that of the 'thoughtful advocate', who 'acknowledges uncertainties, anticipates policy option consequences, and balances consequences of intervention versus no intervention'.[11]

In other words, after reviewing the findings the investigator should always ask 'So what?', should supply facts that can form a useful basis for an answer to this question, and should consider providing a thoughtful answer based on the available information. Needs for further research and new investigative tools should be spelled out in detail, unless the conclusions can be regarded as definitive, with no need for confirmation. Even then there may be suggestions for new lines of study, or new hypotheses to be tested.

To help in formulating recommendations about practical applications and, subsequently, in decisions about their implementation, *action-oriented indices* (based on ancillary data when necessary, as well as on the study findings) may be desirable; these may necessitate new analyses. As examples:

1. If intervention directed at a risk factor is under consideration, then the attributable fraction in the population[12] would be a useful measure; this is an estimate of the proportion of cases in a given population that (under certain assumptions) can be attributed to the risk factor and would be prevented if the risk factor were eliminated. It is a much more helpful basis for decisions than (say) a rate ratio or odds ratio. A large case-control study in New York revealed a weak association between breast cancer and ever taking alcoholic drinks, with an odds ratio (controlling for numerous confounders) of only 1.4, but because of the high prevalence (83%) of drinking, the attributable fraction was appreciable: '25% of breast cancer among these women … is attributable to ever drinking alcohol'.[13]
2. The absolute number of cases that might be caused or prevented is often of more interest than any ratio.
3. At the level of lifestyle changes by the individual, it is less useful to know that there is a statistically significant dose–response relationship between the consumption of fruit and vegetables and cancer, than to know by how much the risk decreases per serving.[14]
4. As a guide to clinical practice, answers to questions about specific subgroups, like 'What is the risk of cardiovascular disease among healthy nonsmoking young women who use combined oral contraceptives?',[15] are more useful than overall 'summary' findings controlling for effects related to health, smoking and age. Even where subgroups are too small to warrant any conclusions, it has been suggested

that full data be published in the journal's electronic space, to make them available for cumulation and use in meta-analyses.[16]

5. If the introduction of a specific preventive procedure is being considered, the preventable fraction in the population (what proportion of cases would be prevented?) can be estimated and translated into terms of (for example) doctor visits, hospital beds, disability, or deaths. Also, it is very easy to estimate the number of people to whom the procedure must be applied in order to prevent one case,[17] and this can be converted to economic terms. Similar indices can be used to express the expected impact of therapeutic procedures.

6. If screening is under consideration, then useful indices include the numbers of tests and positive tests required in a given population to identify one case. Measures of gain in certainty[18] may be helpful with respect to decisions about diagnostic tests.

Whatever recommendations are made, it may be necessary to qualify them by specifying the conditions necessary for their application, and by limiting them to specific populations or circumstances.

An opposite view

Or maybe it is wrong to make practical recommendations? Maybe too few epidemiological researchers really understand the process of policy-making? This is the view of the journal *Epidemiology*, which for many years has discouraged public health policy recommendations in research reports:

> ...it is simply too facile to toss off a policy recommendation in the closing paragraph of a scientific paper without giving the implicit decision analysis the due consideration it deserves. Making good health policy is complicated. ... Our editorial policy is intended to avoid trivializing a complex process and to increase the likelihood that policy discussions are treated with the seriousness and depth of understanding that they deserve.[19]

Two of three invited commentators agreed with this decision. One said that he himself would make a policy recommendation only in the unlikely instance that he had information on all its potentially important consequences, including economic benefits and costs, and could conduct a formal decision analysis (although 'even if I were trained to do such an analysis, the length limitations of a research paper probably would not provide me the space to do so').[20] Another averred that while epidemiologists should have a place at the policy-making table, they should avoid taking positions based on the results of a single study. 'The best science comes from a series of articles...'; it is questionable whether a policy statement 'uttered in the last paragraph of an article in a scientific journal that few if any policy makers will read, will have a significant impact...'.[21]

The third commentator dissented. He cited examples (safer designs of handguns, child restraints in motor vehicles) in which he believed the inclusion of policy comments in scientific reports had had a material influence. 'If epidemiologists can inform policy makers of the comparative effectiveness of policies or of the need for formulation of new policies that would reduce the incidence of disease and injury, it seems counterproductive to silence the voice of epidemiologists...'.[22]

According to studies of what authors actually do, slightly over one-quarter of epidemiological reports (not published in *Epidemiology*) include policy statements, three-quarters of these making recommendations concerning clinical or public health practice and the remainder recommending further research.[23]

Ya pays yer money, ya takes yer choice.

Notes and References

1. Morton LM, Cahill J, Hartge P. Reporting participation in epidemiologic studies: a survey of practice. American Journal of Epidemiology 2006; 163: 197.
2. In large-scale epidemiological surveys in the United Kingdom, people who consented to follow-up or review of their medical records tended to be male and younger. They also tended to have whatever symptom was under investigation, with odds ratios of 1.61 for consent to follow-up, and 1.44 for consent to review of records (Dunn KM, Jordan K, Lacey RJ, Shapley M, Jinks C. Patterns of consent in epidemiologic research: evidence from over 25,000 responders. American Journal of Epidemiology 2004; 159: 1087).
3. Leaverton PE, Sorlie PD, Kleinman JC, Dannenberg AL, Ingster-Moore L, Kannel WB, Cornoni-Huntley JC. Representativeness of the Framingham risk model for coronary heart disease mortality: a comparison with a national cohort study. Journal of Chronic Diseases 1987; 40: 775.
4. In a trial of antimanic treatment, only 17% of consecutively admitted patients met the inclusion criteria (area of residence, age, diagnosis, severity of illness), and there were substantial differences between the included and excluded patients (Licht RW, Gouliaev G, Vestergaard P, Frydenberg M. Generalisability of results from randomised drug trials: a trial on antimanic treatment. British Journal of Psychiatry 1997; 170: 264).

   In a trial of schizophrenia treatment, on the other hand, where only 22% of diagnostically appropriate patients met the eligibility criteria and only 9% entered the study, the authors concluded that the selection bias had little clinical relevance, except for inferences relating to some small subgroups of patients (Robinson D, Woerner MG, Pollack S, Lerner G. Subject selection biases in clinical trials: data from a multicenter schizophrenia treatment study. Journal of Clinical Psychopharmacology 1996; 16: 170).
5. Lloyd-Williams F, Mair F, Shiels C, Hanratty B, Goldstein P, Beaton S, Capewell S, Lye M, Mcdonald R, Roberts C, Connelly D. Why are patients in clinical trials of heart failure not like those we see in everyday practice? Journal of Clinical Epidemiology 2003; 56: 1157.
6. Gartlehner G, Hansen RA, Nissman D, Lohr KN, Carey TS. A simple and valid tool distinguished efficacy from effectiveness studies. Journal of Clinical Epidemiology 2006; 59: 1040.
7. Angell M, Kassirer JP. Clinical research – what should the public believe? New England Journal of Medicine 1994; 331: 189.
8. Taubes G. Epidemiology faces its limits. Science 1995; 269: 164.
9. Pharaoh P. Bed-sharing and sudden infant death. Lancet 1996; 347: 2.
10. Weed DL. Science, ethics guidelines, and advocacy in epidemiology. Annals of Epidemiology 1994; 4: 166.
11. Savitz DA, Greenland S, Stolley PD, Kelsey JL. Scientific standards of criticism: a reaction to 'Scientific standards in epidemiologic studies of the menace of daily life' by A. R. Feinstein. Epidemiology 1990; 1: 78.

12. The simplest formula for the *attributable fraction in the population* is $(R_p - R_u)/R_p$, where R_p is the rate in the population and R_u is the rate in people unexposed to the causal factor. An alternative formula is $P_e(RR - 1)/[1 + P_e(RR - 1)]$, where P_e is the proportion of the population exposed to the factor and RR is the ratio R_e/R_u, where R_e and R_u are respectively the rates in people exposed and unexposed to the causal factor.

   This measure assumes that the risk factor is causal. Its use to indicate the proportion of preventable cases is meaningful only if the factor can be eliminated and it can be assumed that this would reduce the risk. See Rockhill B, Newman B, Weinberg C (Use and misuse of population attributable fractions. American Journal of Public Health 1998; 88: 15).

13. Bowlin SJ, Leske MC, Varma A, Nasca P, Weinstein A, Caplan L. Breast cancer risk and alcohol consumption: results from a large case-control study. International Journal of Epidemiology 1997; 26: 915

14. Colditz GA. Epidemiology – future directions. International Journal of Epidemiology 1997; 26: 693.

15. A review of 74 studies about combined oral contraceptives and cardiovascular disease revealed only five that addressed the cited question, and 14 others that did not, although they probably had the necessary data (Hannaford PC, Owen-Smith V. Using epidemiological data to guide clinical practice: review of studies on cardiovascular disease and use of combined oral contraceptives. British Medical Journal 1998; 316: 984.

16. Editor-in-Chief. Our policy on policy. Epidemiology 2001; 12: 371.

17. The number of people to whom a procedure (preventive or therapeutic) must be applied in order to prevent one case, complication or death is the reciprocal of the difference between the rates or proportions (incidence or mortality) in the study samples exposed and not exposed to the procedure. For example, if the rates are 5 and 3 per 1000 respectively (i.e. 0.005 and 0.003), this number is $1/(0.005 - 0.003)$, or 500. If the calculation is based on person-year rates, then the number obtained is the required number of person-years of exposure.

18. See note 36, Chapter 17.

19. Rothman KJ. Policy recommendations in Epidemiology research papers. Epidemiology 1993; 4: 94.

20. Weiss NS. Policy emanating from epidemiologic data: what is the proper forum? Epidemiology 2001; 12: 373.

21. Greenbaum DS. Epidemiology at the edge. Epidemiology 2001; 12: 376

22. Teret S. Policy and science: should epidemiologists comment on the policy implications of their research? Epidemiology 2001; 12: 374.

23. Jackson LW, Le NL, Samet JM. Frequency of policy recommendations in epidemiologic publications. American Journal of Public Health 1999; 89: 1206. Begier EM, Samet JM. Studies of particulate air pollution and mortality: when do authors comment on the policy implications? Epidemiology 2002; 13: 743.

30

Writing a Report

"'Ouch! Have a heart, Doc!" spluttered shapely Dolores X, the last of my hundred age and sex-matched controls, as I struggled to find her vein. "Do you really have to have my blood to find out whether people with malignant lymphogranuloma have a lot of antibody to some silly old virus?"' may be overdoing it somewhat as an introductory paragraph in a scientific report. But it serves to draw attention to the need for readability – a report should be written so as to attract, or at all events not repel, potential readers. To do this, it need not be written as a farce, a whodunit, or a lyric poem, but it should fulfil the following criteria:

1. The title should clearly explain what the report is about; if necessary, a subtitle can be added for extra clarity. A prospective reader usually looks first at the contents page of a journal, to see which titles 'tickle their fancy'. A journal is 'an open market where each salesman must cry his goods if he wishes to get an audience at his stall'.[1] Some journals now insist on *declarative titles* that include the main finding or message of the report.[2]
2. The abstract should be informative. A reader who has been attracted by the title will usually look at the abstract next, to decide whether the report is worth reading. 'The summary is your advertisement',[3] and should provide a picture in miniature of the whole report. It should include the objectives, specify the study population, and summarize the findings and discussion. Salient numerical details may – even should – be included. Many journals request structured abstracts, with subheadings such as Background, Objectives, Methods (or Design, Setting, Sample, Measures), Results, and Conclusions.
3. The report should be easily intelligible.[4] This requires clarity of language (this is preferable to elegance of style), a logical presentation of facts and inferences, the use of easily understood tables and charts, and an orderly arrangement of the report as a whole.[5] A scientific report may be all Greek to the layman, but it should be easily understood by the readers for whom it is written. A report's style and content should be appropriate for its expected readers; a report written for the general public or political decision makers would obviously differ from one aimed at a professional public.
4 The report should be no longer than is necessary. Unnecessary verbiage should be removed, and the report pruned to the minimum required for clearly communicating what has to be communicated. This process of pruning and condensing is not an easy one (who was it who apologized for sending a long letter by saying that he had not had the time to write a short one?).[6]

Writing a good report may take much time and effort. The most difficult task is usually the preparation of the first draft, since this requires a crystallization of the investigator's ideas on how best to express the facts and inferences; subsequent revisions are usually easier. Comments from colleagues are often useful. Many writers find it helpful to tuck a draft in a drawer – or let it rest in peace on a computer disk – and bring it out for a fresh look after a few weeks.

No investigation is complete until a report has been written. Even if the results are of interest only to the investigator, they should be placed on record, albeit in a short and even handwritten form. If they are of wider interest, they should be made available to a wider audience. Whether they should be published in print (or an electronic publication) is a question for the investigator (and later, of course, an editor or publisher) to decide. Particularly in academic fields, there is a tendency to publish whenever possible, because of the stress laid on the number or weight of publications when decisions are made about hiring, firing, promotion and tenure.

This 'Publish or perish!'[7] motivation apart, publication may often be seen as an obligation. The investigator may feel a duty to communicate the results, 'positive' or 'negative', to others who may be able to replicate them, build their own research efforts upon them, or apply them in action. An editorial in the British Medical Journal relates that Kocher's method of reducing dislocations of the shoulder was regarded as an innovation when it was described in a German medical journal in 1870. His method had been portrayed 3000 years earlier, however, in a wall painting in a tomb in the Nile Valley. 'The moral of this episode,' says the editorialist, 'is clear. Recognition of original work can be ensured only by publication in a reputable journal'.[8]

Succinct advice on the writing of a paper[9] is to be found in a document describing 'uniform requirements for manuscripts submitted to biomedical journals (the Vancouver style)', prepared by a committee of editors. Most journals have sanctioned these guidelines. Some journals, however, have their own requirements, particularly for the format of references – consult the journal's 'advice to contributors'. It is important to select the right journal for the report, and to tailor the content as well as the style of the report to the journal.[10] When choosing a journal,[11] electronic journals, whose contents can be freely accessed on-line, should be kept in mind.[12]

To be useful, a report should not only give the results of the study and the inferences that have been drawn from them, but also enough information about the methods to enable a critical reader to appraise the validity of the findings and conclusions or (ideally) to check the findings by replicating the study. The report should include a description of the study population and its characteristics, information (if relevant) about methods and criteria used for choosing subjects or groups, sampling and randomization procedures, response rates, representativeness of samples, comparability of groups, reasons for nonparticipation and withdrawals, etc. The validity and reliability of questionnaires and other study methods should be described, and operational definitions (including diagnostic criteria) should be specified. Ideally, the description of the methods should be a detailed one; questionnaires (other than standard ones) should be published in full.[13] Unfortunately (or fortunately?) this is usually practicable only in books or dissertations required for university degrees, and as a rule only the highlights can be described. The rest has to be taken on trust.

Checklists are available, indicating what items should be included, or considered for inclusion, in reports of studies of different kinds.[14]

To help the reader to make a judgement about the study, the investigator should make an honest and critical appraisal of it, and point out and discuss the main sources of possible error. Possible biases should be stated and not left for others to reveal.

Where possible, facts should be presented in a form that may be useful to other investigators who prefer to use different categories or indices when measuring variables, e.g. by presenting full frequency distributions rather than 'collapsed' scales and combinations of categories.

Tables and figures should be well enough titled and captioned and (if necessary) have enough footnotes to be reasonably intelligible without reference to the text. The tables should be well constructed, and without anomalies such as totals that do not tally, percentages that do not add up to about 100% (say between 99.8% and 100.2%), and the use of too many decimal places. If percentages are used, no doubt should be left as to what the denominator is (it is often helpful to add '100%' in the requisite place).

Diagrams should clarify and not complicate, and care should be taken that they do not mislead.[15] Graphs may be used as an alternative to tables with many entries. In general, data should not be duplicated in graphs and tables; but a graph may sometimes help to elucidate tabulated data. If curves have been 'smoothed', then the method used should be stated. The recommendations of seven core medical journals are summarized by Puhan *et al.* (2006),[16] who state that the key principles of graph construction are that data symbols should be clearly distinguishable, that the arrangement should facilitate estimation of values and important relationships in the data, and that full explanations should be provided.

The results of statistical procedures should be given in numbers and not just words (and preferably not only in pictures). Until lately, many writers and some editors felt that a sprinkling of P values lent a report an aura of scientific respectability, but the pendulum has now swung away from significance tests towards confidence intervals. The advice in the 'Vancouver style' guidelines lines is:

> When possible, quantify findings and present them with appropriate indicators of measurement error or uncertainty (such as confidence intervals). Avoid relying solely on statistical hypothesis testing, such as the use of P values, which fails to convey important quantitative information.[9]

Many of the copious results produced by statistical software can or should be omitted from the report.[17]

References should be carefully checked. A few small errors are probably inevitable, but an examination of a random sample of references in three public health journals found that in 15% the cited reference 'failed to substantiate, was unrelated to, or even contradicted the author's assertation', and 3% had major citation errors ('reference not locatable'). Minor citation errors were rife.[18] Nonessential self-citations should be avoided.[19]

The report should include a clear statement of the author's views about whether further research is needed (and if so, what); recommendations (if any) about the practical application of the results (see p. 300) – i.e. whether and how they should be applied, and any cautions about their application – should be very explicit. This may not only be helpful to readers who may wish to extend or apply the research, but it may help journalists, assiduously hunting for 'news' in the columns of scientific journals, to avoid exaggerating the importance of findings, overstating health hazards, or suggesting unwarranted changes in lifestyle or health care.

Oral Reports

Study findings are often reported orally, especially to colleagues or students and at scientific meetings. Oral reports are generally very different from written ones; they are much less complete and are often accompanied by more (but simplified) tabular or graphic material, and the sequence of presentation may be altered to maintain interest or stimulate discussion. Just as much care should be taken, however, to present the methods and findings accurately, to point out possible sources of error in the data and the inferences, and if there are recommendations, to make them even handed.

Especial care is needed in reports to journalists. Investigators sometimes make exaggerated claims or statements to reporters (as do their research institutions in press releases), going beyond what is said or will be said in the published study report. 'Preliminary' announcements of results, prior to the study's completion, may be hazardous.

Notes and References

1. Asher R. Why are medical journals so dull? British Medical Journal 1958; ii: 502.
2. The Journal of Clinical Epidemiology, for example, asks for simple declarative titles summarizing the message of the article as succinctly as possible (McGowan J, Tugwell P. Informative titles described article content. Journal of the Canadian Health Libraries Association 2005; 26: 83). The titles often include an active verb (e.g. 'Depression decreases cardiorespiratory fitness in older women'), and resemble the headlines used by journalists, 'who know a thing or two about getting people to read what they write' (Smith R. Informative titles in the BMJ. British Medical Journal 2000; 320: 915).

    Informative titles have been criticized on the grounds that they may be misleading (Goodman NW. Survey of active verbs in the titles of clinical trial reports. British Medical Journal 2000; 320: 914). Goodman found that the use of active verbs like 'prevents' and 'causes' in titles is increasing exponentially, and he uses a regression equation to predict that by 2070, 27.6% (95% CI., 23.5% to 36.1%) of all clinical papers will have one such verb in the title.
3. Dart RA, Galloway A. Memorandum on writing a scientific paper. Johannesburg: Department of Anatomy, University of the Witwatersrand (Roneo); 1934. This inaccessible reference is retained as a tribute to Raymond A. Dart (see http://en.wikipedia.org/wiki/Raymond_Dart).
4. The need for intelligibility was realized by Geoffrey Chaucer in the 14th century when he departed from tradition and wrote a scientific treatise in simple English rather than in Latin, in order to explain the astrolabe to his son: 'This tretis, divided in fyve parties, wole I shewe thee under ful lighte rewles and naked wordes in English; for Latin ne canstow yit but small, my lyte sone. But natheles, suffyse to thee thise trewe conclusiouns in English, as wel as suffyseth to

thise noble clerkes Grekes thise same conclusiouns in Greek, and to Arabiens in Arabik, and to Jewes in Ebrew, and to the Latin folk in Latin' (Chaucer G. A treatise on the astrolabe. Cited by Gordon IS, Sorkin S. The armchair science reader. New York, NY: Simon & Schuster; 1959. p. 294).

5. Keep the language as simple as possible. Instead of impressing, the use of obscure terminology may lead to floccinaucinihilipilification by the reader.

   But excessive linguistic simplicity may be self-defeating, as exemplified by Zongker D (Chicken chicken chicken: chicken chicken. Annals of Improbable Research 2006; 12 (5): 17. Available at http://www.ingentaconnect.com/content/improb/air/2006/00000012/00000005/art00006.

6. It was Blaise Pascal, in 1657 and French. But Cicero and St Augustine both said something very similar, earlier (http://palimpsest.stanford.edu/byform/mailing-lists/exlibris/2003/07/msg00105.html).

7. The pressure to publish is so strong that some investigators are led to falsify data or to pirate papers. *Scientific fraud* is usually undiscovered or (if unmasked) unreported. 'The best estimate today is perhaps that the prevalence of fraud is between 0.25% and 0.5% of research projects' (Lock S. Fraud in medical research. Journal of the Royal College of Physicians of London 1997; 31: 90). For examples, see Broad WJ (Fraud and the structure of science. Science 1981; 212: 137, 264); Broad WJ, Wade N 1982 (Betrayers of the truth. Simon & Schuster, New York), Stewart WW, Feder N (The integrity of the scientific literature. Nature 1987; 325: 207). One researcher who submitted reports containing repeated falsifications received nearly $1 million in cancer research funds.

   In a postal survey in 1998 of all members of the International Society for Clinical Biostatistics, 51% of respondents (i.e. 18% of the sample) said they knew of at least one fraudulent project (fabrication, falsification, suppression of data, or deceptive reporting) in their proximity during the last 10 years; the main motives seemed to be career and power, not financial reward (Ranstam J, Buyse M, George SL, Evans S, Geller NL, Scherrer B, Lesaffre E, Murray G, Edler L, Hutton JL, Colton T, Lachenbruch P. Fraud in medical research: an international survey of biostatisticians. Controlled Clinical Trials 2000; 21: 415).

   In addition to falsification, fabrication, and plagiarism, there are other, less serious and more common, questionable research practices. For example, a postal survey in 2002 of 3600 scientists funded by the US National Institutes of Health revealed that in the previous 3 years between 3.1% and 6.0% had avoided presenting data that contradicted their previous research results (Martinson BC, Anderson MS, de Vries R. Scientists behaving badly. Nature 2005; 435: 737).

   Deceptive reporting is not always fraudulent, but can be due to a misunderstanding of research methods or terminology – an investigation of 3137 so-called 'randomized controlled trials' reported in China in 1994–2005 revealed that only 7% of them were truly randomized (Wu T, Li Y, Liu G, Bian Z, Li J, Zhang J, Xie L, Ni J. Investigation of authenticity of 'claimed' randomized controlled trials [RCTs] and quality assessment of RCT reports published in China. Cochrane Colloquium Proceedings, 2006. Available at http://www.imbi.uni-freiburg.de/OJS/cca/index.php/cca/article/view/1928).

8. Editorial. Where to publish? British Medical Journal 1968; 4: 344.

9. *Advice on writing*: See Hall GM (ed.) (How to write a paper, 3rd edn. London: BMJ Books; 2003). Succinct advice on the writing of a manuscript can be found at http://www.sfedit.net/newsletters.htm.

   The *Vancouver style guidelines* (updated February 2006) are available at http://www.icmje.org. In addition to recommendations about manuscript preparation, the guidelines place emphasis on ethical issues. For example, authorship should be limited to people who meet all three of the following criteria: (1) substantial contributions to conception and design, or acquisition of data, or analysis and interpretation of data; (2) drafting the article or revising it critically for important intellectual content; and (3) final approval of the version to be published.

Also, information that might identify subjects should not be published without informed consent, obtained after the subject has seen the manuscript.

The guidelines say that all *conflicts of interest* should be reported. These exist when an author 'has ties to activities that could inappropriately influence his or her judgment, whether or not judgment is in fact affected. Financial relationships with industry ... either directly or through immediate family, are usually considered to be the most important conflicts of interest. However, conflicts can occur for other reasons, such as personal relationships, academic competition, and intellectual passion'.

10. Guyatt GH, Haynes RB. Preparing reports for publication and responding to reviewers' comments. Journal of Clinical Epidemiology 2006; 59: 900.

11. *Impact factors* of epidemiology and public health journals can be viewed at http://www. epidemiologic.org/2006/10/impact-factors-of-epidemiology-and.html. The impact factor is the number of times the journal is cited (in a given period) per article published.

12. BioMed Central presently publishes over 180 peer-reviewed open-access e-journals (http://?www. biomedcentral.com/browse/bysubject), including several in the fields of public health, epidemiology, and primary care. A fuller list of open-access journals in the health sciences is available at http://www.doaj.org/doaj_func=subject&cpid=20. Some medical open-access journals have a high impact factor (McVeigh ME. Open access journals in the ISI citation databases; 2004. scientific.thomson.com/ts/media/presentrep/essayspdf/openaccesscitations2.pdf).

13. A review of studies that use questionnaires and were published in epidemiology journals in 2005 showed that, in half of those that did not use an identifiable existing questionnaire, there was no mention of a pretest. Only 47% even discussed validation, and in only one-third were any complete questions printed in the article or a referenced article (Rosen T, Olsen J. The art of making questionnaires better. American Journal of Epidemiology 2006; 164: 1145).

To enable readers to evaluate findings, it has been suggested that journal editors should insist on the inclusion of key questions, and that questionnaires be published in the journal's online repository or in another website (Schilling LM, Kozak K, Lundahl K, Dellavalle RP. Inaccessible novel questionnaires in published medical research: hidden methods, hidden costs. American Journal of Epidemiology 2006; 164: 1141).

14. *Checklists of items to be included in reports* include the following:

For observational studies, the most recent recommendations are the STROBE (Strengthening the Reporting of Observational Studies in Epidemiology) recommendations, which (with their explanations) take up 36 pages in Epidemiology (2007; 18: 800–835). The accompanying reservations by prominent epidemiologists (Epidemiology 2007; 18: 789–799) are well worth reading. They express concern about 'any effort to formalize reporting in a field as heterogeneous as observational epidemiology', emphasize the importance of good judgment rather than specific criteria, stress the importance of a well-done study rather than merely a well-written report ('avoid judging an apple by how well it is polished'), and suggest that 'guidelines ... should come with expiration dates'.

For randomized controlled trials: see the CONSORT statement, available (with updates and explanations) at http://www.consort-statement.org.

For meta-analyses of randomized controlled trials: Moher D, Cook DJ, Eastwood S, Olkin I, Rennie D, Stroup DF. Improving the quality of reports of meta-analyses of randomized controlled trials: the QUORUM statement. Lancet 1999; 354: 1896.

For web-based surveys: Eysenback G. Improving the quality of web surveys: the checklist for reporting results of Internet E-surveys (CHERRIES). Journal of Medical Internet Research 2004.

15. For misuses of diagrams, see Huff D, Geis I (How to lie with statistics. New York, NY: W W Norton; 1993).

    Detailed illustrated advice on the construction of bad graphs can be found at http://lilt.il-stu.edu/gmklass/pos138/datadisplay/badchart.htm. The key requirements are data ambiguity (inadequate explanation), data distortion, and data distraction (by using an unnecessarily high ink-to-data ratio).

16. Puhan MA, ter Riet G, Eichler K, Steurer J, Bachmann LM. More medical journals should inform their contributors about three key principles of graph construction. Journal of Clinical Epidemiology 2006; 59: 1017.

17. Cummings P. Reporting statistical information in medical journal articles. Archives of Pediatrics and Adolescent Medicine 2003; 157: 321. For a detailed on-line guide to the presentation of statistical results, see the Statistical Good Practice Guidelines at http://www.rdg.ac.uk/ssc/publications/guides/toptgs.html.

18. Eichorn P, Yankauer A. Do authors check their references? A survey of accuracy in three public health journals. American Journal of Public Health 1987; 77: 1011.

    Similar levels of inaccuracy of quotations and citations of references have been reported in numerous medical, dental and nursing journals. The following advice, given towards the beginning of the 20th century, is apparently not yet followed: 'Take no reference for granted. Verify the reference that your best friend gives you. Verify the reference that your revered chief gives you. Verify, most of all, the references that you yourself found and jotted down. To err is human, to verify is necessary' (Place F Jr. Verify your references: a word to medical writers. New York Medical Journal 1916; 104: 697). We borrowed this reference from Putterman C, Lossos IS (Author, verify your references! or, The accuracy of references in Israeli medical journals. Israel Journal of Medical Sciences 1991; 27: 109), who apparently copied it from Roland CG (Thoughts about medical writing. XXXVII. Verify your references. Anesthesia and Analgesia 1976; 55: 17). Readers are advised to verify this!

19. Although self-citations may be tempting. A seminal study of over half a million citations has shown that the more one cites oneself the more one is cited by others, and this effect increases with time (Fowler JH, Aksnes DW. Does self-citation pay? http://jhfowler.ucsd.edu/does_self_citation_pay.pdf).

31

Rapid Epidemiological Methods

The terms 'rapid epidemiological methods', 'rapid appraisal', and 'rapid assessment' usually refer to simplified procedures that can speed up a study in order to provide real-time results as a basis for programme decisions and action.[1] In a district of Uganda, only 10 days were required to collect, analyse and publish information on the utilization of health services, health-seeking behaviour, immunization coverage, and the nutritional status of children.[2] A 50-page report of the findings of a health survey of children in a town in Myanmar was also issued 10 days after the commencement of field work, as was a 70-page report on surveys of antenatal care and family planning in Thailand.[3]

Since these rapid methods are relatively undemanding and inexpensive, they are usually advocated for use in developing countries. They may, however, be useful wherever manpower, finances or other research resources are limited, as in many studies carried out by practitioners in the context of community health services in developed countries. Some rapid methods (not discussed in this chapter) involve the use of sophisticated and expensive electronic communication and processing techniques.

Simplified methods may provide less detailed or valid information than would be provided by more rigorous methods. They are to an extent 'quick and dirty', and the key question to be asked before using them is whether their results can adequately meet the study's purpose. Can the direction and degree of inaccuracy be estimated, and are the results likely to be useful despite their margin of error? If so, there is no reason not to use simple procedures, particularly if the alternative is to obtain no information at all. Care must be taken, of course, to avoid unnecessary inaccuracy, e.g. by giving due attention to the training of data collectors and by checking completed questionnaires and the coding of data.

We will give separate consideration to four aspects: simplified sampling procedures (especially the use of two-stage cluster samples), simple data collection (including rapid qualitative appraisal), rapid processing, and rapid methods of evaluating care.

Simplified Sampling Procedures

The easiest way to simplify sampling is, of course, to use a *sample of convenience* instead of a probability sample. But the disadvantages are obvious, and this shortcut should be taken only if rough 'ballpark figures' will suffice, or for some qualitative research procedures.

Research Methods in Community Medicine: Surveys, Epidemiological Research, Programme Evaluation, Clinical Trials   J. H. Abramson and Z. H. Abramson   Copyright © 2008, John Wiley & Sons Ltd

Purposive sampling will often satisfy a study's needs. It may be decided, for example, that patients attending a health facility are sufficiently representative of the total community to warrant their use (with reservations) as a study sample for a specific purpose, or that tests and interviews of antenatal clinic attenders and men attending outpatient clinics will provide useful information on the prevalence of sexually transmitted diseases in refugee camps,[4] or that surveillance of influenza can be carried out by watching 'sentinel' populations (e.g. by recording sick absenteeism in selected schools or workplaces).

In some countries, the selection of subjects and controls for telephone interviews can be simplified by random digit dialling (see p. 79), but this is not necessarily cheap or time-saving.

Two-stage cluster sampling

The EPI cluster sampling technique was initially advocated by the WHO's Expanded Programme on Immunization as a rapid, cheap and accurate basis for surveys of immunization coverage, and has since been widely used for descriptive surveys of specific diseases, service coverage, health-service needs, blindness, and other topics.[5] Cluster surveys of this kind should be considered not only when resources are limited, but whenever rapid results are required, especially in emergency situations.[6]

The EPI technique has four advantages: it does not require a detailed sampling frame; it uses clusters of subjects who live close to one another; subjects are selected in the field by a procedure so simple it can be used by health workers with minimal technical support; and it can provide reasonably representative data.

The selection process has two stages. First, communities (villages, urban blocks, neighbourhoods of a city, etc.) are chosen using a random procedure requiring reasonably accurate estimates of population size. Then, clusters are selected in the chosen communities by a method that provides a 'self-weighted' sample. The sample falls short of being a true probability sample, since the second stage does not use random sampling, which would require a census or detailed map for use as a sampling frame. The basic method is simple:

1. *Decide on the number of clusters and determine their size.* The number of clusters will depend on the manpower and time available; the more clusters, the more valid the results – 30 is probably a minimum. Calculate the size of the required sample[7] and divide it by the number of clusters (and round the answer up, to make it a whole number) to determine how many subjects are needed in each cluster. The original EPI recommendation (for surveys of vaccination status) was 30 clusters with seven children in each; 30 clusters of 30 individuals have been suggested for nutritional surveys.
2. *Randomly select the communities where clusters will be sought.* Make a list of the communities (in any order), with their population sizes, and calculate the cumulative population size, as shown in Table 31.1, which displays the communities in an imaginary region. Compute a sampling interval by dividing the total population size by the required number of clusters. In this instance, if 30 clusters are wanted, the sampling interval is 120,300/30 = 4010. Choose a random number between

1 and 4010, and fit it into position in the list to identify a community. If the random number is 1946, which lies between 1100 and 3900, then the first community chosen is F. Now add the sampling interval to 1946 (1946 + 4010 = 5956) and use the result (5956) to select the second community (P). Again, add 4010 (5956 + 4010 = 9966) and select community H. Again, add 4010 (9966 + 4010 = 13,976) and select H again – meaning that two separate clusters are required from community H. And so on. This selects communities with a probability proportional to their size.

3. *Select clusters.* In each selected community, randomly select one household to be the starting point and then use a systematic procedure to select other households, to create a cluster. To choose the starting point, go to a central place and randomly choose a direction, e.g. by spinning a bottle or throwing up a pen or pencil and seeing how it lands (this is sometimes called the 'spin-the-pen' method); then count the number of households between the central point and the edge of the community in that direction, choose one of them at random, and visit it. For subsequent choices, take the unvisited household whose door is closest to the household last visited. Visit each of the chosen households in turn until the number of subjects (say, children of the right age) required in a cluster has been found. This has been called the *random walk* method.

A multistage design may be used in a survey of a very large region, by selecting communities in two (or more) stages, each using the systematic probability-proportional-to-size method described above; that is, first select subregions and then communities. A map-based modification (the 'centric systematic area sample method') has been described, based on division of the survey area into equally sized squares and selection of the communities closest to the centre of each square (the number of the communities to be selected in the square being determined by the number of communities that the survey team can cover in one day), and then investigation of every household in the

Table 31.1 List of communities, showing cumulative population size

Community	Population size	Cumulative population size
D	1,100	1,100
F	2,800	3,900
P	5,000	8,900
S	600	9,500
H	9,400	18,900
E	3,200	22,100
A	3,500	25,600
Q	1,200	26,800
C	4,300	31,100
M	4,900	36,000
G	3,900	39,900
etc.	–	120,300

community.[8] More rigorous sampling procedures can be used, such as selecting communities randomly within each square, or using a finer grid and selecting a single central community in each square.

Computer simulations have shown that the EPI sampling method is usually satisfactory for the rapid appraisal of immunization status or the prevalence of a disease, although the results may be biased and less precise than those based on random sampling, and its accuracy for different diseases varies. The method is less satisfactory if the survey covers a wide range of topics, so that different-sized clusters are required for measuring different characteristics, or if associations (e.g. with nutritional status) are under study. The results in different clusters or subsets of clusters can be compared only if the samples are large. The main deficiencies of the EPI design arise from its failure to use random methods when selecting clusters, and from the use for this purpose of quota sampling; results may be misleading if subjects with similar characteristics tend to live close to one another.

If there is no reason to suspect bias, then the results of a study using the EPI design are dependable. They are of course not precise – no results based on a small sample can be precise. But the degree of imprecision can be assessed (as it can in a study based on random sampling). As an example, a recent study of mortality following the 2003 invasion of Iraq[6] pointed to an estimated 655,000 excess Iraqi deaths between March 2003 and June 2006, presumably as a consequence of the war (95% confidence interval: 393,000 to 943,000). The wide confidence interval expresses the imprecision of the method of study. But, within the stated limits, there is no reason to doubt the accuracy of the findings. In the words of the chief researcher, speaking of a similar earlier study in Iraq,[6] 'Can one estimate national figures on the basis of a sample? The answer is certainly yes (the basis of all census methods), provided that the sample is national, households are randomly selected, and great precautions are taken to eliminate biases. These are all what we did. Now the precision of the results is mostly dependent on sample size. The bigger the sample, the more precise the result'.[9] The summary dismissal of the new study's results by the president of the United States during a news conference[9] ('I don't consider it a credible report.... The methodology is pretty well discredited') seemed to be misguided, although some researchers have expressed doubts about the manner in which the study plan was put in effect.[9]

The use of random selection in the last stage would, of course, mitigate the deficiencies of the EPI method. If a list or map of households in each chosen community is available or can be constructed, then the households to be visited can be selected randomly from this sampling frame; but then this becomes a less 'rapid' method. Simpler suggested remedies are the use of (say) the fifth nearest household instead of the nearest one, and splitting the community into quadrants and selecting a quarter of each cluster from each quadrant, starting at the centre point of the quadrant.

A 'not quite as quick but much cleaner' alternative

A suggested 'not quite as quick but much cleaner' alternative[10] to the EPI cluster survey design, aimed at retaining the advantages of ease and cheapness but making the procedure more rigorous and appropriate even for surveys that make multiple measurements, is based on the preselection of a 'target segment size' – the number of households to be surveyed for each cluster – instead of fixing the number of subjects needed in each cluster. This number is reached by first calculating the required sample size,[7] then (using the best available data) estimating how many households will have to be contacted in order to locate this number of subjects (e.g. children aged under five, or children with diarrhoea in the previous fortnight), and dividing this total number of households by the number of clusters (at least 30). Communities are selected randomly (as in the basic EPI method), and the chosen communities are divided into equal segments, each containing (approximately) the required number of households; this requires a rough sketch map showing the dwellings (households) in the community. A segment of the community is then chosen at random, and all eligible individuals in all the dwellings in the chosen segment are included in the sample. This method, which has been called the 'compact segment sampling' method, ensures that all households in the study population have approximately the same probability of being selected.

A comparison of the 'random walk' and 'compact segment sampling' methods, used in studies of vaccination coverage in the same region at about the same time, revealed markedly similar results. It was concluded that, although the compact segment sampling method was preferable, the EPI random walk method can give accurate results if carried out by experienced workers.[11]

The lot quality technique

The *lot quality technique*, a method developed to assess the acceptability of lots (batches) of manufactured parts coming off an industrial production line, is a promising rapid sampling method that identifies communities with a high (or low) prevalence of the characteristic under study.

The procedure has been shown to be a rapid and reliable way of determining whether trachoma is a public health problem in a community. A systematic or 'random-walk' sample of houses is selected in a village or other community, and then a maximum of 50 children in the sample are examined, stopping as soon as a predetermined number of cases have been found. (This is the number that will correctly identify about 95% of communities with the sought prevalence, calculated from cumulative binomial probabilities.) For example, finding nine cases (and then stopping) would be highly accurate in pointing to a prevalence of 20% or more, whereas finding no cases, or only one, would mean a prevalence of less than 5%. These prevalences would determine the treatment strategy in the different communities.[12]

Simple Data-collection Methods

Data collection may be simplified in various ways. The most obvious ones are to restrict the variables to those that are essential to meet the study's purposes (resulting in very short questionnaires or examinations) and to choose sources that are easily accessible (available records may, despite their deficiencies, contain enough information to obviate the need for a more demanding survey).

If available, simpler procedures can be chosen rather than more accurate but elaborate ones, e.g. a rapid urine test for use in surveys of iodine deficiency[13] or a simple test card for identifying people with low vision.[14] Household food inventories or brief dietary questionnaires may supply enough information on dietary practices, rendering detailed dietary interviews unnecessary.[15] In countries without well-developed death certification, verbal autopsies[16] – questionnaires or structured interviews administered by lay personnel to relatives or friends of the deceased – may provide a degree of information on mortality from gastroenteritis, measles, accidents, HIV-associated conditions and other causes.

It may be decided to use simple proxy measures, e.g. arm circumference or weight-for-height as easy and cheap indices of malnutrition in children.[17]

Other examples[18] are night blindness as a relatively easily measured surrogate for vitamin A deficiency, a history of wheezing or whistling in the chest as a measure for the lifetime prevalence of asthma, a characteristic depigmentation pattern ('leopard skin') as an index of the endemicity of onchocerciasis, and appraisal of the burden of lymphatic filariasis by measuring the rate of infection of insect vectors or by examining men for hydroceles.

If the measures are simple, then it is easy to train health workers or others in their use. Schoolteachers can measure weight and height with adequate precision, assistants can be taught simple cataract recognition, and traditional midwives have been taught to identify low birth-weight babies by using a hand-held scale that shows a coloured signal if the weight is below 2.5 kg. In Tanzania, a simple questionnaire on diseases and symptoms was administered to children by teachers, and a comparison with urine tests showed that reports of haematuria or schistosomiasis had a high validity.[19]

Cross-sectional methods, e.g. for appraising child growth in a community, are obviously faster than longitudinal ones. Simple data on current infant feeding practices can, if appropriately analysed, rapidly provide a picture of the average duration of breast-feeding and the age at introduction of supplements.[20]

Rapid qualitative appraisal

Simple qualitative methods (see p. 147) permit rapid appraisal of knowledge, attitudes and practices relevant to health and health care (*rapid ethnographic assessment*, *rapid assessment procedures*) using procedures for which 'one does not need an advanced degree in anthropology ... One does need ... the ability to develop rapport with people and to accurately record and transmit their views, beliefs and behaviours'.[21]

The basic methods[22] are conversations and informal interviews with members of the public and key informants, focused discussions with small groups of people whose opinions and ideas are of interest, the nominal group technique (described in Chapter 20), and unstructured observations, e.g. of housing conditions or sanitary arrangements or the manner in which mothers prepare infant foods or oral rehydration solutions. Simple guides and checklists are available for use in collecting data on various aspects of health and health care.[21]

Confirmation of validity by *triangulation* (comparing what different methods reveal, to determine their common findings) is an important feature of this approach.

The participation of community leaders, members of the public and providers of health services in qualitative research activities can often be developed into partnerships in the ongoing development of services and improvements in their delivery and utilization.[23]

Rapid Processing

The keys to rapid processing are good planning, prompt entry of data into a computer – preferably at the time of obtaining the data – and appropriate statistical software. Data-entry programs (see Appendix C) that check the data for mistakes as they are entered (possibly even at the time they are collected) can prevent subsequent time-consuming investigations of errors. User-friendly software for statistical analysis can be downloaded from the Internet to facilitate rapid analysis.

The use of computers as survey tools is no longer unusual in developing countries, although special courses and customized programs may be required.[24] As demonstrated in a malaria survey in the Gambia, use of a hand-held computer for collecting and checking questionnaire data can significantly increase both speed and accuracy.[25] In Myanmar, initially computer-illiterate survey personnel learned to operate a spreadsheet program in order to estimate sample sizes and select communities for a two-stage cluster design and calculate and graphically display confidence intervals.[26]

Rapid Methods of Evaluating Care

Longitudinal studies (trials and cohort studies) are time-consuming methods of evaluating care procedures and programmes. But evaluation can be speeded up if it is based on easily obtained cross-sectional data or on inquiries about previous care.

The *lot quality technique* (see above) may be used to monitor the quality of health care. It has been used (especially in developing countries) to assess immunization coverage, family planning, antenatal care, the use of oral rehydration therapy, and health-worker performance.[27]

A simple way of testing the effectiveness of a health programme is to compare the status of people who have and have not been exposed to the programme. In clinics in Lesotho, for example, a children's growth monitoring and nutrition education programme was evaluated by means of a cross-sectional study in which maternal knowledge about infant feeding was measured, and mothers were classified according to whether or not they had previously attended the clinic. Women who had attended were found to be more knowledgeable about the introduction of animal protein foods, the use of oral rehydration salts, and the method of weaning.[28] But an evaluative study based on simple comparison of the findings or changes seen in people who voluntarily or perforce participate or do not participate in a programme is generally not convincing, as the comparison may be confounded by differences (not all of which may be controlled in the analysis) other than the difference in exposure to the programme. The authors correctly limited their conclusion to the statement that previous clinic attendance 'appeared to be' beneficial.

A relatively simple and rapid way of evaluating preventive and therapeutic procedures or programmes is to compare people who have experienced an unfavourable outcome (cases) with controls, to see whether they differ in their prior exposure to the procedure or programme. The unfavourable outcome is generally one that the procedure or programme aims to prevent, as in case-control studies[29] to evaluate immunization procedures, PAP testing, breast cancer screening, aspirin to protect against myocardial infarction, family planning, prenatal and intrapartum care, child health services, and improvements in water supply and sanitation, but it may also be a suspected undesirable side-effect, as in studies comparing the neonatal exposure to vitamin K prophylaxis of children who do and do not develop cancer.[30] Like all case-control studies, these pose problems, with particular reference to the appropriateness of the controls. It is not easy to exclude the possibility that the cases and controls may have initially had differences affecting their prognosis, maybe related to their eligibility, preparedness or ability to undergo the procedure or participate in the programme. There may also be bias due to differences in the recall or reporting of exposure. Therefore, care is required to control for confounding and other biases. But the information required for properly appraising or controlling these biases is generally difficult to obtain, and the conclusions are often equivocal. An inbuilt limitation of this method is its capacity to examine only one outcome, the outcome used to define cases.

Notes and References

1. The evolution and use of *rapid methods* are reviewed by Smith GS (Development of rapid epidemiologic assessment methods to evaluate health status and delivery of health services. International Journal of Epidemiology 1989; 18(suppl. 2): S1), who points out that their introduction was a major factor in the worldwide eradication of smallpox.

    For symposia on the use of rapid methods, see special issues of the International Journal of Epidemiology (Rapid epidemiologic assessment. 1989; 18(supp. 2): S1) and Health Policy and Planning (Rapid assessment methods for the control of tropical diseases. 1992; 7(1): 1). Also, see Scrimshaw SCM, Hurtado E (Rapid assessment procedures for nutrition and primary health care: anthropological approaches to improving programme effectiveness. Los Angeles, CA: UCLA Latin American Center Publications; 1987).

    Rapid assessment is especially important in mass emergencies, where health needs should be appraised within 24–48 hours (Guha-Sapir D. Rapid assessment of health needs in mass emergencies: review of current concepts and methods. World Health Statistics Quarterly 1991; 44: 171).

2. Materia E, Imoko J, Berhe G, Dawuda C, Omar MA, Pinto A, Guerra R. Rapid surveys in support of district health information systems: an experience from Uganda. East African Medical Journal 1995; 72: 15.

3. Frerichs RR, Tar KT. Computer-assisted rapid surveys in developing countries. Public Health Reports 1989; 104: 14.

4. Mayaud P, Msuya W, Todd J *et al.* STD rapid assessment in Rwandan refugee camps in Tanzania. Genitourinary Medicine 1992; 73: 33.
5. For fuller descriptions of *EPI cluster sampling*, see Lemeshow S, Robinson D (Surveys to measure programme coverage and impact: a review of the methodology used by the Expanded Programme on Immunization. World Health Statistics Quarterly 1985; 38: 65) and Bennett S, Woods T, Liyanage WM, Smith DL (A simplified general method for cluster-sample surveys of health in developing countries. World Health Statistics Quarterly 1991; 44: 98).

   Recent descriptive studies illustrate the wide variety of topics for which this sampling method has been used: Gabutti G, Rota MC, Salmaso S, Bruzzone BM, Bella A, Crovari P (Epidemiology of measles, mumps and rubella in Italy. Epidemiology and Infection 2003; 129: 543); Vellinga A, Depoorte AM, Van Damme P (Vaccination coverage estimates by EPI cluster sampling survey of children [18–24 months] in Flanders, Belgium. Acta Paediatrica 2002; 91: 599); Okrah J, Traoré C, Palé A, Sommerfeld J, Müller O (Community factors associated with malaria prevention by mosquito nets: an exploratory study in rural Burkina Faso. Tropical Medicine & International Health 2002; 7: 240); S. Sreevidya S, Sathiyasekaran BWC (High caesarean rates in Madras (India): a population-based cross sectional study. BJOG: An International Journal of Obstetrics and Gynaecology 2003; 110: 106); Morris SS, Carletto C, Hoddinott J, Christiaensen LJM (Validity of rapid estimates of household wealth and income for health surveys in rural Africa. Journal of Epidemiology and Community Health 2000; 54: 381); Mahgoub SEO, Bandeke T, Nnyepi M (Breastfeeding in Botswana: practices, attitudes, patterns, and the sociocultural factors affecting them. Journal of Tropical Pediatrics 2002; 48: 195).

   Bias and precision vary for prevalence studies of different diseases (Katz J, Yoon SS, Brendel K, West KP Jr. Sampling designs for xerophthalmia prevalence surveys. International Journal of Epidemiology 1997; 26: 1041).

   The degree of clustering of a disease within the sample clusters may be of interest; a survey in Tanzania, for example, revealed clustering of trachoma within neighbourhoods in villages, not explained by known risk factors (West SK, Munoz B, Turner VM, Mmbaga BBO, Taylor HR. The epidemiology of trachoma in Central Tanzania. International Journal of Epidemiology 1991; 20: 1088).

   Approximate *incidence rates* can sometimes be derived from prevalence findings based on cluster studies. For example, approximate poliomyelitis incidence rates have been computed from the prevalence of lameness and other symptoms (LaForce FM, Lichnevski MS, Keja J, Henderson RH. Clinical survey techniques to estimate prevalence and annual incidence of poliomyelitis in developing countries. Bulletin of the World Health Organization 1980; 58: 609. Babaniyi O, Parakoyi B. Cluster survey for poliomyelitis and neonatal tetanus in Ilorin, Nigeria. International Journal of Epidemiology 1991; 20: 515. Schwoebel V, Dauvisis A-V, Helynck B *et al.* Community-based evaluation survey of immunizations in Burkino Faso. Bulletin of the World Health Organization 1992; 70: 583).

   Computer simulations to test the accuracy of EPI cluster sampling are described by (among others) Bennett S, Radalowicz A, Vella V, Tomkins A (A computer simulation of household sampling schemes for health surveys in developing countries. International Journal of Epidemiology1994; 23: 1282) and Harris D R, Lemeshow S (Evaluation of the EPI survey methodology for estimating relative risk. World Health Statistics Quarterly 1991; 44: 107).
6. Cluster surveys have a special role in *emergency situations*. In the public health disaster that followed civil disturbances in Rwanda in 1994, for example, when over half a million Rwandans fled to Zaire, such surveys, combined with morbidity surveillance, provided a basis for a well-coordinated programme that was associated with a steep decline in deaths of refugees by the second month of the crisis (Goma Epidemiology Group. Public health impact of Rwandan refugee crisis: what happened in Goma, Zaire, in July, 1994? Lancet 1995; 345: 339).

After Yugoslavia's civil war and disintegration, it took only 2 months to obtain a picture of health services use and related problems (Legetic B, Jakovljevic D, Marinkovic J, Niciforovic O, Stanisavljevic D. Health care delivery and the status of the population's health in the current crises in former Yugoslavia using EPI-design methodology. International Journal of Epidemiology 1996; 25: 341).

Cluster surveys are probably the only practical way to obtain accurate estimates of mortality in national emergency situations: Coghlan B, Brennan RJ, Ngoy P, Dofara D, Otto B, Clements M, Stewart T (Mortality in the Democratic Republic of Congo: a nationwide survey. Lancet 2006; 367: 44); Roberts L, Lafta R, Garfield R, Khudhairi J, Burnham G (Mortality before and after the 2003 invasion of Iraq: cluster sample survey. Lancet 2004; 364: 1857); Burnham G, Lafta R, Doocy S, Roberts L (Mortality after the 2003 invasion of Iraq: a cross-sectional cluster sample survey. Lancet 2006; 368: 1421); Depoortere E, Checchi F, Broillet F. Gerstl S, Minetti A, Gayraud O, Briet V, Pahl J, Defourny I, Tatay M, Brown V (Violence and mortality in West Darfur, Sudan [2003–04]: epidemiological evidence from four surveys. Lancet 2004; 364: 1315).

7. See note 19, Chapter 8.
8. Myatt M, Feleke T, Sadler K, Collins S. A field trial of a survey method for estimating the coverage of selective feeding programmes. Bulletin of the World Health Organization 2005; 83: 20.
9. Comments by Dr Gilbert Burnham in an email to David Edwards (http://www.warmwell.com/_04dec4bbcbias.html), and by George W. Bush (http://edition.cnn.com/2006/WORLD/meast/10/11/_iraq.deaths/index.html).

    See: Death toll in Iraq: survey team takes on its critics. Nature 2007; 446(1 March): 8.
10. Turner AG, Magnani RRJ, Shuaib M. A not quite as quick but much cleaner alternative to the Expanded Programme on Immunization (EPI) cluster survey design. International Journal of Epidemiology 1996; 25: 198.

    See also Brogan D, Flagg EW, Deming W, Waldman R (Increasing the accuracy of the Expanded Programme on Immunization's cluster survey design. Annals of Epidemiology 1994; 4: 302) and Grais RF, Rose AMC, Guthmann JP (Don't always spin the pen: two alternative methods for second stage sampling in cluster surveys in urban zones. Emerging Themes in Epidemiology 2007; 4: 8).
11. Milligan P, Njie A, Bennett S. Comparison of two cluster sampling methods for health surveys in developing countries. International Journal of Epidemiology 2004; 33: 469.
12. Myatt M, Limburg H, Minassian D, Katyola D. Field trial of applicability of lot quality assurance sampling survey method for rapid assessment of prevalence of active trachoma. Bulletin of the World Health Organization 2003; 81: 877.
13. Rendl J, Bier D, Groh T, Reiners C. Rapid urinary iodide test. Journal of Clinical Endocrinology and Metabolism 1998; 83: 1007.
14. Keeffe JE, Lovie-Kitchin JE, Maclean H, Taylor HR. A simplified screening test for identifying people with low vision in developing countries. Bulletin of the World Health Organization 1996; 74: 525.
15. Patterson RE, Kristl AR, Shannon J, Hunt JR, White E. Using a brief household food inventory as an environmental indicator of individual dietary practices. American Journal of Public Health 1997; 87: 272.

    Examples of short dietary questionnaires: Dobson AJ, Blijlevens R, Alexander HM *et al.* (Short fat questionnaire: a self-administered measure of fat-intake behaviour. Australian Journal of Public Health 1993; 17: 1144); Retzlaff BM, Dowdy AA, Walden CE, Bovbjerg VE, Knopp RH (The Northwest Lipid Research Clinic Fat Intake Scale: validation and utility. American Journal of Public Health 1997; 87: 181).

16. *Verbal autopsies* work best for causes of death, like tuberculosis and accidents, that are easy to distinguish from other causes, and for broad groupings of causes. Causes of death are best assigned by physician review of the information, but algorithms based on specific history items provide an alternative approach, with results within 20% of the gold standard for some causes of death (Quigley MA, Chandramohan D, Rodrigues LC. Diagnostic accuracy of physician review, expert algorithms and data-derived algorithms in adult verbal autopsies. International Journal of Epidemiology 1999; 28: 1081). Accuracy may vary in different settings.

17. Arm circumference: see Velzeboer MI, Selwyn BJ, Sargent F, Pollitt E, Delgado H (Evaluation of arm circumference as a public health index of protein energy malnutrition in early child-hood. Journal of Tropical Pediatrics 1983; 29: 135; The use of arm circumference in simplified screening for acute malnutrition by minimally-trained health workers. Journal of Tropical Pediatrics 1983; 29: 159). Weight-for-height may be more useful than arm circumference (Bern C, Nathanail L. Is mid-upper-arm circumference a useful tool for screening in emergency settings? British Medical Journal 1995; 345: 631).

18. *Proxy measures*: Sommer A, Hussaini G, Muhilal T I, Susanto D, Saroso JS (History of night blindness: a simple tool for xerophthalmia screening. American Journal of Clinical Nutrition 1980; 33: 887); Kuehni CE, Brooke AM, Silverman M (Prevalence of wheeze during child-hood: retrospective and prospective assessment. European Respiratory Journal 2000; 16: 81); Edungbola LD, Alabi TO, Oni GA, Asaolu SO, Ogunbanjo BO, Parakoyi BD ('Leopard skin' as a rapid diagnostic index for estimating the endemicity of African onchocerciasis. Journal of Epidemiology 1987; 16: 590); Pani SP, Srividya A, Krisknamoorthy K, Das PK, Dhanda V (Rapid assessment procedures (RAP) for lymphatic filariasis. National Medical Journal of India 1997; 10: 19); Gyapong JO, Adjei S, Gyapong M, Asamoah G (Rapid community diagnosis of lymphatic filariasis. Acta Tropica 1996; 61: 65); Venkataswamy G, Lepkowski JM, Ravilla T, Brilliant GE, Shanmugham CAK, Vaidyanathan K, Tilden RL and the Aravind Rapid Epidemiologic Assessment Staff (Rapid epidemiologic assessment of cataract blindness. International Journal of Epidemiology 1989; 18: S60); Ritenbaugh CK, Said AK, Gaslal OM, Harrison GG (Development and evaluation of a colour-coded scale for birthweight surveillance in rural Egypt. International Journal of Epidemiology 1989; 18: S54).

19. Lengeler C, Mshinda H, de Savigny D, Kilima P, Morona D, Tanner M. The value of question-naires aimed at key informants, and distributed through an existing administrative system, for rapid and cost-effective health assessment. World Health Statistics Quarterly 1991; 44: 150.

20. Ferreira MU, Cardoso MA, Santos AL, Ferreira CS, Szarfarc SC. Rapid epidemiologic assessment of breastfeeding practices: probit analysis of current status data. Journal of Tropical Pediatrics 1996; 42: 50.

21. Scrimshaw SCM, Hurtado E (1987; see note 1).

22. For descriptions and illustrations of *rapid qualitative assessment* methods, see Scrimshaw SCM, Hurtado E (1987; see note 1), the symposia cited in note 1, and Ong BN, Humphris G (Prioritising needs with communities: rapid appraisal methodologies in health. In: Popay J, Williams G (eds), Researching the people's health. London: Routledge; 1994).

23. See, for example, Dale J, Shipman C, Lacock L, Davies M (Creating a shared vision of out of hours care: using rapid appraisal methods to create an interagency, community oriented, approach to service development. British Medical Journal 1996; 312: 1206).

24. The *use of computers* in surveys in developing countries is illustrated by Forster D, Snow B (Using microcomputers for rapid data collection in developing countries. Health Policy and Planning 1982; 7: 67), Bertrand WE (Microcomputer applications in health population surveys: experience and potential in developing countries. World Health Statistics Quarterly 1985; 38: 91), Gould JB, Frerichs RR (Training faculty in Bangladesh to use a microcomputer for public health: followup report. Public Health Reports 1986; 101: 616), Forster D,

Behrens RH, Campbell H, Byass P (Evaluation of a computerized field data collection system for health surveys. Bulletin of the World Health Organization 1991; 69: 107), Frerichs RR (Simple analytic procedures for rapid microcomputer-assisted cluster surveys in developing countries. Public Health Reports 1989; 104: 24), Frerichs RR, Tar KT (1989; see note 3), and Blignaut PJ, McDonald T (A computerised implementation of a minimum set of health indicators. Methods of Information in Medicine 1997; 36: 122).

    However helpful a computer may be, it cannot work magic. A description of one computer program claims that it 'is designed to allow anyone, no matter how knowledgeable or ignorant of statistical and survey methods, to conduct a useful and correctly designed survey. It has everything you need...' (PC Magazine 1989; 8: 254). (Throw away this book!)

25. Forster D *et al.* (1991; see note 24).

26. Frerichs RR (1989; see note 24).

27. Robertson SE, Anker M, Roisin AJ, Macklai N, Engstrom K, LaForce FM. The lot quality technique: a global review of applications in the assessment of health services and disease surveillance. World Health Statistics Quarterly 1997; 50: 199.

28. Ruel MT, Habicht J-P, Olson C. Impact of a clinic-based growth monitoring programme on maternal nutrition knowledge in Lesotho. International Journal of Epidemiology 1992; 21: 59.

29. Most of these case-control studies are cited by Baltazar JC (The potential of the case-control method for rapid epidemiological assessment. World Health Statistics Quarterly 1991; 44: 140) and Smith GS (1989; see note 1).

30. Conflicting results are presented by McKinney PA, Juszczak E, Findlay E, Smith K (Case-control study of childhood leukaemia and cancer in Scotland: findings for neonatal intramuscular vitamin K. British Medical Journal 1998; 316: 173) and Passmore SJ, Draper G, Brownbill P, Kroll M (Case-control studies of relation between childhood cancer and neonatal vitamin K administration: retrospective case-control study. British Medical Journal 1998; 316: 178) and discussed by von Kries R (Editorial: Neonatal vitamin K prophylaxis: the Gordian knot still awaits untying. British Medical Journal 1998; 316: 161).

32

Clinical Trials

Clinical trials are experiments or quasi-experiments that test hypotheses concerning the effects (favourable or unfavourable) of intervention techniques applied to individuals. They may be tests of therapeutic agents, devices, regimens or procedures (therapeutic trials), of preventive ones (prophylactic trials), or of rehabilitative or educational procedures, etc. (Trials of screening and diagnostic tests were discussed on pp. 171–172.)

The main objectives are usually to measure the efficacy and safety of the procedure, and their variation among patients with different characteristics. Attention may also be focused on efficiency, e.g. by comparing the costs of different ways of achieving a similar benefit. Other questions (concerning compliance, satisfaction, etc. – see p. 50) may also be asked, but are usually seen as subsidiary, serving only to explain why the outcome was or was not satisfactory; they may, however, be dominant features in studies that centre on feasibility or acceptability.

A distinction has been made between *explanatory* clinical trials, whose purpose is mainly to provide biological information (e.g. about the way drugs act and the way the body reacts to them) and *pragmatic* or *practical* ones, which aim to test procedures under the conditions in which they would be applied in practice.[1] Pragmatic trials are concerned with effectiveness rather than efficacy (see p. 51).

Clinical trials may be set up not only to appraise the effects of individual-focused procedures, but also (in some instances) to evaluate programmes. The latter use of clinical trials will be discussed in Chapter 33.

The use of case-control studies (instead of trials) to appraise the effects of treatments and other procedures is discussed on p. 320.

Here are seven examples of trials. In the first four the subjects were randomly allocated to the groups that were compared. (For the findings, refer to the notes; no prizes.)

The objectives of the studies were:

1. To compare the incidence of stroke in elderly people with systolic hypertension (and normal diastolic blood pressure) who received medicinal treatment or indistinguishable placebos.[2]
2. To compare the prevalence of symptoms of adenoidal hypertrophy, before and after operation, in children who had only their tonsils removed or who had their adenoids out too.[3]

Research Methods in Community Medicine: Surveys, Epidemiological Research, Programme Evaluation, Clinical Trials   J. H. Abramson and Z. H. Abramson   Copyright © 2008, John Wiley & Sons Ltd

3. To compare the proportions of people with common colds who were cured or improved 2 days after starting treatment with antihistaminic tablets or indistinguishable dummy placebo tablets.[4]
4. To compare the relief of symptoms in patients with angina pectoris after ligation of the internal mammary arteries (an operation designed to increase blood flow to the heart) or a sham operation (in which only a skin incision was made).[5]
5. To compare the progress of two patients with scurvy ('putrid gums, the spots and lassitude, with weakness of their knees'), who were given two oranges and one lemon every day, with the progress of 10 similar patients who were given other treatments.[6]
6. To compare the occurrence of complications in soldiers whose wounds were treated with boiling oil or with a mixture of egg yolks, oil of roses and turpentine.[7]
7. To compare the countenances of four children fed on legumes and water for 10 days (Daniel, Shadrach, Meshach and Abednego) with those of children fed on King Nebuchadnezzar's meat and wine.[8]

Study Designs

The following are the basic study designs. If the intervention is not under the investigator's control (i.e. if decisions on who gets what, and when, are not made by the investigator) then the study is a *quasi-experiment*. (As noted on p. 13, some writers refer to any unrandomized trial as a quasi-experiment; the terminology used is less important than an awareness that careful consideration must be given to the possible biases in all experiments, whether 'true' or 'quasi'.)

1. *Parallel studies*, in which two or more independent groups are studied prospectively and compared.
2. *Externally controlled studies*, in which a single experimental group is studied and the findings are compared with data obtained from other sources.
3. *'Self-controlled' studies*, in which the subjects are their own controls. These may be based on observations before and after a single treatment (*before–after studies*), or *crossover studies*, in which two or more treatments are applied in sequence to the same subjects.

These designs may be combined. Other designs (e.g. factorial, Latin and Greco-Latin squares[9]) may also be used. A *factorial design* permits appraisal of the effects of two or more factors, and also of their joint effects. A simple example is the Physicians' Health Study, which examined the effect of aspirin on cardiovascular mortality and the effect of beta-carotene on cancer incidence; participants were randomly divided into four groups, who were respectively given aspirin and a placebo, beta-carotene and a placebo, aspirin and beta-carotene, or two placebos. Its successor, Physicians' Health Study II, is a randomized, double-blind, placebo-controlled trial that uses a $2 \times 2 \times 2 \times 2$ factorial design to test the effects of beta-carotene, vitamin E, vitamin C, and multivitamins, alone and in combination.[10]

Types of clinical trial

1. Parallel (concurrent controls)
2. External controls
3. 'Self-controlled'

Parallel studies, or trials with *concurrent controls*, compare groups exposed to different interventions. A treated group may be compared with a control group that receives no treatment (or a placebo), or two or more groups who are having different treatments may be compared with each other or with an untreated group. If the allocation of subjects to the groups is random, the study is a *randomized controlled trial (RCT)*. A well-done RCT has a high level of internal validity, and can provide convincing evidence and precise estimates of the effect of an intervention. It is generally regarded as the standard with which other methods of study should be compared, although its internal validity may be achieved at the expense of external validity. The manner in which subjects are selected for a trial may interfere with generalizability, and (as noted on pp. 280–282 in Chapter 28) the results of an RCT are not always more useful than those of a well-done nonexperimental study.

Parallel comparisons require information about the subjects before as well as after the intervention (i.e. they should be 'premeasure–postmeasure' or 'pretest–post-test' studies). This not only permits a check on the comparability of the groups before the intervention, it also makes it possible to take proper account of possible confounders and modifiers in the analysis. Many studies are based on a comparison of the changes observed in different groups; the measurement of change, e.g. in blood pressure or other characteristics, requires baseline data. Trials with no information about prior status ('postmeasure-only' trials or 'post-test' trials) have unknown and possibly serious biases; Daniel's biblical trial (see p. 326) is an example.

In *externally controlled studies* the findings in the experimental group are compared with control data obtained from other sources, e.g. with statistics reported by other medical agencies that did not use the experimental procedure. In a therapeutic trial of this sort, the comparison is usually with cases treated in the past (*historical controls*). This approach may sometimes be of unquestioned validity, e.g. if the disease being treated is one that, according to previous experience, never disappears or is always fatal. Ethical constraints may compel the use of historical controls; a physician who is convinced of the merit of a new treatment and, therefore, cannot ethically use randomization may decide to perform a trial using historical controls.

There may, however, be serious bias in externally controlled studies; the results of treatment may differ because the controls differed from the experimental subjects, or were treated by other clinicians, or at another time (when circumstances affecting the prognosis, such as other components of patient management, were different), or were appraised differently, etc. Even patients treated in the same centre and in the same way, but at different times, may have very different outcomes.[11]

Trials with historical controls may provide the first clues to real breakthroughs in medical science; on the other hand, results may be misleading, and yet make a subsequent RCT ethically unacceptable. Historical controls are sometimes used as a check on the results of a trial using concurrent controls; if the randomized controls fared worse than previous experience would lead one to expect, this needs explaining.

In *self-controlled studies*, use of the subjects as their own controls prevents confounding by many characteristics that may influence the outcome. But there are possible biases in a simple 'before–after' study – those connected with extraneous events or with changes that occur with time, nonspecific effects caused by the performance of the experiment itself, changes in methods of measurement, and regression to the mean (see p. 74); in a parallel study, comparison is made with a control group that is subject to the same effects. However, such studies may be appropriate in some circumstances (e.g. testing a treatment in patients with refractory disease, or appraising the value of supplementary feeding for children in refugee camps).[12]

In a *crossover study* each subject is given the different treatments (or treatment and placebo) under comparison, one after another. Each subject is ghach's[13] own control. The sequence of assignment is generally randomized, so that this is a kind of RCT. A 'washing-out period' may be required between treatments, to permit the effects of the previous treatment to disappear, and the method is not feasible if a treatment has 'protracted "carry-over" effects'. The *N of 1* clinical trial or *single-case experiment*[14] is a special kind of crossover study aimed at determining the efficacy of a treatment (or the relative value of alternative treatments) for a specific patient. The patient is repeatedly given a treatment and placebo, or different treatments, in successive time periods. The trial often leads to a decision to change the patient's treatment. If a number of 'N of 1' trials are conducted on similar patients, then they may provide a basis for generalizations.[15]

Randomization

Randomization is a procedure whereby the assignment of treatments is left to chance. The allocation to groups (representing the *arms* of the study) is decided by tossing a coin or some other strictly random method. This can be justified only if the investigator is in *equipoise*, i.e. genuinely uncertain about which arm of the study is best.

Randomization does not guarantee that the groups will be identical, but it makes misleading results less likely, by ensuring that the only differences between the groups are those that occur by chance. This applies both to known risk and protective factors and to unsuspected ones. Unless the groups are very small, marked differences become unlikely.

The random assignment procedure should be applied to *all* the subjects included in the study – to all the volunteers entering a prophylactic trial, or to all the patients whose diagnosis, clinical condition and other features make them eligible for inclusion in a therapeutic trial, and who have agreed to participate in it (Table 32.1). Exclusion criteria (too old, too ill, etc.) should be laid down in advance and, if possible, applied before the subjects are assigned to groups. If there is an objection to putting a subject

Table 32.1   A typical randomized controlled trial

1.	Eligible? → If not, exclude
2.	Consent? → If not, exclude
3.	Randomize to Groups A and B
4.	Treat (subjects may be blinded to treatment)
5.	Follow up all members of Groups A and B
6.	Compare outcomes or changes in Groups A and B

in any one of the groups, then they should be excluded from the trial before allocation. Such exclusions do not bias the results of the comparison (internal validity), although they may limit the applicability of the results (external validity). The results of a well-conducted RCT can validly be applied to whatever kind of person entered the trial ('no bias is caused by exclusion, even if for silly reasons')[16], but not to anyone else.

Sometimes, as a convenient and theoretically adequate alternative to randomization, a systematic method of assignment is used, such as the allocation of alternate patients to treatment and control groups. Such methods have been criticized on the grounds that they are too easily manipulated by well-meaning clinicians. In a controlled trial of anticoagulant therapy for myocardial infarction, in which the patient's treatment was determined by whether admission occurred on an odd- or even-numbered day of the month, it was found that the physicians (convinced of the value of the treatment) saw to it that more patients were admitted on odd-numbered days.[17]

Another simple and valid alternative to ordinary randomization, convenient only in small trials in which subjects are introduced one by one, is *minimization*. The assignment of each subject is influenced by the distribution of selected prognostic variables in the previously assigned members of the groups, using a random procedure that weighs the scales in favour of a decision that will minimize the differences between the groups with regard to these prognostic factors.[18] It is a method of balanced randomization (see below).

Whichever of these methods of allocation is used, it is wise before drawing conclusions to compare the groups to check whether they were similar before the trial started. In a large-scale trial of the effect of extra milk on the height and weight of schoolchildren, for example, the children allocated to the experimental group turned out to be initially shorter and lighter than the control children.[19]

Randomization may be achieved by tossing a coin or throwing a die, using tables[20] of random numbers or random permutations, or letting a computer[21] do the work.

Since simple randomization may produce groups that (by chance) differ somewhat in size, especially if the number of subjects is small, *balanced randomization* is usually preferred. This imposes a constraint on the randomization process so as to prevent the allocation ratio from diverging (by chance) from the intended ratio of, say, 1:1 or 2:1. Various methods are available for this purpose.[22]

Both simple and balanced randomization (or systematic assignment) may be carried out separately in various strata of the study population, generally using strata that it is believed may influence the outcome of the trial, such as age, severity of the disease, or month (if seasonal factors are deemed important). The purpose of this *prestratification* is to reduce variation between the groups with respect to important prognostic factors that may be confounded with the effects of the treatment. *Matching* may also be used for this purpose. In a multicentre trial, each centre is generally regarded as a stratum.

Balanced randomization may be conducted in successive *blocks* of subjects (a term that comes from agricultural experiments in which a field was divided into blocks, in each of which a number of treatments were tried). The blocks may be the same size as the number of arms of the study, or a multiple of that number. In each block, a constraint is applied to the random selection process to ensure that the same number of subjects (one or more) is allocated to each arm of the study (or to ensure any desired ratio between the number allocated to the arms). This *blocked randomization* procedure is particularly appropriate in clinical trials in which the subjects are not available at the outset, but accrue with the passage of time. There is separate randomization of each pair or set of successively enrolled subjects. The procedure ensures that (after the enlistment of each complete block) the groups are balanced, and it also controls for any effects connected with the passage of time. Blocked stratification may be applied separately in each stratum (usually, in each centre of a multicentre trial).

Matching and prestratification may be useful in small studies, but statisticians disagree about their value in large studies (the collective noun for statisticians is 'a variance of statisticians'). The grounds for opposition are that these procedures complicate the trial unnecessarily, and the effects of important prognostic factors can just as well be taken into account during the analysis, by *post-stratification* ('retrospective stratification') – i.e. stratifying the subjects according to characteristics that are found to be related to the outcome – or other methods.[23]

Group-randomized Trials

In some trials the units are not individuals, but clusters of individuals. This may be for convenience, or because the intervention cannot be applied to individuals but only at a group level, often because it involves the social functioning or physical environment of the group. Examples are villages, towns, schools, classes in schools, work-sites, families, married couples, and general practices.

In these trials, it is the clusters that are allocated to the arms of the study – preferably by randomization – not their individual members.

The analysis of randomized trials of this sort (*group-randomized* or *cluster-randomized* trials)[24] may require special techniques, which treat the groups as the units of analysis and take account of the likelihood that there will be a degree of similarity between the members of the group with respect to the way they are affected by the intervention. Cluster-randomized trials will be discussed in more detail in Chapter 33.

Making the Trial Easier

Randomized controlled trials are often unfeasible, and are always difficult to perform. The constraints include ethical problems, insufficiency of resources or subjects, and the rapid evolution and obsolescence of treatments in some fields. 'It is hard to argue with the concept that every medical therapy should be evaluated in an RCT', says one expert, who also points out that the method 'is slow, ponderous, expensive, and often stifling of scientific imagination and creative changes in treatment protocols', and declares that it 'is a last resort for the evaluation of medical interventions'.[25]

There are a number of designs that try to lessen logistic or ethical difficulties, while still endeavouring to limit potential bias; special precautions are needed in their analysis or interpretation. For example:

1. Assign fewer patients to the less favourable therapy ('response adaptive randomization').[26] In a trial that compares treatments whose success can be adjudged rapidly, each patient's treatment may be determined by the previous patient's result ('Play the winner') or by the cumulative results for all previous subjects (the 'two-armed bandit' method). Or two treatments may be tried in a half or third of the patients, and the more successful of the two can then be used in the remaining subjects.
2. Reduce the number of randomized concurrent controls, but compensate for this by also using historical controls who were treated at the same institution with the same eligibility criteria and methods of appraisal, and use both sets of controls in the analysis.[27]
3. Stop accepting new subjects as soon as there is a definitive answer.[28] A sequential design of this sort is practicable if subjects enter the trial serially and results are available soon. It requires the prior establishment of 'stopping rules', and ongoing analysis. In some studies it is important to set up a rule for stopping the study if the treatment appears to be harmful. Adaptive clinical trial designs permit changes in sample size in midstream, but they require complex sequential interim analyses.
4. Assign all subjects who are at higher risk to the new treatment, and either assign subjects at lower risk randomly, or assign them to the standard treatment (or placebo). Statistical modelling is used to make sense of the results.[29]
5. In a trial comparing a new treatment with the best current standard therapy, randomize the subjects before obtaining their consent.[30] This is Zelen's prerandomized or 'randomized consent' design; see Table 32.2). Give Group A the standard therapy and ask the members of Group B for their consent to the new treatment. If they

Table 32.2 A prerandomized controlled trial

1.	Eligible? → If not, exclude
2.	Randomize to Groups A and B
3.	Consent? (Requested in one or both groups)
4.	If refused, give treatment preferred by subject
5.	Treat (subjects cannot be blinded to treatment)
6.	Follow up all members of Groups A and B
7.	Compare outcomes or changes in Groups A and B

consent, give them the new treatment; if not, give them the standard treatment. (Alternatively, ask the members of Group B to choose between the two treatments.) Then compare the outcomes in Group A (all of whom received the standard treatment) and Group B (some of whom received the new treatment). This is a valid comparison of randomized groups, although the design 'dilutes' the difference between the treatments; but this may be offset by the higher participation rate that may be expected in such studies. The only ethical problem in this *single consent* method is that members of Group A are not offered the experimental treatment. This is overcome in the *double consent* (*double prerandomized*) design, where (in addition) members of Group A are asked for their consent to the standard therapy (otherwise, they are given the new therapy); if they tend to consent, the comparison of Groups A and B remains useful. Randomization comes before consent in many *cluster trials*, where groups, not individuals, are randomized. (The groups may be, for example, the patients of different general practitioners, or children in different classes or schools.) Disadvantages of prerandomized trials are that the subjects cannot be kept unaware of their treatment, and that it becomes difficult to examine the modifying effects of factors that are associated with the patient's decisions; the latter difficulty can be partly overcome by stratifying by selected factors when randomising. Zelen's designs continue to excite debate.

6. In a study in which random allocation is impossible because subjects have already been assigned to treatment groups – for example, if a new treatment is applied in one centre (a clinic or hospital ward) and not in another; the 'usual care' (control) centre – use *prospective individual matching*. That is, base the analysis on the subjects in the two centres who can be individually matched against each other with respect to important prognostic factors. In effect, this turns the trial into a matched cohort study.[31]

7. Let the patient select a form of treatment, and then control for the confounding effects of differences between the groups by using appropriate analytic methods. The potential biases of this kind of quasi-experiment are the same as those of nonexperimental studies, and the results cannot be expected to be as convincing – or necessarily the same – as those of randomized trials. This approach is advocated by opponents of randomization ('One is uncomfortable with a randomized protocol that lets chance dictate the medical care a human being receives'), who also plead for data banks for the accumulation of clinical experience, to provide material for evaluative studies ('One randomised trial with 100 patients can dramatically change physician behavior, whereas the experience of 100,000 patients might be neglected').[32]

Bias in Clinical Trials

Clinical trials may be beset by most of the biases discussed in Chapter 27. But an indication of the main problems that are specific to clinical trials is given by the simple Jadad criteria, which are widely used for assessing the quality of randomized clinical trials (as judged from their reports).[33] Points are given for three items that relate directly to the reduction of bias (maximum score, 5):

1. Randomization: 1 point if mentioned, increased to 2 if an appropriate method of randomization is described, and reduced to 0 if an inappropriate method is described.
2. Double-blinding: 1 point if mentioned, increased to 2 if an appropriate method of double-blinding is described, and reduced to 0 if an inappropriate method is described.
3. Withdrawals and drop-outs: 1 point if described in each of the comparison groups.

The aim of a random allocation to the arms of the study is to reduce confounding caused by differences in prognostic factors, i.e. differences that may affect the probability of developing the outcome under study (*susceptibility bias*). Other devices that may be used for this purpose in the design of trials include restriction (by applying inclusion and exclusion criteria), matching, and prestratification.

Double-blinding (see pp. 146–147) aims to reduce information bias connected with the subject's or investigator's knowing to which group the subject has been assigned (e.g. *reporting bias, observer bias, interviewer bias*). Analyses of large numbers of trials have shown that treatment effects tend to be smaller if the trial is double-blinded.[34,35]

Even in the best run of clinical trials, it is unlikely that all subjects will remain in their assigned groups, doing what the members of the group are supposed to do, for the whole duration of the study. Subjects may stop complying; or (in a therapeutic trial) members of a treatment group may have their treatment stopped or changed during the study, in their own interests, or members of a control group may be put on to treatment (examples of *contamination bias*); or subjects may drop out completely, or be withdrawn from the study because of death, the development of complications, or other reasons (*attrition bias*). In trials of interventions that involve a change in behaviour, there are always subjects who do not make the change, or who change their behaviour although they are in a control group – sometimes as a result of interaction with members of the intervention group (another kind of *contamination bias*). As in cohort studies (p. 262), these withdrawals and drop-outs may cause an imbalance between the arms of the study, and confounding of the results. To overcome this bias, the analysis should be based on a comparison of the subjects originally allocated to each group (*intention-to-treat analysis*). This stringent approach may underestimate the efficacy of the treatment. An *on-randomized-treatment* or *per-protocol analysis* may, therefore, be performed as well, comparing the experience of subjects while they were still on their allocated treatment; but the findings must be interpreted with the realization that possible confounding is uncontrolled. The two analyses may provide minimal and maximal measures of the effect of treatment.

Another bias that may be important is what has been called *allocation-of-interventions bias* or *subversion bias* – an analysis of 250 controlled trials showed that the estimated effect of treatment tended to be much smaller in trials in which the allocation scheme was well concealed.[36] The key question is usually whether there is adequate concealment of the next subject to be entered into the study. If concealment is inadequate, then research-ers can subvert the allocation, trying everything from transillumination of envelopes to searches in office files.[36]

Both the findings of the trial and their generalizability may be influenced by *selec-tion bias*, caused either by the restrictions imposed by investigators and the circum-stances of the study or by the readiness of eligible people to participate (*participation bias*). Participants in therapeutic trials tend to be less affluent, less educated, and more severely ill than nonparticipants, and this may lead to an exaggerated measure of the effects of treatment; whereas participants in trials of preventive measures tend to be more affluent, better educated, and more likely than nonparticipants to have a healthy life-style, and this may underestimate effects, as there may be less room for improve-ment.[37] Selection bias may be caused not only by nonparticipation in the study, but also by nonresponse to subsequent requests for information. This has been shown to bias the conclusions of a randomized trial of different methods of promoting mam-mography.[38]

And, of course, we should not forget the *Hawthorne effect* – the influence of know-ing that one is an experimental subject. This was illustrated in a study of patients undergoing knee arthroscopy under spinal anesthesia.[39] They were randomly assigned to two groups, which were treated identically except that the informed consent form received by one group contained the sentences: 'We are conducting research to evalu-ate the acceptability of loco-regional anesthesia. Therefore you are part of a study and will be followed with particular attention and interest to record which side effects of the anesthesia are least acceptable to you'. Controlling for possible confounders, the patients who knew they were being studied scored better on a psychological well-being questionnaire after the operation, and reported significantly less post-operative knee pain and headache.

Planning and Running a Clinical Trial

For a clinical trial to yield convincing conclusions it must be designed and conducted with meticulous attention to detail. Unless the effects of the intervention are very marked and specific, they can be convincingly attributed to the intervention (and not to extrane-ous factors) only if special precautions are taken. These include the use of appropriately selected controls (discussed in Chapter 7) and 'blind' methods (see p. 146), and (where appropriate) matching and prestratification (see p. 330), as well as suitable methods of analysis.

Study objectives should be formulated precisely, in the form of clear and specific hypotheses (see Chapters 4 and 5). The study population should be defined explicitly (Chapter 6) and eligibility and exclusion rules formulated (as in case-control studies; see p. 92). Attention must be given to intervention allocation methods, the size of the groups (p. 84), the selection and precise definition of variables (Chapters 10–12) (including the outcome variables), the use of reliable and valid methods of data collection (Chapters 15–17), quality control (p. 247), and surveillance of compliance. In deciding on *sample size*, the computation may be based on the numbers required to detect a difference in a single primary outcome or, if the study has more than one main objective, separate calculations may be made for each outcome, and the largest sample size selected; but it is recommended that there should be at least 90% power for each endpoint, to ensure sufficient power for meeting all the objectives simultaneously.[40]

Running a trial is not easy, and is beset with day-to-day problems that can easily overshadow the study's *raison d'etre*; trials 'lack glamour; they strain our resources and patience, and they protract to excruciating limits the moment of truth; ... [but] if ... the alternative is to pay the cost of perpetual uncertainty, have we really any choice?'[41] Successful trial management requires careful attention to the rules of the game,[42] the first of which is 'Thou shalt know and follow thy rules'. A written study protocol[43] is generally desirable, and is essential in multicentre trials.[44] The protocol of a therapeutic trial should include a detailed description of the treatment and its permissible modifications. Aids to the planning of the study and writing of a protocol are available on the Internet (see Appendix C).

The selection of a study population for a trial is determined by the reference population the investigator has in mind; that is, to whom are the results to be applied? This is the basis for sound decisions on the source of subjects and the method of enrolling them, and the formulation of eligibility and exclusion criteria. The results of a trial of the treatment of middle-aged adults with moderate hypertension may not be applicable to patients with mild hypertension, or to the elderly.

The generalizability of results depends on who is studied. The results of a trial conducted on volunteers, such as a trial of immunization performed by comparing outcomes in randomly allocated groups of volunteers, may not be directly applicable to the population at large. In all trials there are selective factors – the subject's wishes, the views of the treating physician, family, etc. – that the investigator cannot control. It is important, therefore, to try to appraise the importance and nature of selection bias by determining what proportion of eligible people enter the trial and how those who enter differ from those who do not. The rules and actual reasons for exclusions should, of course, be recorded, so that it is clear to what kinds of subject the results of the trial do not apply. If many people withhold consent, so that possible non-consent bias is an important consideration, it may be enlightening to follow up and compare the progress of nonrandomized as well as randomized subjects; this may be done by a *comprehensive cohort design* (a cohort study with a randomized subcohort)[45] or by parallel trials, one randomized and one nonrandomized (where patients who are eligible for randomization choose their own treatment).[46]

It may not be easy to recruit subjects to the trial. A review of controlled trials of recruitment found single studies showing that recruitment was raised by telephone reminders, monetary incentives, the absence of blinding and the non-use of placebos, the mailing of a questionnaire together with the invitation, and the use of paper rather than Web-based questionnaires.[47]

In a typical RCT, the sequence of steps is: determine eligibility; request informed consent; assign randomly; treat; and follow up. In a prerandomized study, consent and randomization are reversed. In some studies, e.g. where compliance with the taking of medications is regarded as an essential condition for participation, it may be necessary to have a 'run-in' period before eligibility can be finally determined; this period may precede or follow randomization. In the Physicians' Health Study, which tested the prophylactic effect of aspirin and beta-carotene, all participants eligible for randomization were sent packs of aspirin and a beta-carotene placebo and, after an 18-week run-in period, those who reported side-effects to aspirin or had taken less than two-thirds of their pills were excluded from the trial.[48] In studies where treatment cannot be delayed until all diagnostic test results are available, eligibility may not be certain before treatment is started. In principle, randomization should be done as late as possible, i.e. when eligibility is certain and, in a trial where the initial treatment is the same for all patients, only after the initial treatment phase.

To maintain blindedness, the allocation should, if possible, be done by someone not directly connected with the study, or by the pharmacy preparing drugs and placebo, or otherwise by using serially numbered sealed envelopes.[49]

In randomized trials, clinicians may be asked to consult a list showing how successive subjects should be treated, or to open a sealed envelope specifying the next patient's treatment, or to contact a coordinator and be told what treatment to give. It may not be easy to avoid divergence from the random allocation, even if sealed envelopes are used.[50]

If placebos or alternative pharmacological preparations are given to control subjects, then an attempt should be made to maintain blinding, by ensuring that the preparations are indistinguishable to the senses.[51] They should look the same and their containers should not have distinctive labels, so that clinicians, too, are kept unaware of the treatment. To see whether blindness has been maintained, subjects can afterwards be asked if they know what they were given; and effects can be analysed separately in subjects who did or did not know, or thought they knew, what they were having.

Placebos present special problems in nonpharmacological trials,[52] where it may be difficult or impossible to maintain blinding, since an indistinguishable control intervention may be hard to find or difficult to defend ethically. Innovative solutions that have been found include a placebo acupuncture needle that does not penetrate the skin, and sham surgical operations (with just a small incision).[53] At the very least, whoever is assessing the outcome should remain blinded, if this is possible.

Rules for withdrawals from the randomized treatment should be laid down in advance. 'Escape hatches' must always be provided, to enable patients to be withdrawn whenever this is in their best interests – if, for example, they develop worrisome side-effects, illnesses or complications, or whenever (in a double-blind study) it becomes necessary for the clinician to know what treatment is being administered. Subjects may also be withdrawn because they turn out to be ineligible.

Follow-up should be as complete as possible. Subjects who are withdrawn from the study and those who drop out may be highly selected groups, and if they are numerous their exclusion from the analysis may cause serious bias. Wherever possible, the reasons for drop-outs should be ascertained. In a trial with defined endpoints, such as death, the occurrence of a disease or complication, recovery, etc., the aim should be to follow up every member of every study group until the occurrence of an endpoint, the lapse of a predetermined study period, or the conclusion of the study. Patients who turn out to be misdiagnosed or ineligible for other reasons are exceptions to this rule; they can usually be withdrawn without causing bias.

Every trial needs a 'policeman'[54] – an investigator, coordinator or coordinating committee who will keep an eye on the study, ensure smooth running and the avoidance of bias, and protect subjects' interests. It may be important to check adherence to randomization plans and 'blind' techniques, and monitor patients' compliance and the completeness and quality of data. In some trials, ongoing monitoring of data is undertaken in order to see whether the study can or should be stopped early, e.g. because of harmful effects or unexpectedly large beneficial effects. This function is best performed by an independent individual or committee, not the investigators; 'stopping rules' should be laid down in advance.

In the analysis, use should be made of methods that take account of the duration of the subject's participation and the times of endpoint events or repeated appraisals. Confounding can be reduced by appropriate analytic techniques, e.g. by subdividing the groups so that similar subjects can be compared (stratification). Special methods are needed if clusters, not individuals, were randomized.[24]

Clinical trials often yield inconclusive or inconsistent results because of their small size. Results of different trials, however, can be integrated so as to yield firmer conclusions about the effects of the intervention, their consistency, and the factors that influence them (including characteristics of the subjects, variations in the intervention, and the circumstances and methods of the trial). A *meta-analysis*[55] or overview of this sort requires the use of suitable statistical methods. Meta-analysis may be applied to observational as well as experimental studies. It typically includes an appraisal of the quality of the studies (*qualitative meta-analysis*),[56] a comparison of the studies, an analysis of the factors modifying their findings, and (if there are no important modifying effects) a summary statement of the findings in the various studies. Applied to trials, a meta-analysis might review studies that test a specific effect of a specific intervention, or it might compare the effects of different interventions or the various effects of an intervention.

Notes and References

1. Schwartz D, Flamart R, Lellouch J (Clinical trials. London: Academic Press; 1980) describe in detail how the purpose of a trial (explanatory or pragmatic?) can influence planning, conduct and analysis. In a pragmatic trial, the treatment is administered in the manner in which it would be used in practice, to subjects similar to those to whom it would be applied in practice, and appraised in terms of outcomes that are important to patients, rather than biological effects.

    For an example of how decisions were made in a pragmatic trial in primary care, see the account of the DIAMOND study (the Dutch study of InitiAl Management of Newly diagnosed Dypepsia), in which 'adequate symptom relief at 6 months, according to the patient' was chosen as the outcome because this would affect the decision to stop or continue treatment in everyday practice (Fransen GA, van Marrewijk CJ, Mujakovic S, Muris JWM, Laheij RFJ, Numans ME, de Wit NJ, Sansom M, Janden JBMJ, Kotterus JA. Pragmatic trials in primary care: methodological challenges and solutions demonstrated by the DIAMOND study. BMC Medical Research Methodology 2007; 7: 16).

Also, see Roland M, Torgerson DJ (Understanding controlled trials: what are pragmatic trials? British Medical Journal 1998; 316: 285. Understanding controlled trials: what outcome should be measured? British Medical Journal 1998; 317: 1075).

2. The patients for this study were recruited from 198 centres in 23 European countries. After an average follow-up period of 2 years the incidence of stroke was 42% lower (95% confidence interval, 14 to 63% lower) in the treatment group, 72% of whom continued their treatment throughout. The trial was then stopped on the grounds that it would be unethical to continue it. Total cardiovascular mortality was 27% lower (95% confidence interval, 48% lower to 2% higher in the treatment group) (Staessen JA, Fagard R, Thijs L *et al*. Randomised double-blind comparison of placebo and active treatment for older patients with isolated systolic hypertension. Lancet 1997; 350: 757).

3. Symptoms generally attributed to adenoidal hypertrophy (nasal obstruction, snoring, rhinorrhoea, etc.) were very prevalent in both groups before operation, and were seldom found after operation. They were equally common in both groups, both before and after operation. The study was 'blind', i.e. the examiner did not know the kind of operation (Hibbert J, Stell PM. Critical evaluation of adenoidectomy. Lancet 1978; 1: 657).

4. The proportions who were cured or improved were very similar among patients taking antihistaminic and placebo tablets. This applied to people who started treatment within a day of the onset of symptoms, 1 day after onset, 2 days after, and 3 days or more after onset (Hill AB. Statistical methods in clinical and preventive medicine. Edinburgh: Churchill Livingstone; 1962. pp. 105–119).

5. Internal mammary ligation was performed on 304 'unselected' patients with angina pectoris and/or a history of myocardial infarction, and symptomatic improvement was reported in 95% (Battezzatti M, Tagliaferro A, Cattaneo AD. Clinical evaluation of bilateral internal mammary artery ligation as treatment of coronary heart disease. American Journal of Cardiology 1959; 4: 180). In a randomized trial in 17 patients with angina pectoris, the results (significant improvement in just over half the cases) were very similar in the patients who had this operation and in those who had a sham operation. One patient, previously unable to work because of his heart disease, was almost immediately rehabilitated and returned to his former occupation, and reported 100% improvement after 6 months; his arteries had not been ligated. The patients were told only that they were participating in a trial of the procedure, and the clinicians who appraised progress did not know which operation had been done (Cobb LA, Thomas GT, Dillard DH, Merendino KA, Bruce RA. An evaluation of internal-mammary-artery ligation by a double-blind technic. New England Journal of Medicine 1959; 260: 1115).

6. 'The most sudden and visible good effects were perceived from the use of the oranges and lemons; one of those who had taken them, being at the end of six days fit for duty … The other was the best recovered of any in his condition; and being now pretty well, was appointed nurse to the rest of the sick' (who remained sick as ever). The trial was not blind, the sample sizes were decided arbitrarily, the allocation of treatments was not strictly random, and no significance test was done. But the observed difference was significant ($P = 0.022$) by Fisher's exact test, Fisher being a statistician who was born about 130 years later (Lind J. The prophylaxis, or means of preventing this disease, especially at sea. In: Anonymous, A treatise of the scurvy. Edinburgh: Sands, Murray and Cochran; 1753 pp. 137–177).

7. This experiment was forced on Ambroise Paré one day in 1537, when he ran out of boiling oil. The next morning the soldiers he had treated with boiling oil 'were feverish with much pain and swelling about their wound', whereas the others had 'but little pain, their wounds neither swollen nor inflamed'; cited by Bull JP (The historical development of clinical therapeutic

trials. Journal of Chronic Diseases 1950; 10: 218). The trial was not blind, the treatments were not allocated at random, and statistical significance was not tested; but the difference was so convincing that Paré determined 'never again to burn thus so cruelly the poor wounded'; and boiling oil is eschewed to this very day in the treatment of arquebus wounds.

8. 'At the end of ten days their countenances appeared fairer and fatter in flesh than all the children which did eat the portion of the king's meat' (The Book of Daniel 1: 15). Methodological flaws in this biblical clinical trial are: sample too small, duration too short, no randomization, no control of extraneous factors such as physical activity, ill defined endpoint, no information about countenances at start of trials.

9. Latin and Greco-Latin squares are too complicated to explain here. It takes 22 pages in Fleiss JL (The design and analysis of clinical experiments. New York, NY: Wiley; 1986. pp. 241–262).

10. Christen WG, Gaziano JM, Hennekens CH. Design of Physicians' Health Study II – randomised trial of beta-carotene, vitamins E and C, and multivitamins, in prevention of cancer, cardiovascular disease, and eye disease, and review of results of completed trials. Annals of Epidemiology 2000; 10: 125.

11. Pocock SJ (Randomised clinical trials. British Medical Journal 1977; 1: 1661) found variations of up to 46% in the death rates of control groups (who had the same treatment) used by the same investigators in different cancer chemotherapy trials.

12. Taylor WR. An evaluation of supplementary feeding in Somali refugee camps. International Journal of Epidemiology 1983; 12: 433.

13. 'Ghach' is an epicene (genderless) pronoun that avoids the sexist use of 'his', 'he', and 'him' and obviates the need to say 'his or her', 'he or she', or 'him or her'. It is to be found in a list of about 100 such words conveniently assembled by Dennis Baron (professor of English and linguistics at the University of Illinois at Urbana-Champaign), and available on the Internet at http://www. english.uiuc.edu/-people-/faculty/debaron/essays/epicene.htm. 'Ghach' is the Klingon epicene pronoun, transliterated by the linguistics expert Marc Okrand (Okrand M. The Klingon Dictionary, 2nd edn. Simon & Schuster; 1992).

14. *Single-patient trials*, like RCTs, are applications of Pickering's counsel to clinicians: 'If we take a patient afflicted with a malady, and we alter his conditions of life, either by dieting him, or by putting him to bed, or by administering to him a drug, or by performing on him an operation, we are performing an experiment. And if we are scientifically minded we should record the results' (Pickering G. Physician and scientist. Proceedings of the Royal Society of Medicine 1949; 42: 229).

   A typical *N of 1* trial is based on successive pairs of treatment periods, a treatment being given in one period and another treatment (or a placebo) in the other; the sequence within each pair is decided randomly; where possible, 'blind' methods are used. The greater the number of time periods, the more convincing the results. The method is appropriate for chronic, stable conditions and treatments that act fast and stop acting soon after they are discontinued.

   Methods are described by (among others) Guyatt G, Sackett D, Adachi J, Roberts R, Chong J, Rosenbloom D, Keller J (A clinician's guide for conducting randomised trials in individual patients. Canadian Medical Association Journal 1988; 139: 497) and Johannessen T, Petersen H, Kristensen P, Fosstvedt D (The controlled single subject trial. Scandinavian Journal of Primary Health Care 1991; 9: 17).

   The uses, strengths and weaknesses of these trials are briefly reviewed by Janosky JE (Use of the single subject design for practice based primary care research. Postgraduate Medical Journal 2005; 81: 549).

15. A *series of N-of-1 trials*: a method of combining the trials is presented by Zucker R, Schmid H, McIntosh MW, D'Agostino RB, Selker HP, Lad J (Combining single patient [*N*-of-1] trials to

estimate population treatment effects and to evaluate individual patient responses to treatment. Journal of Clinical Epidemiology 1997; 50: 401).

Notcutt W, Price M, Miller R, Newport S, Phillips C, Simmons S, Sansom C (Initial experiences with medicinal extracts of cannabis for chronic pain: results from 34 'N of 1' studies. Anaesthesia 2004; 59: 440) say merely that their results permit generalization and open the way to other studies.

16. Peto R, Pike MC, Armitage P *et al*. Design and analysis of randomised clinical trials requiring prolonged observation of each patient. I. Introduction and design. British Journal of Cancer 1976; 34: 585. Design and analysis of randomised clinical trials requiring prolonged observation of each patient.II. Analysis and examples. British Journal of Cancer 1977; 35: 1.

17. Wright IS, Marple CD, Beck DF. Myocardial infarction: its clinical manifestations and treatment with anticoagulants. New York, NY: Grune & Stratton; 1954. pp. 9–11.

18. Because *minimization* ensures the similarity of the groups compared in a trial, its protagonists say that 'if randomisation is the gold standard, minimisation may be the platinum standard' (Treasure T, MacRae KD. Minimisation: the platinum standard for trials. British Medical Journal 1998; 317: 362). Except in very large studies, minimization permits the control of more prognostic factors than stratification (Scott NW, McPherson GC, Ramsay CR, Campbell MK. The method of minimization for allocation to clinical trials: a review. Controlled Clinical Trials 2002; 23: 662). Simple instructions are provided by Altman DG (Practical statistics for medical research. London: Chapman & Hall, 1991. pp. 443–445). For software, see Appendix C.

A more elaborate alternative to minimization takes account of the relative importance of different prognostic factors (Gicquel S, Marion-Gallois R. Randomization with *a posteriori* constraints: description and properties. Statistics in Medicine 2007; 26: 5033).

19. 'Student'. Biometrika 1931; 23: 398.

20. *Using random numbers*. If all the subjects are known in advance, random sampling methods (see p. 79) can be used to assign them randomly.

If candidates are continuously enrolled during the trial, or if balanced randomization is desired, blocks of subjects can be randomized separately. If the subjects are paired, single-digit random numbers can be used as substitutes for tossing a coin; an even number might mean 'Treat the first member of the pair', and an odd number 'Treat the second'. A similar method can be used for allocating successive cases in a list or series; successive random numbers are used, odd and even numbers being interpreted as 'Group A' and 'Group B' respectively. If the required allocation is 2:1, numbers 1 to 6 might be used for one group, and 7 to 9 for the other (zeros being ignored). If subjects are to be allocated equally to three groups, 1–3 might be taken to mean Group A, 4–6 Group B, and 7–9 Group C (zeros ignored).

Random permutations are easier to use than random numbers, because each number appears once only. Fleiss JL (The design and analysis of experiments. New York, NY: Wiley; 1986) supplies a table (Table A.7) and instructions (pp. 47–51).

For software, see Appendix C.

21. See Appendix C.

22. Simple instructions for *balanced randomization*, using allocation ratios of 1:1, 1:2 or 1:1:1, are given by Peto *et al*. (1976; see note 16). To obtain a balanced 1:1 allocation to two groups (A and B), for example, list all 30 of the possible arrangements of three As and three Bs (AAABBB, AABABB, etc.) and then (using random numbers) choose which of these sequences will be applied to each successive set of six subjects.

When allocating patients to three treatments, the groups can be kept equal by ensuring that three of each successive nine patients go into each group. This might be done by denoting treatment A as 1, 2 or 3, treatment B as 4, 5 or 6, and treatment C as 7, 8 or 9. One-digit random numbers are then chosen. Going from left to right in the top line of the table on p. 86, the first number is 9. This means that the first case should go into Group C. The second number is 6 and the third 2, i.e. the second case should be put in Group B and the third in Group A. The fourth number, 2, is ignored, as we have already had a 2. The next number is 7, so the fourth case goes into Group C. And so on for the whole series of nine cases; the final sequence is C, B, A, C, B, C, A, A, B (Hill AB. A short textbook of medical statistics. London: Hodder & Stoughton; 1977. pp. 303–304).

23. Altman DG (1991; see note 18, pp. 466–471) discusses the analysis of controlled trials briefly, and Fleiss (1986; see note 20) does so at greater length.

24. *Cluster-randomised trials*: Kerry SM, Bland JM (Analysis of a trial randomised in clusters. British Medical Journal 1998; 316: 54); Campbell MK, Mollison J, Steen N, Grimshaw JM, Eccles M (Analysis of cluster randomized trials in primary care: a practical approach. Family Practice 2000; 17: 192); Campbell MJ (Cluster randomized trials in general [family] practice research. Statistical Methods in Medical Research 2000; 9: 81); Raudenbush SW (Statistical analysis and optimal design for cluster randomised trials. Psychological Methods 1997; 2: 173); Murray DM, Varnell SP, Blitstein JL (Design and analysis of group-randomized trials: a review of recent methodological developments. American Journal of Public Health 2004; 94: 423).

25. Bailar JC III. Introduction. In: Shapiro SH, Louis TA (eds), Clinical trials: issues and approaches. New York, NY: Marcel Dekker; 1983. pp. 1–12.

26. *Response-adaptive randomization* has been little used in practice. See Berry DA, Eick SG (Adaptive assignment versus balanced randomisation in clinical trials: a decision analysis. Statistics in Medicine 1995; 14: 231), Rosenberger WF, Lachin JM (The use of responsive-adaptive designs in clinical trials. Controlled Clinical Trials 1993; 14: 471), and Hu F, Rosenberger WF (Optimality, variability, power: evaluating response-adaptive randomisation procedures for treatment comparisons. Journal of the American Statistical Association 2003, 98: 671), who find that the 'play-the-winner' rule is the best variant.

27. Pocock SJ (The combination of randomised and historical controls in clinical trials. Journal of Chronic Diseases 1976; 29: 175) suggests combining the data for the randomized and histori-cal controls in different ways, based on varying degrees of mistrust of the historical data. In a review paper, Louis TA, Shapiro S H (Critical issues in the conduct and interpretation of clinical trials. Annual Review of Public Health 1983; 4: 25) warn that the inclusion of historical controls 'can compromise a trial's validity, even if the investigators are convinced that it is valid'.

28. Armitage P. Sequential medical trials, 2nd edn. Oxford: Blackwell; 1975. The stopping rule may be less extreme for harmful than for beneficial effects (DeMets DL, Ware JH. Asymmetric group sequential boundaries for monitoring clinical trials. Biometrika 1982; 69: 661) – 'The optimal sample size of a clinical trial is defined as the minimum number of subjects required to confidently determine the actual effect size of the primary endpoint, while ensuring that there is enough data to also determine the relative safety of the test treatment', says Golub HL (The need for more efficient trial results. Statistics in Medicine 2006; 25: 3231). The proceedings of a workshop on adaptive clinical trials will be found in Statistics in Medicine 2006; 25(19).

29. Finkelstein M O, Levin B, Robbins H (Clinical and prophylactic trials with assured new treat-ment for those at greater risk: I. A design proposal. American Journal of Public Health 1996; 86: 691). Finkelstein MO, Levin B, Robbins H (Clinical and prophylactic trials with assured new treatment for those at greater risk: II. Examples. American Journal of Public Health 1996; 86: 696). Mosteller F (Editorial: The promise of risk-based allocation trials in assessing new treatments. American Journal of Public Health 1996; 86: 622).

30. For explanations of *Zelen's designs*, see Zelen M (A new design for randomised clinical trials. New England Journal of Medicine 1979; 300: 1242. Randomised consent designs for clinical trials: an update. Statistics in Medicine 1990; 9: 645).

For discussions and debates, see 'Variance and dissent' section, New England Journal of Medicine (1983; 36: 609), Homer CSE (Using the Zelen design in randomised controlled trials: debates and controversies. Journal of Advanced Nursing 2002; 38: 200), and Torgerson D

(The use of Zelen's design in randomised trials. British Journal of Obstetrics and Gynaecology 2004; 111: 2).

Commenting on a study of self-poisoners, a British Medical Journal editorial says 'Some research ethics committees still take the view that Zelen designs are unethical, but a conventional random allocation design [in this study] would probably have resulted in a severely underpowered trial, which is itself unethical' (Hatcher S, Owens D. Do get in touch. British Medical Journal 2005; 331: 788). Similarly, it was concluded that a Zelen design provided the best guarantee for obtaining valid results in a study of heroin addicts (Schellings R, Kessels AGH, ter Riet G, Sturmans F. The Zelen design may be the best choice for a heroin provision experiment. Journal of Clinical Epidemiology 1999; 52: 503). In a study of the value of screening patients with idiopathic venous thromboembolism for hidden cancer, a Zelen design was used because the investigators did not wish to upset members of the control group about the possibility of cancer, and then refrain from examining them (Piccioli A, Lensing AWA, Prins MH, Falanga A, Scannapieco GL, Ieran M, Cigolini M, Ambrosio GB, Monreal M, Girolani A, Prandoni P, Old Uncle Tom Cobley and all (Extensive screening for occult malignant disease in idiopathic venous thromboembolism: a prospective randomised clinical trial. Journal of Thrombosis and Haemostasis 2004; 2: 884).

31. Charplentier PA, Bogardus ST, Inouye K. An algorithm for prospective individual matching in a non-randomised clinical trial. Journal of Clinical Epidemiology 2001; 54: 1166.

32. Weinstein MC. Allocation of subjects in medical experiments. New England Journal of Medicine 1974; 291: 1278.

33. Jadad AR, Moore RA, Carroll D, Jenkinson C, Reynolds DJM, Gavaghan DJ, McQuay HJ. Assessing the quality of reports of randomised clinical trials: is blinding necessary? Controlled Clinical Trials 1996; 17: 1.

For fuller discussions, see Jüni P, Altman DG, Egger M (Assessing the quality of randomised controlled trials. In: Egger M, Smith GD, Altman DG (eds), Systematic reviews in health care: meta-analysis in context, 2nd edn. London: BMJ Books; 2001. pp. 87–108) and a review by Gluud LL (Bias in clinical intervention research. American Journal of Epidemiology 2006; 163: 493), which provides references to numerous other measures of quality, and reports that studies with inadequate randomization tend to give more positive results.

34. Colditz GA, Miller JN, Mosteller F. How study design affects outcomes in comparisons of therapy. I. Medical. Statistics in Medicine 1989; 8:441.

35. In trials of interventions aimed at changing lifestyles there are always subjects who fail to change their habits, or who change them despite being in a control group (Schulz KF, Chalmers I, Hayes RJ. Empirical evidence of bias: dimensions of methodological quality associated with estimates of treatment effects in controlled trials. Journal of the American Medical Association 1995; 273: 408).

36. Schulz KF. Subverting randomisation in controlled trials. Journal of the American Medical Association 1995; 274: 1456.

37. McKee M, Britton A, Black N, McPherson K, Sanderson C, Bain C. Methods in health services research: interpreting the evidence: choosing between randomised and non-randomised studies. British Medical Journal 1999; 319: 312.

38. Partin MR, Malone M, Winnett M, Slater J, Bar-Cohen A, Caplan L. The impact of survey nonresponse bias on conclusions drawn from a mammography intervention trial. Journal of Clinical Epidemiology 2003; 56: 867.

39. De Amici D, Klersy C, Ramajoli F, Brustia L, Politi P. Impact of the Hawthorne effect in a longitudinal clinical study: the case of anaesthesia. Controlled Clinical Trials 2000; 21: 103.

40. Borm GF, Houben MGJ, Welsing PMJ, Zielhuis GA. An investigation of clinical studies suggests those with multiple objectives should have at least 90% power for each endpoint. Journal of Clinical Epidemiology 2006; 59: 1.

41. Fredrickson DS. The field trial: some thoughts on the indispensable ordeal. Bulletin of the New York Academy of Medicine 1968; 44: 985.

42. Margitic SE, Miles NL. Ten commandments of successful trial management. Preventive Medicine 1998; 27: 84.

43. For a specimen protocol outline, see Friedman LW *et al.* (Fundamentals of clinical trials. Boston, MA: John Wright; 1983. p. 6). For general advice, see Guyatt G (Preparing a research protocol to improve chances of success. Journal of Clinical Epidemiology 2006; 59: 893).

44. The organization of multicentre trials is described by Friedman LW *et al.* (1983; see note 43, p. 211) and Stanley K, Stjernsward J, Isley M. (The conduct of a cooperative clinical trial. Recent Results in Cancer Research no 77. Berlin: Springer-Verlag, 1981). For statistical aspects, see Fleiss JL (1986; see note 20, p. 176).

45 Olschewski M, Schumacher M, Davis KB. Analysis of randomised and nonrandomised patients in clinical trials using the comprehensive cohort follow-up study design. Controlled Clinical Trials 1992; 13: 226.

46. Marcus SM. Assessing non-consent bias with parallel randomised and nonrandomised clinical trials. Journal of Clinical Epidemiology 1997; 50: 823.

47. Authors of nearly 60% of randomized trials published in the British Medical Journal and Lancet said they had not met their recruitment targets, or had needed to extend their recruitment period (Watson JM, Torgerson DJ. Increasing recruitment to randomised trials: a review of randomised controlled trials. BMC Medical Research Methodology 2006; 6: 34).

48. Lang JM, Buring JE, Rosner B, Cook N, Hennekens CH. Estimating the effect of the run-in on the power of the Physicians' Health Study. Statistics in Medicine 1991; 10: 1585.

49. Altman DG, Schulz KF. Concealing treatment allocation in randomised trials. British Medical Journal 2001; 323: 446.

Use of an automated e-mail reply system for announcing a subject's allocation has been proposed by Cunningham A (A review finds that the autoreply e-mail function avoids problems of subject allocation concealment. Journal of Clinical Epidemiology 2006; 59: 567).

50. One investigator, scarred by his experiences in collaborative (i.e. multiclinic) clinical trials, cautions that 'consecutive numbering of envelopes alone is inadequate protection against tampering with randomisation. The envelopes, if used, should be serially numbered, opaque, and sealed with water-insoluble glue to prevent steaming them open, and all nonopened envelopes should be returned to the coordinating center which should check the integrity of the seal. Still better, the coordinating center should issue an assignment only after the clinic has identified the eligible patient by name' (Ederer F. Practical problems in collaborative clinical trials. American Journal of Epidemiology 1975; 102: 111).

Says one sceptic who believes that one reason for the positiveness of positive clinical trials is that clinicians are able to get around these efforts at secrecy: 'If I am left with 20 patients and two times 10 sealed envelopes, I can see to it that my preferred treatment wins' (Knipschild P. The false positive therapeutic trial. Journal of Clinical Epidemiology 2002; 55: 1191).

51. Methods used to establish blinding, to avoid unblinding, and to keep assessors of outcomes in the dark are reviewed in detail by Boutron I, Estellat C, Guittet L, Dechartres A, Sackett DL, Hrobjartsson A, Ravaud P (Methods of blinding in reports of randomized trials assessing pharmacological treatments: a systematic review. PLoS Medicine 2006; 3(10): e425).

The success of blinding should be assessed in a preliminary study, or early in the study, before there is evidence of efficacy (Boutron I, Estellat C, Ravaud P. A review of blinding in randomized controlled trials found results inconsistent and questionable. Journal of Clinical Epidemiology 2005; 58: 1220).

It would be heresy to question the use of placebos in control groups. But it is interesting that a meta-analysis of 156 clinical trials in which randomly allocated placebo groups and no-treatment groups were compared showed an overall significant difference only in reports of pain, not in any other outcomes (Hrobjartsson A, Gotzsche PC. Is the placebo powerless? Update of a systematic review with 52 new randomized trials comparing placebo with no treatment. Journal of Internal Medicine 2004; 256: 91).

52. Methods of blinding used in trials of nonpharmacological treatments are reviewed in detail by Boutron I, Guittet L, Estellat C, Moher D, Hrobjartsson A, Ravaud P (Reporting methods of blinding in randomized trials assessing nonpharmacological treatments. PLoS Medicine 2007; 4(2): e61).

53. In view of the risks of sham surgery, anaesthesia, and prophylactic antibiotics, Macklin R (The ethical problems with sham surgery in clinical research. New England Medical Journal 1999; 341: 992) concludes: 'The placebo-controlled trial may well be the gold standard of research design, but unlike pure gold, it can be tarnished by unethical applications'. Heckerling PS (Placebo surgery research: a blinding imperative. Journal of Clinical Epidemiology 2006; 59: 876) states that the risks must be 'minimized … and reasonable in relation to the importance of the knowledge that is expected to result', but that placebo surgery studies are ethical only if the investigators measuring outcome are blinded to treatment allocation.

54. Mainland D. The clinical trial – some difficulties and suggestions. Journal of Chronic Diseases 1960; 11: 484.

55. *Meta-analysis.* Egger M, Smith GD, Altman DG. Systematic reviews in health care: meta-analysis in context, 2nd edn. BMJ Books; 2001. Egger M, Smith GD, Sterne JAC. Systematic reviews and meta-analysis. In: Detels R, McEwen J, Beaglehole R, Tanaka H (eds), Oxford textbook of public health, 4th edn, vol 2. Oxford University Press; 2002. pp. 455–475. Abramson JH. Meta-analysis: a review of pros and cons. Public Health Reviews 1990; 18: 1. For a state-of-the-art review with 281 references, see Sutton AL, Higgins JPT (Recent developments in meta-analysis. Statistics in Medicine 2007; DOI: 10.1002/sim.2934).

    Meta-analyses are difficult to do well, and should not be undertaken lightly. Meta-analysis software is reviewed by Sterne JAC, Egger M, Sutton AJ (Meta-analysis software. In: Egger M, Smith GD, Altman DG; see note 33, pp. 336–346). For free software, see Appendix C.

56. Elizabeth Barrett Browning's sonnet, 'How do I love thee? Let me count the ways...' has no connection with a literature search that identified 86 different tools for assessing the quality of observational studies, not all of which included 'the three most fundamental domains … appropriate selection of participants, appropriate measurement of variables, and appropriate control of confounding' (Sanderson S, Tatt ID, Higgins JPT. Tools for assessing quality and susceptibility to bias in observational studies in epidemiology: a systematic review and annotated bibliography. International Journal of Epidemiology 2007; 36: 666).

33

Programme Trials

Programme trials are experiments or quasi-experiments that test hypotheses concerning the effects of health programmes. The programme may be one directed at a specific problem or population category (e.g. mass screening, antismoking, clean air, prevention of AIDS, care of stroke patients or the elderly), or it may be an organizational form – a programme trial may appraise day-care hospitals, health centres, the work of a category of health personnel (nurse practitioners, chiropodists, village health workers), etc.

A programme trial endeavours not only to appraise outcomes, but to determine whether these can be attributed to the intervention rather than to extraneous factors. The aim is to obtain generalizable knowledge, applicable to settings like the one in which the trial was performed, about the value of a *type* of programme. In these respects a programme trial differs from a simple programme review (see p. 25), which is an observational study (generally descriptive, sometimes with an analytic component) that aims to appraise the implementation and/or outcome of a specific programme provided for a specific group or community, without using the rigorous methods required to assess whether the outcome can be ascribed to the programme.

Most studies of public health interventions are nonexperimental or quasi-experimental.[1] But their importance should not be minimized – nonexperimental or quasi-experimental studies are more practicable than true experiments, and may provide useful and sometimes generalizable lessons. Quasi-experiments that have controls and those that have measurements made before the intervention are, of course, more convincing than those that do not.[1]

Programmes are sometimes evaluated by using a case-control design, as explained on p. 320. In the Netherlands, for example, the value of a cancer screening programme was confirmed by a study of women who died of breast cancer and matched survivors, comparing their history of participation in the programme.[2]

Objectives of Programme Trials

The objectives of evaluative studies were listed in Chapter 5. The main focus of a programme trial is usually the outcome of care, and its variation in different population groups or different circumstances. There may also be interest in economic efficiency. Appraisals of performance, compliance, satisfaction, facilities and settings usually

Research Methods in Community Medicine: Surveys, Epidemiological Research, Programme Evaluation, Clinical Trials   J. H. Abramson and Z. H. Abramson   Copyright © 2008, John Wiley & Sons Ltd

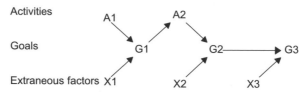

Figure 33.1   Goal attainment model.

have the specific purpose of explaining effectiveness or its lack, although some trials focus on feasibility or acceptability.

Effectiveness can be convincingly demonstrated only if the outcomes used as criteria are clearly desirable ones – i.e. worthwhile 'end-results' in their own right, or stepping-stones to such end-results. In instances where the benefits to be expected from an activity are certain (e.g. immunization), a measure of its performance may be used as a criterion of effectiveness.

The outcomes selected for appraisal are generally those that the programme tries (explicitly or implicitly) to achieve. The goal attainment model[3] is illustrated in Figure 33.1. Every programme goal (G2) may imply one or more subgoals or intermediate goals (G1) that must be achieved if the programme goal is to be attained. Activities (A1 and A2) are performed in order to achieve the goals. As an example, attaining a reduced prevalence of hypertension (G2) as a result of antihypertensive treatment (A2) requires the achievement of an intermediate goal, the identification of hypertensives in the population (G1), as an outcome of screening activities (A1). These activities (A1 and A2), which aim at achieving goals G1 and G2, constitute the programme. (This is, of course, an oversimplification; most programmes comprise a number of longer, branched, and interconnecting chains.) It may also be possible to define 'ultimate goals' or end results (G3) that may result from the operation of the programme, but without further programme activities, e.g. a reduction in mortality from stroke.

Any outcome that is inherently desirable – in this instance, G2 or G3 – is a satisfactory criterion of effectiveness in a programme trial. But extraneous factors (X1, X2 and X3) may contribute to each outcome, and their possible confounding effects must be controlled.

A trial may, of course, aim to appraise undesired as well as desirable outcomes.

A trial that appraises an outcome may become more meaningful if it also opens the programme's 'black box' by examining the performance of activities and the attainment of intermediate goals leading up to the outcome. Success in attaining the desired outcome can be convincingly attributed to the programme only if the programme activities were performed satisfactorily, and failure to achieve the outcome may be explained by failure to perform these activities. A randomized controlled trial indicating that a programme providing extensive health examinations produced no change in mortality over the next 20 years,[4] for example, would be more meaningful if information was provided on the extent to which the examinations led to the provision of therapeutic and preventive care.

Here are three examples of programme trials. The study objectives were:

1. To compare the changes in attitudes to smoking and the prevalence of smoking among boys in the 10th to 12th grades in two schools, one with an antismoking

programme and one without; controlling for grade, membership of sports teams, parents' smoking habits, and other variables.[5]

This is clearly a quasi-experiment. There may be differences between the two schools, and the same precautions against confounding must be taken as in an observational cohort study. Randomization would not help – the two schools will have the same differences, whatever the assignment, and these must be taken into account in the analysis.

2. To compare the incidence of diarrhoea in children's day-care centres in which a hand-washing programme was introduced (hand-washing after toilet activities and before handling food or eating) with the incidence in control day-care centres.[6]

This is a true experiment, if the day-care centres can be randomized. (It would then be a cluster-randomized trial.) The results would be strengthened by a comparison of actual behaviour in the various centres.

3. To compare the incidence of trachoma (an eye disease spread by eye discharges) in Tanzanian villages in which mass treatment with an antibiotic ointment was followed by an intensive educational programme to encourage face-washing, and in villages that received mass treatment only.[7]

Here, too, randomization and measurements of behaviour would be desirable.

Study Designs

Programme trials may be individual-based or group-based.

In the former, individuals are allocated (preferably randomly) to groups that are exposed (or not exposed) to the programme under study. These trials do not differ in their design from clinical trials that examine treatments applied to individuals, as described in Chapter 32.

In group-based trials, the experimental units are groups, or even total communities (*community trials*), that are exposed (or not exposed) to the programme. They may be undertaken to test aetiological hypotheses, not only to evaluate programmes. A classic example is Goldberger's demonstration of the nutritional origin of pellagra, based on experimental changes of diet in orphanages and a mental hospital.[8]

The basic experimental or quasi-experimental designs are the same for programme trials as for clinical trials (see p. 327), i.e. parallel, externally controlled, and 'self-controlled' (including crossover) studies. Individual-based (clinical) and parallel, externally controlled and 'self-controlled' group-based trials will be discussed in more detail below.

Since investigators may not have the power to decide in which groups or communities programmes will be established, or when, many programme trials are quasi-experiments. But an increasing number of group-based trials are based on clusters that are randomly allocated to the intervention and control arms of the study. These cluster-randomized trials will be given separate consideration below (p. 351).

Clinical Trials to Evaluate Programmes

It is sometimes feasible to conduct a randomized clinical trial in which some individuals are allocated to a programme and others are used as controls, or individuals are allocated to different programmes.

For example, in a trial of breast cancer screening, members of the Health Insurance Plan of New York were randomly allocated to two groups; some women were offered four annual screening examinations (clinical and mammographic) and others continued to receive their usual medical care. Rates of mortality and other endpoints in the two groups were compared. This demonstrated a considerably lower rate of breast cancer mortality in the next 18 years in the group assigned to the screening programme, among women aged 50 or more.[9]

As another example, rates of compliance with antihypertensive drug treatment were compared in workers randomly allocated to treatment by industrial physicians during working hours, or by their family doctors. This trial also compared the rates of compliance among men exposed and not exposed to an educational programme (slide–audiotape and booklet) about hypertension. No differences in compliance were found; an unexpected finding was that there was a dramatic increase in absenteeism among workers who were told they had hypertension, especially in the group exposed to the educational programme.[10]

Trials of this kind cannot be 'blind'. Bias caused by the Hawthorne effect (see p. 74) may be reduced if an alternative programme is offered to the control subjects. In a trial that showed the effectiveness of physical fitness classes as a way of preventing recurrences of low back pain in hospital workers, for example, a 'back school' (providing instruction on the prevention of back strain) was arranged for the control subjects.[11]

As in other clinical trials, more than one outcome may be studied. In a trial in Seattle, for example, individuals were randomly assigned to a prepaid health maintenance organization or to insurance plans requiring the payment of a fee-for-service, and the outcomes that were compared included changes in blood pressure, functional visual capacity, cholesterol, smoking habits, weight, physical functioning, role functioning, bed-days, serious symptoms, mental health, and other indices of general health.[12]

In trials where there are nonparticipants, outcomes should, of course, be measured in the total groups, including their nonparticipant members. Nonparticipants are likely to differ from participants, and their exclusion may introduce bias. As an example, if women who did not accept the offer of breast screening made in the Health Insurance Plan study were excluded from the analysis, the results indicated that screening produced a sizeable (but spurious) reduction in mortality from causes other than breast cancer.[9] The crucial comparison in such a study is not between those who participate in the programme and those who do not, but between the randomized groups (intention-to-treat analysis; see p. 333).

In trials of programmes that require active participation by the subjects, the extent of participation in the trial (as well as in the programme) may have an important bearing on the conclusions. This applies to community as well as clinical trials. In a trial of worksite smoking cessation programmes, where workers at a large installation who consented to participate were randomly allocated to different programmes, the proportions of the randomized groups who quit smoking (measured 12 months later) ranged from 16 to 26% (as compared with a spontaneous quit rate of 5%). But about 64% of the smokers at the plant had not expressed interest in the smoking cessation project, and another 25% had expressed interest but did not agree to participate.[13] Although the results led to a decision to offer the best of the programmes on a regular basis, the overall impact on smoking habits was likely to be small.

When a programme trial is conducted in a single health service, randomization of individuals is generally difficult or impossible. Making a programme available to some patients and not others may be ethically unacceptable, or resented by the patients; this difficulty can sometimes be overcome if the programme is introduced in stages (a shortage of resources may justify this) and will eventually be available to everyone. In a small practice, where patients know and talk to one another, there is likely to be 'contamination' that may interfere with the evaluation of programmes that call for changes in behaviour.

Parallel Group-based Trials

In parallel group-based trials, two or more independent groups or communities are studied prospectively and compared (see the three illustrative studies on p. 346–347).[14] More groups are preferable to fewer, even if they are smaller. If it is intended to apply the findings to a reference population, then the groups should be representative of that population, but this is seldom feasible. As in clinical trials, randomization (see p. 328) is the best way of reducing bias in these trials, although this may not prevent marked differences if there are few groups. Randomization is of no importance if only two communities are compared: the communities have the same differences, whatever the assignment, and these must be taken into account in the analysis.

Published examples of trials in which randomization was performed include studies with a random allocation of towns (to study the effect of fluoridation of water supplies), factories (programmes for the control of cardiovascular risk factors), villages (fly control measures), families (for the provision of primary care by nurse practitioners or physicians), general practices, and orthodontic clinics (an antismoking program). *Cluster-randomized trials* of this sort, and some of the specific issues that arise in their design and analysis, will be given separate consideration below.

Unfortunately, randomization may not be feasible, since investigators seldom have the power to decide where or when programmes will be established. Most community trials of programmes are quasi-experiments, in which the control groups are purposively selected to be as similar as possible to the intervention groups. The greater this similarity, and the more convincingly it can be demonstrated, the more persuasive are the conclusions. Similarity to the intervention group and the feasibility of obtaining satisfactory data are the main considerations when choosing control groups. There is often a very restricted choice concerning controls.

As in clinical trials, follow-up in programme trials should be complete; people who do not actively participate in the programme should not be excluded.

Postmeasure-only studies, where the findings in an intervention group (after exposure to a programme) are compared with those in a control population, are useful only if it can be assumed that the groups were similar before the institution of the programme.[15] A mobile coronary-care service, for example, was evaluated by comparing case fatality rates in two demographically similar communities in Northern Ireland, one of which had such a service. Fatality was higher in the community without a mobile service, although hospital facilities and hospital treatment were similar. The difference could not be attributed to differences in severity or other characteristics of the cases. The results would have been more convincing, however, if there had been direct evidence that the risk of dying was the same in both communities before the service was instituted or, as the authors point out, if this risk was later found to decrease in the control community when such a service was started there (but later results have not yet been published).[16]

The minimal requirement is generally a *premeasure–postmeasure* design, with 'before' and 'after' measurements in both populations. The longer the time-series the better, as this permits a fuller comparison of trends in both populations. A long follow-up may also permit the cumulation of enough outcome events (diseases and deaths) to permit comparisons of incidence and mortality. On the other hand, long-term comparisons are beset with problems, as the differences in intervention may be attenuated by changes in health care and other influences affecting outcomes, or blurred by changes in the composition of the groups and by difficulties with follow-up. Several controlled community cardiovascular risk reduction trials have failed to show substantial effects on health, and this has been attributed to the spread of interventions and educational messages to the comparison populations,[17] either from the intervention populations ('contamination') or because of wider societal, institutional or cultural changes.

As an illustration, in 1975–76 an appreciably steeper decrease in the prevalence of cardiovascular risk factors was demonstrated in a Jerusalem population exposed since 1970 to such a programme (the CHAD programme) than in a neighbouring community receiving ordinary medical care from another agency. Risk-factor status continued to improve in the exposed population, but it did so in the comparison population also, and in 1985–87 the differences were smaller than in 1975–76. Risk-factor control had improved very considerably in the comparison population, partly as a result of a policy decision stimulated by the success of the CHAD programme, and partly as a result of greater nationwide awareness by the media, public, and medical profession of the importance of these risk factors. Among other changes, by 1975–76, 70% of hypertensives in the comparison community were under control. No one was very surprised that a 23-year follow-up of mortality revealed no significant differences between the populations.[18]

A feasible manoeuvre if a service is expanding to a progressively larger population is to compare the 'before' data for each newly admitted chunk with the contemporaneous 'after' data for the population admitted previously (on the assumption that the populations were initially similar), and later with its own 'after' data. In a study in South Africa, this technique showed that a reduction in infant mortality could be attributed to a health centre's efforts.[19] In a city in the United States, it demonstrated that a programme for increasing the availability of medical care (by providing services free) apparently led to increased sickness, as measured by self-appraisals of health, the number of symptoms, and limitation of activities because of poor health.[20] A more ambitious multiple-group time-series design (i.e. the use of serial observations in different communities as a basis for both inter-community and within-community comparisons) has been used in community trials of cardiovascular disease prevention programmes.[21]

Cluster-randomized trials

The main advantage of trials based on randomly allocated clusters is that they permit the evaluation of interventions that are administered at a group level rather than the individual level. This might be, for example, a health education or screening programme in a family practice, or an organizational innovation in the practice, or an educational intervention directed at health professionals in the hope of improving the health of the individuals they serve. By comparing clusters, these trials also reduce the possibility of being misled by the spread of effects to individuals at whom the intervention was not targeted, e.g. because of 'contamination' of other members of the cluster in an educational programme, or because of herd immunity in an immunization programme.

Cluster-randomized trials are generally parallel trials, but they may also have a crossover design.

The clusters may be stratified before randomization. In a study of general practices, for example, this might serve to ensure a balance between general practices of different sizes. Clusters may also be matched.

Ethical issues require special consideration in cluster-randomized trials, since it is generally impracticable to obtain informed consent for inclusion in the trial from every individual subject.[22]

If the trial outcome is measured at a group level, so that the clusters are the units of analysis, a cluster-randomized trial can be handled as if it were a simple randomized trial, with no need for special precautions when deciding on sample size or when analysing the results. This applied, for example, to a trial of safety-education packages delivered to families, in which the outcomes were the possession and use of safety equipment and safe practices at home.[23]

But if outcomes are measured at an individual level, then account must be taken of the likelihood that there will be a degree of similarity between members of the same cluster, and this has to be taken into account both in designing and in analysing the study.

To decide on sample size,[24] i.e. the required number of clusters (given their average size) or the required size of clusters (given their number), what is needed, in addition to the requirements for computing sample size for a simple random study (see p. 84), is a measure of the degree of homogeneity of clusters with respect to the study variables. This measure is the *intracluster correlation coefficient* (ICC), and use is usually made of a value observed in a previous study of similar variables in similar clusters.[25] Small differences in the ICC can have a strong effect on the trial's power to detect significant effects.

It is recommended that there should be at least four clusters in every arm of the trial.[26]

The effect of clustering should, of course, always be taken into account in the analysis, since ignoring it may lead to spuriously significant results and unduly narrow confidence intervals for the effects of intervention. (But a review of cluster-randomized trials in primary health care published between 1997 and 2000 revealed that this was done in only 59% of them.)[26]

An especially complicated (multilevel) type of analysis may be required if it is wished to appraise the effects on the outcome both of variables measured at the cluster level and of variables measured at the individual level.[27]

Externally Controlled Community Trials

In an externally controlled community trial the investigator limits the investigation to groups or communities that are exposed to the programme, and compares the findings with data obtained from other sources. National data may be used, or published reports of surveys or trials in other populations. The validity of such studies is often in serious doubt. Definitions and study methods may be different, the study population may differ in its characteristics or circumstances from the population from which the control data are derived, and the data may refer to different times.

'Self-controlled' ('Before–After') Community Trials

In 'self-controlled' community trials, observations before and after the institution of the programme are compared. The group or community is its own control. As in clinical trials of this sort, the main biases (see p. 332) are those connected with extraneous events or changes that occur between the observations, nonspecific effects caused by the trial itself, and changes in methods of measurement. 'Before–after' experiments of this sort, without external controls, are common in public health. 'Infant mortality dropped after the introduction of the programme' is adduced as evidence of effectiveness, although the same change might have occurred without the programme. Salutary testimony to the weakness of this reasoning is provided by McKeown's demonstration that although the introduction of specific immunization procedures and antibiotic treatment was followed by reductions in rates of mortality from tuberculosis, pneumonia, whooping cough, measles and other infective diseases, these changes were continuations of trends that had been observed for many years prior to the introduction of these procedures.[28]

To be reasonably convincing, the 'before–after' trial should be replicated in different populations or at different times – does infant mortality invariably or almost invariably drop when the programme is instituted? It is also helpful to examine data for a number of years before the institution of the programme – is there evidence of a change in the time trend?

It is also helpful if a 'before–after' study can be extended to an examination of what happens when the programme is withdrawn. It must be very rare, however, for an investigator to have the power or ethical justification for a decision to discontinue a programme that has shown an apparent effect. Such studies, therefore, are generally opportunistic quasi-experiments. In a rare example of a quasi-experimental crossover community trial, the effects of a programme to encourage the performance of Pap smears were observed in two Indian communities in the United States: one in which such a programme was instituted in 1978 and one in which it was discontinued in the same year.[29]

A Word of Caution

Programme trials are important. Their topics are seldom trivial, and their practical implications may be prodigious. The importance of careful planning and rigorous methods of study and analysis can, hence, not be underestimated. The fact that most programme trials are quasi-experimental community trials, where the investigator does not have the power to make decisions on the allocation of study groups or (in some instances) on the collection of data, does not mean that the rules can be relaxed. On the contrary, the appraisal of bias and its analytic control become especially important.

Two major principles have been specified for the use of quasi-experimental designs.[30] The first requires that 'all plausible alternative explanations of the relationship between cause and effect or treatment and outcome be specified, and evidence to counter these rival explanations considered or demonstrated'. The second is that of 'assessing the consistency of findings from studies across times and across research settings, methods, and populations'.

The provision of sound scientific evidence about the value of health-care programmes cannot ensure that policy for health care will be based on sound scientific evidence, or indeed that there will be *any* policy for health care.[31] But the provision of unsound scientific evidence can hardly improve matters.

Notes and References

1. An analysis of studies dealing with preventive interventions published in six community health journals in 1992 revealed that 30% were randomized controlled trials; a further 29% could and should have been RCTs (Smith PJ, Moffatt MEK, Gelskey SC, Hudson S, Kaita K. Are community health interventions evaluated appropriately? A review of six journals. Journal of Clinical Epidemiology 1997; 50: 137).

    This distribution is influenced by publication bias – programme evaluations are often of interest only to those concerned with the particular programme reviewed, and are much less likely to be published than programme trials. If a paper's 'subject is of local interest only or is not generalizable' the American Journal of Public Health rejects it on sight (Northridge ME, Susser M. Annotation: seven fatal flaws in submitted manuscripts. American Journal of Public Health 1994; 84: 718).

2. Collette HJA, Day NE, Rombach JJ, De Waard F. Evaluation of screening for breast cancer in a non-randomised study (the DOM project) by means of a case-control study. Lancet 1984; 1: 1224

3. The classic paper on the evaluation of programme effectiveness, which presents the *goal attainment model*, is by Deniston OL, Rosenstock LM, Getting VA (Evaluation of program effectiveness. Public Health Reports 1968; 83: 323).

4. The investigators concluded that general health examinations 'are of little value in preventing diseases leading to death'. In this programme (in Stockholm in the early 1970s) people with a need for intervention were referred for care, but there was no follow-up. The unanswered question is whether mortality remained unaffected despite appropriate care, or because of insufficient care (Theobald H, Bygren LO, Carstensen J, Hauffman M, Engfeld P. Effects of an assessment of needs for medical and social services on long-term mortality: a randomised controlled study. International Journal of Epidemiology 1998; 27: 194).

5. Using an increased awareness that 'smoking is dangerous to health' as a criterion, this programme was effective. Using changes in smoking habits as a criterion, it was ineffective (Monk M, Tayback M, Gordon J. Evaluation of an antismoking program among high school students. American Journal of Public Health 1965; 55: 994. Reprinted in Schulberg HC, Sheldon A, Baker F (eds). Program evaluation in the health fields. New York, NY: Behavioural Publications; 1969. pp. 345–359).

6. This study was done in suburban Atlanta, Georgia. During the 35 weeks of the trial the incidence of diarrhoea in the centres where hands were washed was half that in the control centres. Before the hand-washing programme was started the incidence was higher in the experimental than in the control centres (Black RE, Dykes AC, Anderson KE. American Journal of Epidemiology 1981; 113: 445).

7. Three pairs of villages (matched for maternal education, cleanliness of children's faces, and baseline prevalence of trachoma) participated in this study. The face-washing programme was administered to randomly chosen households in one randomly chosen village in each pair. The programme increased the prevalence of clean faces and reduced the incidence of severe trachoma in two villages but not in the third, in which there was 'a very strong ethos of disapproval for families who tried to be better than other families or "put on airs"' (West S, Munoz B, Lunch M, Kayongoya A, Chilangwa Z, Mmbaga BBO, Taylor HR. Impact of face-washing on trachoma in Kongwa, Tanzania. Lancet 1995; 345: 155).

8. Goldberger J, Waring CH, Tanner WF. Pellagra prevention by diet among institutional inmates. Public Health Reports 1923; 38: 2361. Reprinted in Pan-American Health Organization and Buck C (The challenge of epidemiology: issues and selected readings. WHO; 1990. pp. 726–730).

9. Shapiro S. Periodic screening for breast cancer: the HIP Randomised Controlled Trial. Health Insurance Plan. Journal of the National Cancer Institute Monographs 1997; 22: 27.

10. Sackett DL, Haynes RB, Gibson ES *et al.* Randomised clinical trial of strategies for improving medication compliance in primary hypertension. Lancet 1975; 1: 1205. Haynes RB, Sackett DL, Taylor DW, Gibson ES, Johnson AL. Increased absenteeism from work after detection and labeling of hypertensive patients. New England Journal of Medicine 1978; 299:741.

11. Donchin M, Woolf O, Kaplan L, Floman Y. Secondary prevention of low back pain. Abstracts: Kyoto, Japan, May 15–19, 1989. International Society for the Study of the Lumber [*sic*] Spine, Toronto. p. 18.

12. This study (part of the Rand Health Insurance Study) found that the outcome differed for poor and well-off individuals who had health problems at the outset (Ware JE Jr, Brook RH, Rogers WH *et al.* Comparison of health outcomes at a health maintenance organisation with those of fee-for-service care. Lancet 1986; i: 1017).

13. Omenn GS, Thompson B, Sexton M *et al.* A randomised comparison of worksite-sponsored smoking cessation programs. American Journal of Preventive Medicine 1988; 4: 261.

14. The design of programme trials is discussed by Hoffmeister H, Mensink GBM (Community-based intervention trials in developed countries. In: Detels R, McEwen J, Beaglehole R, Tanaka H (eds), Oxford textbook of public health, 4th edn, vol 2. The methods of public health. New York, NY: Oxford University Press, 2002. pp. 583–598) and in the same volume by Wu Z (Community-based intervention trials in developing countries. pp. 599–620).

15. The lack of baseline information about mortality, morbidity, growth and nutritional status is a serious problem in trials of new patterns of grass-roots primary health care in developing countries. Even discounting ethical considerations, it is difficult to collect such data before community health workers, on whom these care programmes are usually based, start to function.

    In the Narangwal project in India, for example (an important controlled study of the comparative effectiveness of nutritional care, medical care, and their combination), no 'before' measurements were available in the villages studied. Information on births and deaths was not collected in a uniform way until the second year of the project. The validity of the conclusions rests on the assurance that the villages were similar in such features as size, education, the distribution of occupational groups, and access to previously available health services (Kielmann AA, Taylor CE, Parker RL. The Narangwal Nutrition Study: a summary review. American Journal of Clinical Nutrition 1978; 31: 2040).

16. Mathewson ZM, McCloskey BG, Evans AE, Russell CJ, Wilson C. Mobile coronary care and community mortality from myocardial infarction. Lancet 1985; 1: 441.

Later data have not been published, according to Moore W, Kee F, Evans AE, McCrum-Gardner, Morrison C, Tunstall-Pedoe H (Pre-hospital coronary care and coronary fatality in the Belfast and Glasgow MONICA populations. International Journal of Epidemiology 2005; 14: 422).

17. Feinleib M. Editorial: New directions for community intervention studies. American Journal of Public Health 1996; 86: 1696.

18. Abramson JH, Gofin J, Hopp C, Schein MH, Naveh P. The CHAD program for the control of cardiovascular risk factors in a Jerusalem community: a 24-year retrospect. Israel Journal of Medical Sciences 1994; 30: 108.

19. Kark SL, Cassel J. The Pholela Health Centre: a progress report. South African Medical Journal 1952; 26: 101, 132. Kark SL. The practice of community oriented primary health care. New York, NY: Appleton-Century-Crofts; 1981. pp. 243–245.

20. Diehr PK, Richardson WC, Shortell SM, LoGerfo JP. Increased access to medical care: the impact on health. Medical Care 1979; 17: 989.

21. Salonen JT, Kottke TE, Jacobs DR Jr, Hannan PJ. Analysis of community-based cardiovascular disease prevention studies – evaluation issues in the North Karelia project and the Minnesota Heart Health program. International Journal of Epidemiology 1986; 15: 176.

22. *Ethical issues* in cluster-randomized trials are discussed in note 18, Chapter 1.

23. Clamp C, Kendrick D. A randomised controlled trial of general practitioner safety advice for families with children under 5 years. British Medical Journal 1998; 316: 1576.

24. For software, see Appendix C.

25. For examples of intraclass correlation coefficients found in primary care practices, see Campbell M, Grimshaw J, Steen N [Sample size calculations for cluster randomised trials. Changing Professional Practice in Europe Group (EU BIOMED II Concerted Action). Journal of Health Services Research and Policy 2000; 5: 12], Elley CR, Kerse N, Chondros P, Robinson E (Intraclass correlation coefficients from three cluster randomised controlled trials in primary and residential health care. Australian and New Zealand Journal of Public Health 2005; 29: 461), and Cosby RH, Howards M, Kaczorowski J, Willan AR, Sellors JW (Randomizing patients by family practice: sample size estimation, intracluster correlation and data analysis. Family Practice 2003; 20: 77).

A database of ICCs calculated in different settings is available at http://www.abdn.ac.uk/hsru/epp/cluster.shtml.

26. Eldridge SM, Ashby D, Feder GS, Rudnicka AR, Ukoumunne OC. Lessons for cluster randomized trials in the twenty-first century: a systematic review of trials in primary care. Clinical Trials 2004; 1: 80.

27. For further discussions of cluster-randomized trials and their analysis, see Campbell MJ (Cluster randomized trials in general (family) practice research. Statistical Methods in Medical Research 2000; 9: 81), Campbell MK, Mollison J, Steen N, Grimshaw JM, Eccles M (Methods of cluster randomized trials in primary care: a practical approach. Family Practice 2000; 17: 192), and Murray DM, Varnell SP, Blitstein JL (Design and analysis of group-randomized trials: a review of recent methodological developments. American Journal of Public Health 2004; 94: 423).

28. McKeown T. The role of medicine: dream, mirage or nemesis? Oxford: Blackwell; 1979.

29. Freeman WL. In: Nutting PA (ed.), Community-oriented primary care: from principle to practice. Washington, DC: Health Resources and Services. Administration, Public Health; 1987. pp. 410–416. In both communities the Pap screening rate was considerably higher when the programme was operative.

30. Patrick DL. Sociological investigations. In: Holland WW, Detels R, Knox G (eds), Oxford textbook of public health, vol 3. Oxford: Oxford University Press; 1985. Chapter 11.

31. Do situations exist in which there is health policy without scientific evidence? In fact there are only a few situations in which there is any kind of policy' (Ibrahim MA. Epidemiology and health policy. Rockville, MD: Aspen; 1985. p. 183).

34

Community-Oriented Primary Care

This chapter is written for practitioners of primary health care (doctors, nurses, health educators, managers and others) who try to 'treat the community as a patient' by appraising the health needs of a population and establishing *community programmes* to deal with these in a systematic way, as well as caring for the needs of its individual members and their families.

This kind of integrated practice, which has been termed *community-oriented primary care* (COPC),[1] requires the systematic collection and use of information as a basis for the planning, implementation, monitoring and evaluation of these programmes.

The community orientation is expressed in a cyclic process (see Figure 34.1),[2] – analogous to *the examination → diagnosis → treatment → follow-up → reassessment* cycle in the care of a patient. In this cycle, activities are continuously influenced by epidemiological and other information. It is an *evidence-based* approach to health care, its 'evidence' being information about the community as well as the results of studies and trials conducted elsewhere.

Without this use of local information, a community orientation is likely to remain a well-meaning aspiration rather than a means of effecting demonstrable improvements in health. Studies of population health, it has been said, 'can be both the *alpha* and *omega* of health care by being the vehicle for both the discovery of need and the evaluation of the outcome of care and treatment'.[3]

A distinction is made (in Figure 34.1) between a *preliminary examination* aimed at 'getting to know' the community and deciding which of its health problems merit detailed study and possible action, and a more detailed investigation (*community diagnosis*) of selected problems. If a convincing *case for action* is revealed, then these explorations may lead to the development of a *programme* or programmes to deal with these problems. Subsequent *monitoring* of programme implementation, *surveillance* of changes in the community's status, and systematic *evaluation* of the programme permit *re-examination* of the situation, leading to decisions about the continuation or modification of the programme and about new issues for study or action.

COPC programmes can deal with selected health problems of the whole population served or of defined subgroups, and may involve health promotion, primary or

Research Methods in Community Medicine: Surveys, Epidemiological Research, Programme Evaluation, Clinical Trials   J. H. Abramson and Z. H. Abramson   Copyright © 2008, John Wiley & Sons Ltd

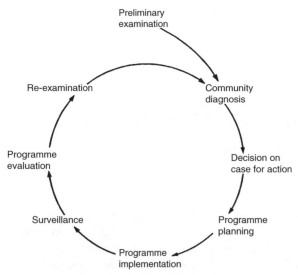

Figure 34.1   The COPC cycle.

secondary prevention, curative, alleviative or rehabilitative care, or any combination of these activities. They may focus on specific disorders or specific risk or preventive factors, may involve individual or family counselling or clinical care, group or community health education, and other activities, and may require community action or inter-agency cooperation.

The prime purpose for which information is collected in COPC is to promote the health of the individuals and community served by the practice, by developing intervention based on the answers to what Kark has called the cardinal questions of community medicine:[4]

1. What is the state of health of the community?
2. What are the factors responsible for this state of health?
3. What is being done about it by the health-care system and by the community itself?
4. What more can be done, what is proposed, and what is the expected outcome?
5. What measures are needed to continue health surveillance of the community and to evaluate the effects of what is being done?

The information collected can also serve to promote community development and the community's involvement in its own care, which may be defined as further aims of COPC. Meetings with community leaders, designed to learn their opinions about health problems and their solutions (see Chapter 20), can stimulate interest and promote community action, as can surveys and feedbacks (using meetings, newsletters, local broadcasts, etc.) of survey findings. Community self-surveys, or surveys in which the community participates,[5] can be especially fruitful in this regard.

Studies in a COPC framework can also provide generalizable new knowledge.[6] There are opportunities for research on, for example, the aetiology, natural history and care of disorders handled in the primary care context, growth and development, and the effects of family processes and psychosocial factors on health and health care. Also – and this is possibly the most important research challenge facing COPC practitioners today – COPC itself can be evaluated: How feasible are specific kinds of COPC programmes in different populations and different health-care systems? How effective are they in comparison with non-community-oriented care? What is their extra cost? And what hospital or other costs do they save?

COPC takes different forms, partly because health-care systems vary and communities' needs vary, and partly because its practitioners sometimes give emphasis to some of its components, often at the expense of others. Epidemiological study of the community can be seen as an essential basis of COPC (as we and, it is to be hoped, you do), or given little consideration. Community involvement or community development can be seen as the end-all and be-all, or regarded as an optional extra. Doctors, nurses and other clinical workers may be the main actors in community programmes, or their work may go on behind the scenes, largely uninterrupted by the community programmes.

This chapter will discuss the application in COPC of the principles and techniques described in previous chapters, with which the reader is now assumed to be familiar. (If not, return to Square 1.) Separate consideration will be given to the definition of the community, the preliminary examination ('getting to know the community'), community diagnosis, evaluation, and some aspects of data collection in COPC.

Defining the Community

The community may be easy or hard to define. Its definition is easiest if the COPC practice cares for the residents of a specific neighbourhood (whether or not they constitute a true community in the sociological sense), workers in specific places of employment, children in specific schools, or other specific groups. People registered as potential users of the services of a given general practitioner, group practice, neighbourhood health centre or health maintenance organization may also be regarded as a 'community' for whose welfare the practice is responsible.

Defining the community is most difficult where there is no explicit responsibility for a specific population. In such instances, the aggregate of people who seek care, or those who have sought care recently, or those who seek care repeatedly, or some defined group of them, may be regarded as the 'community' for COPC purposes. A family physician who does not have a list of registered patients might define the 'community' as all the members of families of which any single member is an active patient. A mapping procedure can determine the census tracts in which the practice's patients reside, to facilitate definition of the community for the purpose of obtaining relevant census-based sociodemographic data.[7]

However defined, this community – the target population for health care – is the study population for survey purposes. The criteria for inclusion require clear formulation. If the community is defined geographically, then decisions are required about the inclusion of transient residents, such as migrant seasonal labourers and their families, and expectant mothers or ill people who come to live with relatives. Information may be required about the target population as a whole or (for specific purposes) about defined subgroups for whom programmes are contemplated or provided, such as infants and their parents, people with a specific disease, or specific high-risk groups. Samples are sometimes used (see Chapter 8 and p. 313), but sampling is obviously an unsatisfactory technique in surveys that aim (as do many surveys in COPC) not only to obtain information at a group level, but also to identify individuals who need care, with a view to offering them this care.

If the community is too large to be studied accurately, then one approach is to start data collection in an 'initial defined area' and then gradually expand this defined segment, as was done in the rural area of Zululand in which COPC was born.[8]

In addition to this prime definition of the community as the target population for whose health care the practice is responsible, it may sometimes be decided to designate the community of which the members of the target population (or a large number of them) form a part for study. If a COPC practice serves part of the population of a town, for example, then it may be also decided to seek information about the town as a whole, in order to learn about available facilities and services, environmental hazards, patterns of leadership and communication, and other relevant 'ecological' factors, and to find census and other easily accessible data that can be applied (even if with reservations) to the target population. This extension may also permit the collection of information required for the planning and evaluation of programmes, e.g. health education projects, that are not restricted to members of the practice's target population, but in which the practice participates, in cooperation with public health or other agencies.

Getting to Know the Community

A general descriptive picture of the community can serve several purposes, the main ones being to identify health problems that merit detailed study and possible action (an 'assessment of needs')[9] and to learn about their possible causes and the resources and circumstances that may be relevant to their solution.

Getting to know the community and its problems is unquestionably a first step; but it is a continuing process, often slow and gradual, and not a one-time transitory activity. Subsequent stages of the COPC process are generally started as soon as they have a sufficient basis, without waiting for a full community picture.

The preliminary examination of the community generally makes use of 'rapid' methods (see Chapter 31), using easily available sources and qualitative research procedures (see p. 147). A search may be made for published reports and ready-made statistics concerning the target population or its area of residence, based on data collected locally, or on small area analysis[10] of information collected at a broader regional or national level. Informal discussions may be held with *key informants* – community members and professionals – concerning their interests and concerns and their perception of the community's problems and ways of solving them. Key informants – people who are believed to know the community well – can be identified by their organizational positions or their reputations. They are people whom others say 'know a lot about this community'; once found, they can be asked to suggest other key informants, in a 'snowball' procedure. Key informants may be able to report on the presence of diseases with obvious manifestations, but are unlikely to be helpful in estimating prevalence or identifying cases.[11] If practicable, more ambitious ways of enlisting community participation in the learning process may be considered.[12]

In addition, easily available clinical and administrative records – especially the practice's own records – may be gathered and analysed in order to obtain information about the use of services, reasons for attendance, infant growth patterns, causes of hospitalization, mortality and its causes, etc. In drawing conclusions from these analyses, it is usually necessary to consider the effects of selection bias, the lack of standardized criteria and methods, incomplete recording, and other shortcomings of the data.

A household health survey is sometimes practicable, especially if the COPC practice is a new one, when the survey can also serve to introduce the public to the services offered to them. It can provide information not available from other sources. As examples, a household survey conducted in a COPC context in the Bronx, New York, revealed that almost half the respondents had no personal health provider, and over half were using hospitals as their primary source of medical care;[13] and in Jerusalem, a survey in a primary care practice revealed numerous cases of coronary heart disease, diabetes, and hypertension who were not known to the practice, and provided the first systematic picture of the prevalence of obesity and smoking.[14]

Home visits provide an excellent opportunity for becoming acquainted with the community, as does direct observation in the field ('using the five senses and touring the community's streets, houses, workplaces, parks, schools, restaurants, stores and service institutions').[15]

Use of a combination of these methods is recommended.[16]

It is important to obtain information about the size and demographic characteristics of the population. Not only is this an essential basis for disease rates and other community health indices, but it also carries its own implications for health and health care. Even the simplest of data, concerning only the population's age and sex distribution, may be of help in planning the allocation of resources. Mobility, too, should be appraised – if there is much flux in the population, then this will have obvious implications for the planning of services.

Demographic information may be available from the registration system used by the practice for administrative or fiscal purposes, from other records (e.g. an age–sex register) maintained as a routine in the practice, or from official sources (national census, population register, school registers, etc.). If not, a basic demographic survey may be required; this is often combined with a health survey. Sometimes, the best that can be done is to use estimates derived from census data for a broad area that includes the practice population, or (by extrapolation) from information about the patients who use the service in a given period.[17]

Consideration should be given to the establishment of a register of the target population, which may be useful not only as a basis for analyses, but also as a sampling frame and a tool for use in the provision of care – for example, as a checklist for identifying elderly people or infants who are not receiving care. Maps, whether drawn by hand or by a computer-driven geographic information system, may also be helpful, particularly for subsequently detecting clustering and high-risk areas by plotting the locations of cases of communicable or other diseases.[18]

'Getting to know the community' is a preliminary stage, in the sense that it must start before the 'community diagnosis' stage can commence, but it can continue in parallel with other stages of the COPC cycle, merging into the surveillance stage in which the community picture is updated – both by continued use of the methods of the preliminary description phase and by special procedures, such as the reporting of births and deaths and other demographic changes.

The more intensive (and selective) 'community diagnosis' stage can start as soon as a need for concentrating on specific issues emerges.

No rules can be laid down concerning the scope of the community appraisal. This must obviously depend on the COPC practice's focus of interest and its resources. A case can be made for the routine collection of a standard set of basic data, but the major part of the data should be selected to meet the practice's specific requirements.

The checklist in Appendix A (p. 383) may be helpful. It is not presented as a blueprint for a study, but as a reminder of topics that may be thought relevant.

Community Diagnosis

In the context of COPC, the community health diagnosis provides detailed information about selected health problems and their determinants. It can be broad or narrow in its scope, and may deal with only a single subgroup of the population, or with a single topic. The topic or topics are generally chosen on the basis of the preliminary examination of the community, but may also be expressions of a national or institutional health policy, not based on local findings. The community diagnosis may be descriptive, analytic, or both.

The community diagnosis may have three main purposes:

1. It permits a decision on the case for action directed at specific problems – is a community programme justified? This particular purpose falls away if programmes are not based on a local appraisal of the community's needs, but are established 'centrally', by policy decisions of health authorities, health maintenance organizations, primary care trusts, or other agencies.
2. It helps in the planning and implementation of programmes.
3. It provides baseline data for the subsequent measurement of changes.

The study procedures that are required may also serve the needs of patient care more directly. A prevalence survey, for example, can identify individuals who need care, and provide a register of cases for use as a framework for the organization and monitoring of a programme.

The community diagnosis may include qualitative elements, especially as a basis for the *case for action*, which depends on the importance of the problem, the feasibility of intervention, and the likelihood that intervention will be effective. Appraisal of the importance of the problem may require detailed epidemiological data on its extent (incidence, prevalence) and impact (e.g. complications, disability, mortality) in the specific community, but it may be obvious without such data. If the problem is regarded as important, then the decision on whether a programme is justified will depend largely on information about the community's felt needs and demands, its readiness and capacity to participate in the programme, attitudes and practices relevant to health care, and the nature and extent of the care presently given. Information on the use and availability of time, manpower and other resources, and evidence of the value of the proposed care procedures and programmes also play an important part in decisions about the case for intervention.

One way of bringing these elements together so as to permit comparisons of alternative approaches to the problem, or of programmes to handle competing problems, is to compute a *priority score*.[19] This is the sum of ratings allotted to different elements, such as:

1. The *relative importance* of the problem: 1, low; 2, moderate, 3, high. This rating is based on the nature, extent and impact of the problem, and is founded both on the epidemiological picture in the community and on general knowledge about the effects of the disorder or risk factor under consideration.
2. The *feasibility and cost* of intervention: 1, low feasibility and/or high cost; 2, intermediate; 3, high feasibility and low cost. This rating is based on practical considerations, including the availability of trained and interested personnel, facilities and other resources, and the possible participation of volunteers or community bodies or other agencies.
3. The *predicted effectiveness* of intervention (if implemented): 1, ineffective; 2, moderate; 3, very effective. This rating is based both on an appraisal of local factors that may influence effectiveness (the community's interest, probable compliance, etc.) and on the results of evaluative studies elsewhere, with respect to undesired as well as desired effects.

Despite the arbitrary features of such a score (subjectivity of ratings, equal weight given to each component), it serves to emphasize that the presence of a problem is not in itself enough to warrant intervention at the community level.

The other purposes of the community diagnosis necessitate more detailed epidemiological investigation. This may include measurement of the occurrence or distribution of the disease (or other problem) and its known risk and protective factors and risk markers, and the identification of groups requiring special care because of their high risk or prevalence of disease or complications, or a high case fatality rate, or poor access to care, poor compliance, poor use of services, etc. Consideration may be given to the study of causal relationships – specifically, what is the importance in this community of the various known causes of the problem? (But a creative mind may also find opportunities for research into new causes.) The community diagnosis may include measures of impact on bed disability, time lost from work, etc., as well as attributable, prevented or preventable fractions.

The diagnosis may also include the identification of *community syndromes*,[20] i.e. sets of associated diseases or other health characteristics that are causally interrelated or have shared or related causes. It may be more effective or efficient to design a programme to handle such a syndrome as a whole, rather than dealing separately with each component.

If the problem under consideration is hypertension, for example, then the community diagnosis might include answers to the following questions: What are the frequency distributions of systolic and diastolic pressures in the community? What is the prevalence of hypertension? How does it vary in different population subgroups? How common are complications? What contribution do hypertension and hypertension-related diseases make to mortality? How strong is the association with overweight in this community? How prevalent is overweight? What are the community's attitudes to hypertension and overweight? How many of the hypertensives smoke cigarettes or have other risk factors for coronary heart disease? What proportion of the community has been screened for hypertension? How many of the known hypertensives are under treatment? Do they take their medication? How many are under adequate control? Do people with borderline hypertension have regular blood pressure checks?

The value of the community diagnosis is generally enhanced if it includes appraisal of the care currently given, asking such questions as: What services are available? How adequately are they used? What are the current care procedures? What is the quality of care? How effectively is the problem prevented or treated?

If the community diagnosis is to provide a useful baseline for the subsequent measurement of change and, hence, for appraising the effectiveness of intervention, then the minimal requirement is information on the incidence or prevalence of the problems at which the programme is directed. Adequate outcome evaluation may be difficult or impossible if appropriate initial data are not available. In order to permit a process evaluation (is the programme running well? – see p. 52) it is also advisable to include measures that will provide baselines for appraising the attainment of the programme's activities and intermediate goals (see p. 346).

In COPC, community diagnosis is often a slow and gradual process, based as it generally is on information continuously collected in the clinical situation, supplemented from time to time by surveys performed outside this situation. If the population is small, then it may be necessary to cumulate several years' experience before satisfactory data, especially on mortality and disease incidence, are available. Moreover, some studies, e.g. of predictors of mortality in the community, are intrinsically long term. At some point, however, and usually sooner rather than later, it is decided that there is enough information to permit the planning and introduction of an intervention programme. This does not halt the process of community diagnosis, which merges imperceptibly into the phase of health surveillance. During this phase, continued appraisal of specific problems and monitoring of the operation of specific programmes are combined with ongoing general surveillance (broad or narrow in its scope) of the community's health and health care, designed to detect and measure changes in the community's health status and its exposure to risk and protective factors.

Evaluation

In COPC, evaluation is always motivated by concern with the welfare of the specific community served. This kind of evaluation, aimed mainly at determining whether the programme is running well and whether its outcomes are satisfactory, is what we have called a *programme review* (see p. 23). Evidence may also be sought that the outcomes can be attributed to the intervention (rather than to other factors), using an experimental or quasi-experimental design (see Chapter 33). This may require study of a control population as well. If such a *programme trial* is contemplated, then it may be wise to attempt to reduce bias – or accusations of bias – by obtaining the assistance of impartial independent co-investigators and (for data obtained outside the ordinary clinical context) of independent observers.

The evaluation may embrace the COPC practice as a whole, or it may be limited to a specific programme or programmes, or specific aspects of programmes. All the basic evaluative questions listed on p. 50 may be asked. Questions about the process and outcome of care usually focus on the activities and goals specified in the programme plan. The scope of the inquiry may vary from simple monitoring procedures (Are people with borderline hypertension having regular blood pressure checks? Are hypertensive patients taking their medication?), through a fuller evaluation including the measurement of immediate outcomes and the detection of obvious undesirable effects (What proportion of the known hypertensives has been brought under control? How many of the patients treated with hypotensive drugs complain of impaired sexual functioning?), to a comprehensive appraisal that may include the measurement of long-term outcomes (Have the frequency distributions of systolic and diastolic pressures or the prevalence of hypertension in the community changed? Has the incidence of stroke or other defined complications fallen?).

It may be helpful to find simple indicators that can be used as surrogates for full evaluations. In COPC projects in Minneapolis, for example, the chlamydia rate in female adolescent patients was used as an indicator of the effects of a programme for preventing teenage pregnancies and sexually transmitted diseases (it dropped from 52 to 29 per 1000 over a 2-year period), and the proportion of prenatal patients screened for HIV (which rose from 17 to 67%) was used as a measure of the success of an HIV screening programme.[21]

Real-time information about activities and intermediate outcomes may be useful as a trigger for immediate corrections to the intervention plan and the way it is implemented, and as a basis for prompt reports to the community. An evaluation of community health promotion programmes has shown that feedbacks on the immediate impact (without waiting to measure long-term changes) can stimulate the development of partnership with the community.[22]

Programmes that aim to change community behaviour can be expected to extend over a long period (marathons rather than sprints), and the evaluation of such programmes, or any evaluation that measures long-term outcomes, will be a long-term affair, fusing with the continuing surveillance of changes in the community picture.[23]

For practitioners with a crusading interest in the extension of COPC, the importance of evaluative studies cannot be overemphasized. Pleading for a 'vibrant and compelling data base with which to make a case for COPC', Rogers[24] has pointed out that it may not be enough to demonstrate effects on mortality or morbidity rates. 'Such statistics ... lack immediacy and emotional impact... A community or a nation will willingly and instantly spend millions to rescue a trapped coal miner ... but it is much harder to get that same community or nation to spend similar sums to reduce infant mortality rates ... As with olives or oysters, a taste for vital statistics is an acquired one'. He suggests that new yardsticks, such as measures of the restoration of crippled people to full functioning, may be needed to excite compassion and interest.

Data Collection in COPC

The collection of information that is accurate enough to be useful for epidemiological purposes is far from easy, and a COPC practice ordinarily has limited resources to devote to this task. Attention should, therefore, be concentrated on data that are of obvious relevance to the practice's needs. There is no point in creating a database that is a cemetery for the interment of useless information, even if some of it will occasionally be exhumed for annual reports or other ritual observances. While the collection of some routine 'basic data' may be considered, the data set should in the main be custom-made to meet the practice's specific needs, particularly those related to its community health programmes.

Data collection in COPC has special features because of the clinical context. First, information is collected to fulfil a double function, meeting the practice's dual responsibilities for individual and community care. When a baby is weighed or a disease is diagnosed – whether in the course of ordinary clinical care or in a special survey – the result may be used both in caring for the individual and at a group level. An audit of records of the performance and results of investigations and the provision of specific advice and other care procedures may provide a basis for decisions both about individual patients and about the overall programme. Second, a good deal of the information needed for community diagnosis and surveillance and programme evaluation can be collected in the course of clinical care, either as part of the ordinary diagnostic investigation and surveillance of patients, or by adding tests and questions to clinic procedures. In a practice where periodic health examinations are conducted, these provide an especially useful opportunity for the collection of such information.

The use of clinical data for epidemiological purposes demands methods that are no less rigorous than those in any epidemiological study, and this may not be easy to achieve. The information to be analysed should be as valid and complete as possible. Careful preparations are needed. Operational definitions of diseases and disabilities should be standardized (especially if diagnoses are made by more than one clinician) – at least for the conditions selected for epidemiological study; for these it may be wise to record the presence or absence of each diagnostic criterion, to permit ongoing or spot checks of conformity with the definition. Standardized procedures should be laid down for the collection of data, especially if questions are asked or examinations done by more than one person. Written instructions that specify the procedures and operational definitions are desirable, especially if there are frequent changes of personnel. Record forms should be convenient to use, and should permit easy retrieval of data for the purposes of analysis. The use of personal computers in the clinic may of course facilitate the whole process. Quality control procedures and tests of validity and reliability should be instituted where necessary – even simple checks on the completeness of recording may yield startling findings.[25]

The integration of epidemiological data collection into a clinical context has both advantages and disadvantages. The clinical situation provides opportunities for doing elaborate tests, for asking questions about delicate matters, and for long-term follow-up. But it may also produce bias. Not only may patients seeking care not be representative, but their illness or apprehension may affect their responses or measurements, and they may tend to give answers they think their health advisers expect. Moreover, observations may be biased by the clinician's prior knowledge of the patient (see *halo effect*, p. 146); this bias may be reduced by the use of standardized objective measures and by making measurements (say of blood pressure) without first referring to the patient's previous values.

Bias caused by the nonrepresentativeness of patients is likely to diminish in time, as more and more of the target population attend for care. In some subgroups, coverage may become so high that the bias can be ignored; this may occur with infants and their mothers, pregnant women, the elderly, and hypertensives or other groups for whom periodic health examinations or special care programmes are organized. Often, however, there is a need for supplementary survey procedures; nonattenders may be identified and invited to attend, or visited at home, or asked to respond by mail or telephone.

The information required in COPC may be collected not only in the clinical situation, but by any appropriate and practicable method. It may be obtained by special surveys, conducted in the clinic context or outside it. These may range in scope from a small follow-up study of a group of patients to a comprehensive community health survey.[26] A community survey can provide information that clinical records cannot or do not; it can appraise the health status and needs of people who have not sought care, it can measure the use of other health services by the practice population, and it may provide the COPC practice with a considerable amount of new information about its patients. Response rates are generally high in surveys performed by or under the auspices of a COPC practice that has a good relationship with the community.

Feedback of the results to the community can be regarded as an important element of a community health survey – which takes us full circle, back to the opening sentence of this book: 'The purpose of most investigations in community medicine ... is the collection of information that will provide a basis for action....' And how can this be done better than by stimulating the community itself to take the action required to improve its health? – in accordance with the principle of the WHO 'Health for All' policy[27] that

> Health for all will be achieved by people themselves. A well informed, well motivated and actively participating community is an element for the attainment of the common goal.

Notes and References

1. *Community-oriented primary care*. Selected bibliography (in chronological order):

    Kark SL. The practice of community-oriented primary care. New York, NY: Appleton-Century-Crofts; 1981.

    Kark SL, Abramson JH (eds). Community-focused health care. Israel Journal of Medical Sciences 1981; 17: 65.

    Abramson JH, Kark SL. Community oriented primary care: meaning and scope. In: Connor E, Mullan F (eds), Community oriented primary care: new directions for health services delivery. Washington, DC, National Academy Press; 1983. pp. 21–59.

    Connor E, Mullan F (1983; see above).

    Nutting PA (ed.). Community oriented primary care: from principle to practice. Washington, DC: Health Resources and Services Administration, Public Health Services, 1987.

    Abramson JH. Community-oriented primary care – strategy, approaches and practice: a review. Public Health Reviews 1988; 16: 3.

    Tollman S. Community-oriented primary care: origins, evolution, applications. Social Science and Medicine 1991; 32: 633.

    Kark SL, Kark E, Abramson JH, Gofin J (eds). Atencion primaria orientada a la comunidad [APOC]. Barcelona: Ediciones Doyma SA; 1994.

    Tollman S, Friedman I. Community-orientated primary health care – South African legacy. South African Medical Journal 1994; 84: 646.

    Gillam S, Plamping D, McClenaham J, Harries J, Epstein L. Community-oriented primary care. London: King's Fund; 1994.

    Nevin JE, Gogel MM. Community-oriented primary care. Primary Care 1996; 23: 1.

    Gillam S, Miller R. COPC – a public health experiment in primary care. London: King's Fund; 1997.

    Rhyne R, Bogue R, Kukulka G, Fulmer H. Community-oriented primary care: health care for the 21st century. Washington, DC: American Public Health Association; 1998

    Kark S, Kark E. Promoting community health: from Pholela to Jerusalem. Johannesburg: Witwatersrand University Press; 1999.

    Strelnick AH. Community-oriented primary care: the state of an art. Archives of Family Medicine 1999; 8: 550.

    Longlett SK, Kruse JE, Wesley RM. Community-oriented primary care: historical perspective. Journal of the American Board of Family Practice 2001; 12: 54.

    Lenihan P, Iliffe S. Community-oriented primary care: a multidisciplinary community-oriented approach to primary care? Journal of Community & Applied Social Psychology 2001; 11: 11.

    Cashman SB, Bushnell FK L, Fulmer HS. Community-oriented primary care: a model for public health nursing. Journal of Health Politics, Policy and Law 2001; 26: 617.

    Geiger J. Community-oriented primary care: a path to community development.. American Journal of Public Health 2002; 92: 1713.

    Epstein L, Gofin J, Gofin R, Neumark Y. The Jerusalem experience: three decades of service, research, and training in community-oriented primary care. American Journal of Public Health 2002; 92: 1717.

Gillam S, Schamroth A. The community-oriented primary care experience in the United Kingdom. American Journal of Public Health 2002; 92: 1721.

Mullan F, Epstein L 2002 Community-oriented primary care: new relevance in a changing world. American Journal of Public Health 92: 1748;

Iliffe S, Lenihan P, Wallace P, Drennan V, Blanchard M, Harris A. Applying community-oriented primary care methods in British general practice: a case study. British Journal of General Practice 2002; 52: 646.

Pickens S, Boumullian P, Anderson RJ, Ross S, Phillips S. Community-oriented primary care in action: a Dallas story. American Journal of Public Health 2002; 92: 1728.

Iliffe S, Lenihan P. Integrating primary care and public health: learning from the community-oriented primary care model. Journal of Health Services 2003; 33: 85.

Sloand E, Groves S. A community-oriented primary care nursing model in an international setting that emphasized partnerships. Journal of the American Academy of Nurse Practitioners 2005; 17: 47.

Moosa SAH. Community-oriented primary care (COPC) in district health services of Gauteng, South Africa. South African Family Practice 2006; 48: 9.

Gofin J, Gofin R. Atencion primaria orientada a la comunidad: un modelo de salud publica en la atencion primaria. Revista Panamericana de Salud Pública 2007; 21: 179.

2. The COPC cycle shown in Figure 34.1 (from Abramson [1988; see note 1]), which was based on the cybernetic planning cycle pictured in Knox EG (Epidemiology in health care planning. Oxford: Oxford University Press, 1979. p. 13), has several variants. For example, *preliminary examination* may be omitted, and *decision on case for action* may be replaced by *prioritization → detailed problem assessment.*

3. Acheson RM, Hall DJ. Epilogue. In: Acheson RM, Hall DJ, Aird L (eds), Seminars in community medicine, vol 2: Health information, planning, and monitoring. London: Oxford University Press; 1976. pp. 145–164.

4. Kark SL (1981; [see note 1], p. 11).

5. *Community-based participatory research*, conducted 'with the participation of those affected by the issue being studied, for the purposes of education and taking action or affecting social change' – i.e. 'research *with* rather than *on* communities' – may enhance organized community action aimed at the prevention of disease and promotion of health (Leung MW, Yen IH, Minkler M. Community-based participatory research: a promising approach for increasing epidemiology's relevance in the 21st century. International Journal of Epidemiology 2004; 33: 499). But 'for academics, dilemmas arise … because it is time-consuming and unpredictable, unlikely to lead to a high production of articles in refereed journals, and its somewhat "messy" nature means it is less likely to attract competitive research funding' (Baum F, MacDougall C, Smith D. Participatory action research. Journal of Epidemiology and Community Health 2006; 60: 854).

For an example of a health survey that was planned by community leaders working with public health researchers, and that provided the first accurate picture of the community's health status, see Benjamins MR, Rhodes DM, Carp JM, Whitman S (A local community health survey: findings from a population-based survey of the largest Jewish community in Chicago. Journal of Community Health 2006; 31: 479).

6. Hannaford PC, Smith BH, Elliott AM. (Primary care epidemiology: its scope and purpose. Family Practice 2005; 23: 1) spell out the wide variety of issues that primary care practitioners have an opportunity to investigate.

7. Mullan F, Phillips RL Jr, Kinman EL. Geographic retrofitting: a method of community definition in community-oriented primary care practices. Family Medicine 2004; 36: 440.

8. *Initial defined area*: Kark SL. An approach to public health. In: King M (ed) Medical care in developing countries. Nairobi: Oxford University Press, 1966. Chapter 5. Kark SL (1981 [see note 1], pp 199–200). In the words of Nutting (1987; [see note 1], p. xxi: 'starting with a "bite-size" subset of the community'.

9. See Trompeter T (Community responsive primary care: a basic guide to planning and needs assessment for community and migrant health. Washington, DC: National Association of Community Health Centers; 1992) and other references on needs appraisal (see note 11, Chapter 2).

10. *Small-area analysis* derives community-specific information from broad databases, such as census, hospital discharge and cancer incidence data sets, with the idea of providing 'good data for good care' (Millman ML. Consensus conference on small area analysis: summary. In: Consensus conference on small area analysis: proceedings. DHHS publication HRS-A-PE 91-1(A). US Public Health Service; 1991. pp. 3–7).

   In two of the other useful papers in the above publication, Nutting PA (Community-oriented primary care and small areas analysis; 1991. pp. 85–88) points out that the information needed by a COPC practice can be helpful even if obtained by methods that are 'perhaps not rigorous enough for publication in the New England Journal', and Lashof JC, Hughes DC (Small area analysis and program evaluation; 1991. pp. 143–151) stress the value of having data both about users of services (the 'clinic population') and about the total target population.

   Computer-produced maps may be helpful for displaying the distribution of health indicators (Williams RL, Flocke SA, Zyzanski SJ, Mettee TM, Martin KB. A practical tool for community-oriented primary care community diagnosis using a personal computer. Family Medicine 1995; 27: 39) and comparing morbidity data for the COPC practice and the total area (Mettee TM, Martin KB, Williams RL. Tools for community-oriented primary care: a process for linking practice and community data. Journal of the American Board of Family Practice 1998; 11: 28).

   Data derived from small-area analysis have obvious limitations if only part of the people living in the area are in the practice population. This has been shown for estimates of the socio-economic characteristics of general practices (Buckingham K. Using census information to estimate GP practice morbidity. Public Health 1996; 110: 191).

   Hospital admission rates do not necessarily reflect the prevalence of specific diseases. A study of 22 small areas in an English district showed moderate positive correlations only for respiratory disease and depression, and none for digestive disease, musculoskeletal disorders, or obesity (Payne JN, Coy J, Patterson S, Milner PC. Is use of hospital services a proxy for morbidity? A small area comparison of the prevalence of arthritis, depression, dyspepsia, obesity and respiratory disease with inpatient admission rates for these disorders in England. Journal of Epidemiology and Community Health 1994; 48: 74).

11. Gyapong JO, Webber RH, Bennett S (The potential role of peripheral health workers and community key informants in the rapid assessment of community burden of diseases: the example of lymphatic filariasis. Tropical Medicine and International Health 1998; 3: 522) found that key informants could report on the presence of elephantiasis and hydroceles, but underreported their prevalence.

    Thorburn MJ, Desai P, Durkin M (A comparison of efficacy of the key informant and community survey methods in the identification of childhood disability in Jamaica. Annals of Epidemiology 1991; 1: 255) found that only a small fraction of children with disabilities were correctly identified by key informants.

12. Methods of *participatory research* are reviewed by Cornwall A, Jewkes R (What is participatory research? Social Science and Medicine 1995; 141: 1667). A detailed illustration of the use of participatory methods, and numerous references to other studies applying these methods, are provided by Vallely A, Shagi C, Kasindi S, Desmond N, Lees S, Chiduo B, Hayes R, Allen C, Ross D (The benefits of participatory methodologies to develop effective community dialogue in the context of a microbicide trial feasibility study in Mwanza, Tanzania. BMC Public Health 2007; 7: 133).

13. Taylor BR, Hayley D. The use of household surveys in community-oriented primary care health needs assessments. Family Medicine 1996; 28: 415.

14. Abramson JH, Epstein LM, Kark SL, Kark E, Fischler B. The contribution of a health survey to a family practice. Scandinavian Journal of Social Medicine 1973; 1: 33.

15. Mettee TM. Community diagnosis: a tool for COPC. In: Nutting PA (ed.) (1987; see note 1, pp. 52–59).

16. Four methods of collecting data on health needs were compared in a study of a neighbourhood in Edinburgh: rapid participatory appraisal, a postal survey, analysis of routinely available small-area statistics, and collation of information held in the practice. The methods were found to be complementary, serving different purposes – 'a composite method may be most informative' (Murray SA, Graham LJ. Practice based health needs assessment: use of four methods in a small neighbourhood. British Medical Journal 1995; 310: 1443).

17. The number of people who use a service during (say) a year can be roughly estimated from information about those who attend during a short survey period, and whether and when they attended previously (Laska E, Lin S, Meisner M. Estimating the size of a population from a single sample: methodology and practical issues. Journal of Clinical Epidemiology 1997; 50: 1143).

    But extrapolations from users to the total target population, e.g. by 'using a fudge factor of about 30 percent to account for non-attenders', are unlikely to be accurate (Hearst N. The denominator problem in community-oriented primary care. In: Nutting PA (ed.) (1987; see note 1, pp. 71–75).

18. *Maps* may be particularly useful in the surveillance of outbreaks and in the identification of environmental hazards. As an example, in a county of South Carolina where children were screened for raised blood lead levels, a computer-based geographic information system was used to identify the areas with the highest risk of exposure to lead (Roberts JR, Hulsey TC, Curtis GB, Reigart JR. Using geographic information systems to assess risk for elevated blood lead levels in children. Public Health Reports 2003; 118: 221).

    Information about *geographic information systems* can be found at http://erg.usgs.gov/isb/pubs/gis_poster and http://www.gis.com.

19. The *scoring scheme* in the text is recommended by Vaughan JP, Morrow RH. (Manual of epidemiology for district health management. Geneva: World Health Organization; 1989). An alternative 'priority score' is the sum of the scores (1–3) allocated to six criteria: prevalence/incidence, severity of problem, effective intervention, acceptability/feasibility, community involvement, and costs and resources (Gillam S *et al.* 1994; see note 1).

20. The *community syndrome* concept was introduced by Kark SL (Epidemiology and community medicine. New York, NY: Appleton-Century-Crofts; 1974. Section 4), who emphasized its potential importance for the development of community health programmes.

    For an example of a study designed to detect community syndromes, see Abramson JH, Gofin J, Peritz E, Hopp C, Epstein LM (Clustering of chronic disorders – a community study of coprevalence in Jerusalem. Journal of Chronic Diseases 1982; 35: 321.

21. Baker NJ, Harper PG, Reif CJ. Use of clinical indicators to evaluate COPC projects. Journal of the American Board of Family Practice 2002; 15: 355.

22. Cheadle A, Beery W, Wagner E *et al.* Conference report: community-based health promotion – state of the art and recommendations for the future. American Journal of Preventive Medicine 1997; 13: 240.

23. The 'marathon' metaphor is used in a paper that points out the importance of measuring change at various milestones in the race between the effects of a health promotion programme and the effects of social, cultural, organizational and policy changes extrinsic to the programme) Green LW. Community health promotion: applying the science of evaluation to the initial sprint of a marathon. American Journal of Preventive Medicine 1997; 13: 225).

An example of a long-term evaluation in a COPC context: Abramson JH, Gofin J, Hopp C, Schein M, Naveh P (The CHAD program for the control of cardiovascular risk factors in a Jerusalem community: a 24-year retrospect. Israel Journal of Medical Sciences 1994; 30: 108).

24. Rogers DE. Community-oriented primary care. Journal of the American Medical Association 1982; 248B: 1622.

25. Checks have found primary care practices where less than half the contacts with patients were recorded (Weitzman S, Bar-Ziv G, Pilpel D, Sachs E, Naggan L. Validation study on medical recording practices in primary care clinics. Israel Journal of Medical Sciences 1981; 17: 21), and where diagnoses were recorded for as few as 9% of episodes (Dawes KS. Survey of general practice records. British Medical Journal 1972; 3: 219), or over half the patients did not live at their registered addresses (Hannay DR. Accuracy of health-centre records. Lancet 1972; 2: 371).

26. A tutorial on the use of **Epi Info** (see Appendix C) in a community health survey is available at http://www.cdc.gov/epiinfo/communityhealth.htm

27. World Health Organization. Targets for health for all. Copenhagen: World Health Organization; 1985.

35

Using the Web for Health Research

Today it is the rare investigator who is not adept at the use of the Internet for reviewing the literature (see Chapter 1), finding statistical programs (see Appendix C) and other tools, and collecting information (or who is not sceptical about the accuracy of a good deal of the information to be found there).[1] This chapter, therefore, will not deal with these uses of the Internet. Nor will it deal with the use of e-mails or other Internet-based communication methods for purposes connected with a study, e.g. to publicize the study or encourage participation or send questionnaires or provide a feedback report of results, or for communicating with co-investigators or granting agencies, or submitting reports to journals for publication.

The focus of the chapter is on Web-based studies, i.e. surveys or trials that use data that are collected on the World Wide Web.

Web-based Surveys

Typical Web-based surveys use self-administered questionnaires that are accessed on the World Wide Web (instead of being supplied on paper or shown on a computer screen by a local data-entry program), with responses that are then transmitted electronically to a database.

The main problem besetting the use of the Internet for health research is of course selection bias. Not everyone uses the Web, not every Web user will access a specific site in which questions are asked, and not every visitor to that site will respond. The study sample of a survey based on responses by surfers who happen to visit a site has been called 'the ultimate convenience sample'.[2] Making generalizations from such a survey requires a leap of faith.

A study of symptoms and attitudes of middle-aged women, for example, based on questionnaires completed by visitors to a women's-health website who defined themselves as experiencing perimenopausal or menopausal symptoms[3] can be of only limited value. At best it can, like a qualitative study, draw attention to the wide range of symptoms experienced around the menopause, or suggest hypotheses about associations. But the specific findings that 89% of respondents felt tired or worn out, or that the number of

Research Methods in Community Medicine: Surveys, Epidemiological Research, Programme Evaluation, Clinical Trials J. H. Abramson and Z. H. Abramson Copyright © 2008, John Wiley & Sons Ltd

symptoms was significantly correlated ($P < 0.001$) with an anxiety index, or that only 66% of women had discussed hormone replacement therapy with their health providers, cannot safely be generalized. They relate only to self-selected women with symptoms who visited a particular website and took the trouble to answer the questionnaire they found there.

For some purposes, this selection bias may be regarded as an advantage, since it can mean access to specific subgroups. A questionnaire provided at a website about atopic eczema, for example, provides an opportunity to survey patients with minimal variants of the disease, not severe enough for patients to see their doctor.[4]

Although the quantitative results of Web surveys based on casual surfers have limited value, the surveys can serve the same important purposes as qualitative surveys (see Chapter 15). They may be extremely helpful, by throwing light on (for example) beliefs, perceptions and practices concerning health and health care.

Other types of Internet research that may be seen as, or have the same uses as, qualitative research include studies of newsgroups, mailing lists, chat rooms, discussion and feedback boards on websites, and blogs – performed with or without the investigator's active involvement in the communications. There have been numerous studies of messages sent to online support groups set up for individuals with various disorders and their caregivers.[5] A study of three Internet discussion groups about diabetes, for example, pinpointed the main concerns of patients and their families, and their satisfaction with the discussion groups.[6]

Ethical issues must of course be addressed in such studies.[7] A group member is quoted as saying 'When I joined this, I thought it would be a support group, not a fishbowl for a bunch of guinea pigs. I certainly don't feel at this point that it is a safe environment, as a support group is supposed to be, and I will not open myself up to be dissected by students or scientists'.[8]

There are widespread differences of opinion as to what constitutes appropriate online ethical conduct.[7] Consideration should be given to the subjects' perceptions of privacy, the potential harm that a breach of privacy might cause, how anonymity and confidentiality can be maintained, and the need for informed consent. Informed consent requires the provision of simply phrased information about the study and its purpose, its sponsors, any risk of harm or discomfort or breaches of anonymity or confidentiality, and the use to which the information will be put. An 'I agree' button may be provided, although this may not necessarily mean informed consent – there is no knowing whether clicking on it means that the information about the study has even been read.

Web-based surveys have obvious advantages compared with other types of survey. These include speed, low cost (in one comparison, less than one-quarter the cost of a postal survey),[9] an attractive interface, ease of use, and adaptability (offering different questions, even in different languages, to different individuals), and maybe, because of the absence of an interviewer, a reduced tendency to give socially desirable replies. Sample size has little effect on cost, and it might well be decided to invite (say) all students in a college to participate, instead of a random sample, to avoid insufficient representation of small subgroups.

The main disadvantage is selection bias, caused by the need for respondents to be computer literate and have access to computers and the Internet (requirements that may be related to income, education, age, and other characteristics), to visit the specific Web page, and then to be motivated to complete the questionnaire. The response rate among surfers who visit the Web page and view the questionnaire is usually low, which of course aggravates the potential for bias. Most comparisons have shown lower response rates (among students invited to participate) for Web surveys than for postal surveys.[10] Response may be improved by sending an e-mailed invitation with an embedded hyperlink to the Web-site containing the questionnaire; but not much else can be done to raise the response rate.[11]

Moreover, populations or subgroups who do have relatively high response rates may be more likely to be surveyed and, if surveyed, to have their results published, leading to a form of publication bias.

If a Web-based study is to achieve external validity as a source of quantitative information that can be generalized to a wider reference population, then the effects of self-selection must be allayed. Ideally, the respondents should be recruited by the investigator, as in studies that are not Web-based. If this has been done, then participation can be restricted to invited subjects by password protection. This approach is easy if the investigator has a list of the members of the reference population, as is possible in studies of (say) workers in a factory or students in a college, or if there is a population registry or a list of the patients in a practice. But the need for Internet access is a constraint even in such instances. Failing selection by the investigator, respondents can be screened, either before or after completion of the questionnaire, by imposing criteria based on selected demographic or other criteria.

Alternatively, information about the respondents can be collected in the hope that this will permit adjustment of the results, by weighting, so as to reduce the effect of known confounders. When adjustment was made for various socioeconomic variables in a Swedish epidemiological study of a population-based sample, the bias in associations between smoking, myocardial infarction, parity, physical activity, and body mass index was small, and relative risks were similar for responders to Web and paper questionnaires.[12] Even if adjustment is not done, information about the respondents may permit interpretations of the findings to be tempered by a better understanding of the possible biases ('The impact of our results would be strengthened if we knew more about the population').[3]

Selection bias may not always be important. An epidemiological study of 31,671 cats vaccinated by veterinarians with World Wide Web access, for example, based on Web-based survey forms filled in by the veterinarians over a 1–3-year follow-up period, which revealed rates of 11.0 and 0.3 per 10,000 vaccine doses for postvaccinal inflammatory reactions and vaccine-site-associated sarcomas respectively, seems unlikely to have been influenced by self-selection of cats or vets.[13]

Apart from selection bias, the accuracy of the information – possible information bias – may require consideration. This may be because of badly worded questions or inadequate explanations, or there may be deliberate untruths, either mischievous or connected with the respondent's apprehensions about the confidentiality of the answers. Perceptions of privacy may differ; the computer may be regarded as 'more private' or 'less private'. Computer literacy may also play a part; not everyone is adept at using a keyboard and mouse; and, especially for people less at home with computers, there may be what has been called a 'Big Brother effect',[14] with a tendency to give socially desirable answers.

The above considerations also apply to the numerous psychological tests and surveys placed on the Web by researchers who wish to analyse the responses.[15] These may be health related (attitudes and perceptions concerning diseases, health care, clinical research, etc.). Student researchers sometimes seem almost desperate in their pleas for participants ('By participating you have the opportunity to win a £30 online gift voucher!' or 'Really really need some participants for a senior thesis').[15] Some psychological researchers claim that Web-based tests can be better than those conducted in student laboratories, despite their selection bias, because the results are 'more representative' – 'more than 80% of all psychological studies are conducted with students as participants, while only about 3% of the general population are students'.[16] Although studies comparing Web studies of subjects recruited through the Web with those conducted in student laboratories have shown surprising agreement, significant differences have sometimes been found.[17]

A promising development is the provision of both an online questionnaire and a postal questionnaire, permitting the members of the selected study sample to choose either. In a large-scale epidemiological study conducted in the United States in 2001 (when almost 60% of households were connected to the Internet), over 50% of respondents chose the Web. It was estimated that each Web participant saved the study about $50, although T-shirts or $5-dollar phone-cards were given as incentives. But despite this use of Web and paper questionnaires in concert, the study's overall response rate was only 37%.[18]

Web-based Trials

Web-based trials are, in principle, no different from Web-based surveys, except that the subjects are allocated to treatment and control groups, and the data collection instruments may be data-entry forms filled in by the researchers, and not necessarily self-administered questionnaires. 'Before' and 'after' data, or serial data to assess change, may be submitted for each study subject. Selection bias should not be more of a problem than in trials not using the Web, unless the subjects themselves are required to fill in the reports. The important requirement is that the subjects should be selected, and allocated to treatment and control groups, by the investigators.

This use of the Web really comes into its own in multicentre trials, where it has been referred to as a new paradigm, providing widened possibilities for the recruitment of both investigators and subjects. An example is a clinical trial of hypertension treatment,[19] conducted at over 800 sites in various countries, mainly primary care physician practices that recruited subjects from their hypertensive patients. For many of the investigators, this was their introduction to clinical research; all that was needed at each site was a computer with an Internet browser. Contact with the study centre was two-way. The Web was used not only to transmit data (including data from external laboratories) to a central database, but to supply the sites with information about the requirements for subject recruitment, informed consent processes, definitions, the study protocol, and so on, and to automatically assign each eligible subject to a treatment or control group.

The subjects recruited for a trial by the investigators, and allocated to treatment and control groups, can be asked to fill in the Web-based reports themselves, as in a double-blind controlled trial of a widely used herbal remedy for the common cold (*Echinacea*), in which 148 students with early symptoms were randomly given the remedy or a placebo, and asked to complete a Web-based questionnaire about symptoms every day for 10 days.[20] The study gave no evidence that the remedy was efficacious.

Similarly, a randomized controlled trial of a Web intervention programme to reduce depression was performed by randomizing samples of depressed and nondepressed members of a health organization (63% of whose members had Internet access) to two groups, one of which was directed to the Web intervention programme. Both groups filled in Web-based questionnaires over a 32-week period. The study failed to find an effect for the Web intervention programme, possibly because of insufficiently frequent visits to the website. A subsequent trial, in which reminders to use the website were sent by postcards and by phone, found a modest positive effect.[21]

In a randomized placebo-controlled trial of the effect on labial herpes of an ointment (sent by mail), where the subjects, who were recruited through newspaper and e-zine advertisements directing them to a website, agreed to use the website to make daily reports during episodes, thus avoiding the need for daily clinic visits, reports were provided on only 67% of the days in question.[22]

The sampling frame can, of course, be a Web source, provided that the randomization is done by the researchers, and that it is realized that the findings may be applicable only to users of the Web. For example, a controlled comparison of Web-based smoking cessation programmes was done by inviting visitors to a smoking cessation website to participate in an interactive computer-tailored programme, and then randomizing them to two alternative programmes. A follow-up survey revealed a significant difference between the results of the two programmes, suggesting that one of them was preferable, at least for visitors to the website in question – or, more specifically, for the self-selected 2% of visitors to the website who enlisted for either programme.[23] But the low response rate to the follow-up survey (35%) threw doubt even on that inference.

When given a choice between supplying follow-up data via the Web or by fax, physicians participating in a therapeutic trial in Japan were more likely to use the Web-based system if they were 55 years or younger (odds ratio = 1.9), or regular users of computers (odds ratio = 4.2).[24]

Technical Aspects

Creating a Web-based study is not easy. It is not enough merely to draft a set of questions. Much more than that is needed before the document can be uploaded to an Internet server to make it available online.[25]

The layout and format of the questions must be decided, and provision must be made for the entry of responses, using text boxes, check boxes, select buttons, radio buttons, drop-down lists, etc., and for the collection of responses and their transmission to a database. Skip mechanisms will usually be needed, to permit branching and jumping to other questions or another page, or to allow subsequent questions to be tailored, depending on the responses that have been made. Instructions, help, warnings and reminders can be offered, using alert boxes and pop-up windows.

Validity checks can be built in, i.e. checks for unacceptable or inconsistent data (with error messages), for incomplete data (with reminder prompts), and for duplicate entries (using passwords, or cookies to detect entries coming from the same computer).

Instructions may be included for the creation of a code book and data file, and for data manipulation and processing, including the creation of new variables, tabulations, and analytic procedures.

Other optional features include a requirement for logging in with a password to restrict access, a mechanism for obtaining informed consent, the automatic collection of data about date and time and the computer used, a back-up recovery process to permit the completion of interrupted sessions, protection against viruses and other malicious software, counts of responses and nonresponses and drop-out rates, and the sending of 'thank-you' and reminder e-mails.

Consideration must be given to possible differences in the appearance of the questionnaire when different operating systems, Internet browsers, and screen settings are used, and to the effect of the presence or absence of Java enablement.

A website for large-scale clinical trials may be expected to supply information and enhance communication among investigators as well as providing randomization, data-entry facilities, reminders, and other essential requirements for the performance of the trial.[26]

All this must be planned and put into effect in advance, and that is not simple. Setting up a Web-based study requires considerable expertise. Appropriate software for doing the job is readily available (see Appendix C), but few researchers will have the know-how required to adapt it to the needs of their study, or the time and patience to learn how to do so.[27] It will be necessary to create and appropriately format HTML (Hyper Text Markup Language) pages and CSS (Cascading Style Sheets) Web forms. This can be done with a simple text editor, but a basic knowledge of HTML and CSS is very useful in using the software effectively and customizing the look and feel of the form. Validation routines using JavaScript can be used to reduce problems of invalid data and multiple submission.[25] Even for an expert, the process is laborious and time consuming,[28] and cooperation with computer mavens is usually essential.

Even with the best of planning, glitches may be expected, calling for expert help. An epidemiological study of high-school students in Texas, for example, was beset by losses of connection to the Internet and, in one school, by a major computer virus infection.[29]

Notes and References

1. A vivid demonstration of the unreliability of Internet information is provided by a meta-analysis of interventions for preventing or treating alcohol hangover. A literature search revealed only 15 randomized controlled trials, and these provided no compelling evidence of effectiveness; the effective expedients are apparently abstinence and moderation. But a Google search revealed over 325,000 Web pages that mentioned hangover cures (Pittler MH, Verster JC, Ernst E. Interventions for preventing or treating alcohol hangover: systematic review of randomized controlled trials. British Medical Journal 2006; 331: 1515).

2. Lakeman R. Using the Internet for data collection in nursing research. Computers in Nursing 1997; 15: 269.

3. Conboy L, Domar A, O'Connell E Women at mid-life: symptoms, attitudes, and choices, an Internet based survey. Maturitas 2001; 38: 129.

4. Eysenbach G, Diepgen TL. Epidemiological data can be gathered with World Wide Web. British Medical Journal 1998; 316: 72.

5. White M, Forman SM. Receiving social support online: implications for health education. Health Education Research 2001; 16: 693.

6. Zrebiac JF, Jacobson AM. What attracts patients with diabetes to an internet support group? A 21-month longitudinal website study. Diabetic Medicine 2001; 18: 154.

7. Eysenbach G, Till JE. Ethical issues in qualitative research on internet communities. British Medical Journal 2001; 323: 1103.

8. King SA. Researching Internet communities: proposed ethical guidelines for the reporting of results. The Information Society 1996; 12: 119. Actually, the Helsinki declaration does not in so many words interdict the dissection of guinea pigs in fishbowls, but that's just splitting hares.

9. Kwak N, Radler B. A comparison between mail and Web surveys: response pattern, respondent profile, and data quality. Journal of Official Statistics 2002; 18: 257.

10. In one comparison of responses to a postal questionnaire and a Web questionnaire by two large, randomly selected samples of students, the response rate (after two follow-up reminders) was 42.5% for the mail survey and 27.4% for the Web survey (Kwak and Radler; see note 9). In another such comparison, the rates were 22.0% and 17.1% (Sax LJ, Gilmartin SK, Bryant AN. Assessing response rates and nonresponse bias in Web and paper surveys. Research in Higher Education 2003; 44: 409).

11. In a randomized trial comparing responses by students (all of whom had Internet access) who were sent either a paper questionnaire or an e-mailed invitation to complete a Web questionnaire, with an embedded hyperlink to take them directly to the website, the response rates were 32% for the mailed questionnaire and 50% for the Web questionnaire (Wygant S, Lindorf R. Surveying collegiate Net surfers – Web methodology or mythology. Quirks Marketing Research Review: article no 5615; 1999).

    A meta-analysis of *factors influencing response rates* in 68 Web-based surveys found that the main factors associated with better response were prior contact with sampled people, follow-up contacts with nonrespondents, and personalized contacts (Cook C, Heath F, Thompson RL. A meta-analysis of response rates in Web- or Internet-based surveys. Educational and Psychological Measurement 2000; 60: 821). Simple questionnaires may have higher response rates than 'fancy' ones, and short questionnaires than long ones, and cash or other incentives may be helpful; but findings are contradictory. Sending follow-up reminders by e-mail may help. See Madge C (Online questionnaires: sampling issues; 2006. Available at http://www.geog.le.ac.uk/orm/questionnaires/quessampling.htm) and Umbach PD (Web surveys: best practices, New Directions for Institutional Research 2004; 121: 23).

Provision of a paper-questionnaire option may increase response; in a large epidemiological study of a population sample in Sweden, the response rate was 70% when a choice between Web and paper questionnaires was offered, and much lower when only Web questionnaires were offered (Ekman A, Dickman PW, Klint A, Weiderpass E, Litton J-E. Feasibility of using web-based questionnaires in large population-based epidemiological studies. European Journal of Epidemiology 2006; 21: 103).

12. Ekman *et al.* (2006; see note 11).

13. Gobar GM, Kass PH. World Wide Web-based survey of vaccination practices, postvaccinal reactions, and vaccine site-associated sarcomas in cats. Journal of the American Veterinary Medical Association 2002; 220: 1477.

14. 'On each landing … the poster with the enormous face gazed from the wall … Big Brother is watching you, the caption beneath it ran'. From George Orwell's novel '1984'.

15. Archives containing over 600 Web-based psychological experiments and surveys are maintained by the University of Zurich (http://genpsylab-wexlist.unizh.ch/browse.cfm?action=browse and http://genpsylab-wexlist.unizh.ch/browse.cfm?action=browse&modus=survey)

16. 'Some say that psychological science is based on research with rats, the mentally disturbed, and college students. We study rats because they can be controlled, the disturbed because they need help, and college students because they are available' (Birnbaum MH (ed.). Psychology experiments on the Internet. San Diego, CA: Academic Press; 2000. pp. 89–117). 'The existing science of human behavior is largely the science of the behavior of sophomores' (McNemar Q. Opinion-attitude methodology. Psychological Bulletin 1942; 43: 289. Cited by Reips U-D (The Web experiment method: advantages, disadvantages, and solutions. In Birnbaum (2000, *op. cit.* pp. 89–117)).

17. Birnbaum MH. Human research and data collection via the Internet. Annual Review of Psychology 2004; 55: 803.

18. Smith B, Smith TC, Gray GC, Ryan MAK. When epidemiology meets the Internet: Web-based surveys in the Millennium Cohort Study. American Journal of Epidemiology 2007; 166(11): 1345.

19. Marks RG, Conlin M, Ruberg SJ. Paradigm shifts in clinical trials enabled by information technology. Statistics in Medicine 2001; 20: 2683.

Readers of this book who, like its authors, are never quite sure of what *paradigms* are, may find the explanation given by Rychetnik L, Hawe P, Waters E, Barratt A, Frommer M (A glossary for evidence based public health. Journal of Epidemiology and Community Health 2005; 58: 538) helpful. ('A paradigm encapsulates the commitments, beliefs, assumptions, values, methods, outlooks, and philosophies of a particular "world view"… many areas of public health research and action … reflect paradigms that are alternatives to post-positivism, for example, critical theory, constructivism, and participatory paradigms…').

Or maybe not.

20. Barrett BP, Brown RL, Locken K, Maberry R, Bobula JA, D'Alessio D. Treatment of the common cold with unrefined *Echinacea*: a randomized, double-blind, placebo-controlled trial. Annals of Internal Medicine 2002; 137: 939.

21. Clarke G, Reid E, Eubanks D, O'Connor E, DeBar LL, Kelleher C, Lynch F, Nunley S. Overcoming depression on the Internet (ODIN): a randomized controlled trial of an Internet depression skills intervention program. Journal of Medical Internet Research 2002; 4(3): e14. Clarke G, Eubanks D, Reid E, Kelleher C, O'Connor E, DeBar LL, Lynch F, Nunley S, Gullion C. Overcoming depression on the Internet (ODIN) (2): a randomized trial of a self-help depression skills program with reminders. Journal of Medical Internet Research 2005; 7(2): e16.

22. Formica M, Kabbara K, Clark R, McAlindon T. Can clinical trials requiring frequent participant contact be conducted over the Internet? Results from an online randomized controlled trial evaluating a topical ointment for herpes labialis. Journal of Medical Internet Research 2004; 6(1): e6.

23. Etter J-F. Comparing the efficacy of two Internet-based computer-tailored smoking cessation programs: a randomized trial. Journal of Medical Internet Research 2005; 7(1): e2.

24. Rahman M, Morita S, Fukui T, Sakamoto J. Physicians' choice in using Internet and fax for patient recruitment and follow-up in a randomized controlled trial. Methods of Information in Medicine 2004; 43: 268.

25. Shaw R. Technical guide to producing online questionnaires; 2006. Available at http://www.geog.le.ac.uk/orm/technical/techcontents.htm.

26. Santoro E, Nicolis E, Franzosi MG. RES3/417: The development of a clinical trial web site: a proposal for a model. Journal of Medical Internet Research 1999; 1(suppl. 1): e79.

27. The University of Leicester offers an intensive online training program (Exploring online research methods in a virtual training environment: an online research methods training package for the social science community. Available at http://www.geog.le.ac.uk/orm/index.htm).

    For referenced guidelines to the design of a Web-based survey, see Umbach PD (Web surveys: best practices. New Directions for Institutional Research 2004; 121: 23).

28. The author of a review of literature on Web survey implementation, who is a research analyst, writes 'On one occasion I did not have the assistance of a programmer and was forced to build the page myself. While the latest software makes programming Web pages relatively easy, all of them require some writing of code to maximize the functionality of Web data collection. After more than forty hours of programming, I had a functioning Web-based survey' (Umbach PD, 2004; see note 27).

29. Cooper CJ, Cooper SP, del Junco DJ, Shipp EM, Whitworth R, Cooper SR. Web-based data collection: detailed methods of a questionnaire and data gathering tool. Epidemiological Perspectives and Innovations 2006, 3: 1. Available at www.epi-perspectives.com/content/3/1/1.

Appendix A

Community Appraisal: A Checklist

Information on the following topics may be helpful in the appraisal of a community's health needs and ways of meeting them. Some of the items in this list are relevant only to a true community; this may be the community served by a COPC practice (see Chapter 34) or the community from which the practice's patients, or many of them, are drawn. Other items are relevant to any target population of a community-oriented practice, however this is defined.

The items in the list are not exhaustive or mutually exclusive, and they are not arranged in order of importance. Some of the information is qualitative.

1. *Definition of the community/population*
   - eligibility criteria, exclusions
2. *Demographic characteristics*
   - population size
   - distribution by age, sex, social class, economic status, educational level, occupation, religion, ethnic group, race, marital status, parity
   - population mobility
   - trends of change in size and demographic composition
   - vital statistics:
     - mortality, birth and fertility rates
     - life expectancy
3. *General information*
   - history of the community
   - physical and climatic characteristics of the neighbourhood
   - economic activities, economic development, occupations
   - affluence/poverty: prevalence of unemployment, household crowding, and other indices of deprivation
   - social attributes: social structure, cohesiveness, social networks, family values and living patterns, formal and informal leadership, political structure
   - community organizations
   - key informants

Research Methods in Community Medicine: Surveys, Epidemiological Research, Programme Evaluation, Clinical Trials   J. H. Abramson and Z. H. Abramson   Copyright © 2008, John Wiley & Sons Ltd

4. *Facilities and services*
- housing, water supply, fluoridation, sanitation, roads, transportation, walkability, shops, schools, libraries, sports facilities, places of worship
- availability of healthy foods
- available health services (including traditional healers)
- information about health services: location, personnel, facilities, fiscal arrangements, accessibility, coverage, quality and effectiveness of care
- health insurance: types and coverage
- other welfare services
- current health and welfare programmes: mother and child health, immunization, family planning, elderly, screening, control of specific diseases, meals-on-wheels, etc.
- discontinued health programmes and the reasons for their failure
- inter-agency and inter-sectoral cooperation in health-related services

5. *Utilization of services*
- consultation rates and reasons for attendance
- use of antenatal, child care, dental and other specific services
- hospitalization rates and reasons for hospitalization
- differential use of services by various groups
- barriers to use of services: language, cultural, geographic, financial

6. *The community's involvement in its own health care*
- the community's interests and concerns: felt needs, expectations of services, demand for services, satisfaction with services
- organized action groups and their activities
- actual and potential participation by community bodies and volunteers in activities run by health agencies
- self-care

7. *Health-relevant knowledge, attitudes and practices*
- lifestyle: e.g. diet, infant feeding, family planning, smoking, drinking, drugs
- knowledge about disease causation, prevention of common diseases, and health maintenance and promotion
- health and illness behaviour
- compliance with medical advice
- trends of change in health-relevant behaviours

8. *Health and disease status*
- causes of death
- common or important diseases (including behavioural and emotional disorders) and disabilities: incidence and prevalence rates, sickness absenteeism
- nutritional status
- growth and development of children
- distribution of health-relevant characteristics, such as weight and blood pressure
- trends of change in health status

9. *Risk and protective factors*
   - prevalence of personal risk factors for important disorders (smoking, obesity, teenage pregnancy, etc.)
   - environmental health hazards
   - immunization status
   - measures of impact of risk and protective factors (attributable, prevented or preventable fractions)

Appendix B

Random Numbers

53 74 23 99 67	61 32 28 69 84	94 62 67 86 24	98 33 41 19 95	47 53 53 38 09
63 38 06 86 54	99 00 65 26 94	02 82 90 23 07	79 62 67 80 60	75 91 12 81 19
35 30 58 21 46	06 72 17 10 94	25 21 31 75 96	49 28 24 00 49	55 65 79 78 07
63 43 36 82 69	65 51 18 37 88	61 38 44 12 45	32 92 85 88 65	54 34 81 85 35
98 25 37 55 26	01 91 82 81 46	74 71 12 94 97	24 02 71 37 07	03 92 18 66 75
02 63 21 17 69	71 50 80 89 56	38 15 70 11 48	43 40 45 86 98	00 83 26 91 03
64 55 22 21 82	48 22 28 06 00	61 54 13 43 91	82 78 12 23 29	06 66 24 12 27
85 07 26 13 89	01 10 07 82 04	59 63 69 36 03	69 11 15 83 80	13 29 54 19 28
58 54 16 24 15	51 54 44 82 00	62 61 65 04 69	38 18 65 18 97	85 72 13 49 21
34 85 27 84 87	61 48 64 56 26	90 18 48 13 26	37 70 15 42 57	65 65 80 39 07
03 92 18 27 46	57 99 16 96 56	30 33 72 85 22	84 64 38 56 98	99 01 30 98 64
62 95 30 27 59	37 75 41 66 48	86 97 80 61 45	23 53 04 01 63	45 76 08 64 27
08 45 93 15 22	60 21 75 46 91	98 77 27 85 42	28 88 61 08 84	69 62 03 42 73
07 08 55 18 40	45 44 75 13 90	24 94 96 61 02	57 55 66 83 15	73 42 37 11 61
01 85 89 95 66	51 10 19 34 88	15 84 97 19 75	12 76 39 43 78	64 63 91 08 25
72 84 71 14 35	19 11 58 49 26	50 11 17 17 76	86 31 57 20 18	95 60 78 46 75
88 78 28 16 84	13 52 53 94 53	75 45 69 30 96	73 89 65 70 31	99 17 43 48 76
45 17 75 65 57	28 40 19 72 12	25 12 74 75 67	60 40 60 81 19	24 62 01 61 16
96 76 28 12 54	22 01 11 94 25	71 96 16 16 88	68 64 36 74 45	19 59 50 88 92
43 31 67 72 30	24 02 94 08 63	38 32 36 66 02	69 36 38 25 39	48 03 45 15 22
50 44 66 44 21	66 06 58 05 62	68 15 54 35 02	42 35 48 96 32	14 52 41 52 48
22 66 22 15 86	26 63 75 41 99	58 42 36 72 24	58 37 52 18 51	03 37 18 39 11
96 24 40 14 51	23 22 30 88 57	95 67 47 29 83	94 69 40 06 07	18 16 36 78 86
31 73 91 61 19	60 20 72 93 48	98 57 07 23 69	65 95 39 69 58	56 80 30 19 44
78 60 73 99 84	43 89 94 36 45	56 69 47 07 41	90 22 91 07 12	78 35 34 08 72
84 37 90 61 56	70 10 23 98 05	85 11 34 76 60	76 48 45 34 60	01 64 18 39 96
36 67 10 08 23	98 93 35 08 86	99 29 76 29 81	33 34 91 58 93	63 14 52 32 52
07 28 59 07 48	89 64 58 89 75	83 85 62 27 89	30 14 78 56 27	86 63 59 80 02

Research Methods in Community Medicine: Surveys, Epidemiological Research, Programme Evaluation, Clinical Trials   J. H. Abramson and Z. H. Abramson   Copyright © 2008, John Wiley & Sons Ltd

```
10 15 83 87 60    79 24 31 66 56    21 48 24 06 93    91 98 94 05 49    01 47 59 38 00
55 19 68 97 65    03 73 52 16 56    00 53 55 90 27    33 42 29 38 87    22 13 88 83 34

53 81 29 13 39    35 01 20 71 34    62 33 74 82 14    53 73 19 09 03    56 54 29 56 93
51 86 32 68 92    33 98 74 66 99    40 14 71 94 58    45 94 19 38 81    14 44 99 81 07
35 91 70 29 13    80 03 54 07 27    96 94 78 32 66    50 95 52 74 33    13 80 55 62 54
37 71 67 95 13    20 02 44 95 94    64 85 04 05 72    01 32 90 76 14    53 89 74 60 41
93 66 13 83 27    92 79 64 64 72    28 54 96 53 84    48 14 52 98 94    56 07 93 89 30
```

Reproduced with permission from Fisher RA, Yates F. Statistical tables for biological, agricultural and medical research. London: Longman; 1974.

Appendix C

Free Computer Programs

The Internet offers a great number of free computer programs that can be used in the planning, performance, and analysis of observational and analytic studies and trials. Some can be downloaded and run on one's own computer, and some are online programs – interactive statistical calculating pages on the Internet that perform calculations when data are entered. Some of these interactive pages are also downloadable. Most of the downloadable programs are suitable for PCs, and some for Macs. Some are Windows programs, some of the older ones are DOS programs, which can be run in a command prompt window (a 'DOS box') in Windows, and some will run in Linux.

The following list of selected programs may be useful. It does not pretend to be comprehensive. Prominence is of course given to the **WinPepi** programs, for a reason that will not escape percipient readers. We have tried to list only programs of good quality, but can take no responsibility.

The list comprises four main sections: (1) Preparing for the study; (2) Tools; (3) Analysis – online lists of free statistical software, and selected multipurpose software; and (4) Programs for specific tasks.

If a statistical program to meet a specific need is not found in Section 4, then the options (assuming that one knows what one is looking for) are to search the lists of free programs in Section 3a, and to explore the lists of tests and other procedures offered by the multipurpose programs listed in Section 3b, such as **WinPepi**, **OpenEpi**, and **OS4**. This is particularly easy with **WinPepi**, since an alphabetical list of its procedures can be viewed at http://www.brixtonhealth.com, or accessed by clicking on 'Finder' in any **WinPepi** program. With the other programs, it is necessary to open them and see what options they offer, or go to their websites or consult their manuals.

The Web addresses (URLs) at which the software is currently to be found (in September 2007) are listed at the end of this appendix.

An obvious additional recourse is Google or some other Internet search engine. A Google search for 'logistic regression free download', for example, will reveal at least one free logistic regression program (currently the 19th search result, among the 797,000 hits reported).

Research Methods in Community Medicine: Surveys, Epidemiological Research, Programme Evaluation, Clinical Trials   J. H. Abramson and Z. H. Abramson   Copyright © 2008, John Wiley & Sons Ltd

The list is arranged as follows:

1. Preparing for the study
   a   Reference management
   b   Sample size and power
   c   Planning a clinical trial
   d   Web-based surveys
2. Tools
   a   Data entry and data management
   b   Random numbers and random sampling
   c   Randomization
   d   Calculators
   e   *P* values
   f   Spreadsheets
   g   Graphs
   h   Epidemic curves
   i   Card indexes
   j   Text editors
3. Analysis: general
   a   Online lists of free statistical programs
   b   Selected multipurpose programs
4. Analysis: specific tasks
   a   Descriptive statistics
   b   Bivariate analyses
   c   Stratified analyses
   d   Multiple linear regression
   e   Multiple logistic regression
   f   Cox regression analysis
   g   Multiple Poisson regression
   h   Analysis of variance
   i   Misclassification
   j   Measuring validity
   k   Measuring reliability
   l   Appraising synergism
   m   Assessing a scale
   n   Multiple comparisons
   o   Cluster samples
   p   Capture–recapture procedure
   q   Standardization (direct and indirect)
   r   Regression to the mean
   s   Survival analysis
   t   Meta-analysis
   u   Multilevel studies
   v   Imputation

w   Bayesian analysis

x   Appraisal of unmeasured confounders

5. Web addresses (URLs)

1. Preparing for the Study

1a. Reference management

BiblioExpress is a simple reference manager without the full capabilities of commercial reference managers, but able to store, arrange, sort, format and export references that have been entered by hand.

Zotero[1] is more than just an excellent reference manager. It not only stores, arranges, formats, and exports references, it also automatically captures citations from most Web pages – it finds citation information on the page and (with a mouse click or two) puts it into standard bibliographic form and stores it. Citations can also be entered by hand. It also permits the storage and management of notes, documents, snapshots of Web pages, and URLs, and it conducts searches through this material – it is an information manager, not only a reference manager. Numerous extra functions are planned.

Zotero is an add-on to the free browser **Firefox**, and it can be used only if **Firefox** is open. It has been translated into several languages, and a plea has been put out for a translation into Klingon.[2]

1b. Sample size and power

Numerous programs that compute required sample sizes and estimate the power of tests are included in Pezzullo's lists (see below), most of them appropriate when planning studies that aim to estimate or compare means, proportions, or rates.

Versatile programs that are also applicable to studies with other objectives include the following:

Describe and **Compare2** (which are **WinPepi** programs).

PS: power and sample size calculation

Lenth's Java applets for power and sample size (interactive page; downloadable).

OpenEpi (online).

In a *cluster sample*, the number and size of clusters required to estimate a rate or proportion can be computed by **Describe**.

Compare2 and **Sampsize**[3] can compute the number and size of clusters required in a cluster-randomized trial for comparisons of rates or mean values. A manual for **Sampsize** in pdf format is available at http://www.abdn.ac.uk/hsru/epp/sampsize.

1c. Planning a clinical trial

The **Trial Protocol Tool** (**TPT**) is a software library for use in planning pragmatic clinical trials. It gives a step-by-step account of how to design a trial, together with reference material, statistical calculators, a protocol template, protocols of well-designed trials, and access to Web resources.[4]

1d. Web-based surveys

The code required for a dynamic Web survey system can be downloaded from the School of Rural Public Health Free Web Survey Project Download Site. It covers design of the survey form, display of the form, the building of external control files, the creation of a code book and data tables and the entry of data into the data tables, data summaries, cross-tabulations, and form counts.[5]

For a list of other software packages and a comparison of their features, see http://|websurveytoolbox.org/FeatureTable.html. The highest rated of these, with respect both to ease of use of the package and the look and feel of the questionnaire, is the **Web Survey Toolbox**.

LimeSurvey is claimed to be 'refreshingly easy', but not everyone may find it so. The authors promise enhanced user friendliness and easier installation in future versions.

Programming expertise is needed to customize these packages to specific study needs.

2. Tools

2a. Data entry and data management

EpiData and **Epi Info** simplify the production of data sets. They help in the design of a questionnaire or data entry form, and can apply rules and calculations during entry of data to the computer, e.g. by restricting data to certain values, controlling the sequence (e.g. jumping over 'female' questions if the subject is a male), and applying calculations (calculation of age, summation of scales, etc.). They permit subsequent recoding, the creation of new variables, and merging of data sets. They also permit subsequent analyses based on the data set. A tutorial on the use of **Epi Info** in a community health survey is available at http://www.cdc.gov/epiinfo/communityhealth.htm.

EpiSurveyor simplifies the creation of data entry forms to be used with mobile handheld devices – currently for Palm-operating-system-based devices only, but soon (we are promised) for others also, including non-Palm mobile phones and Windows Mobile handhelds – enabling their use in the field and transfer of data to a desktop or laptop computer for analysis.

WinIDAMS offers facilities for creating data files and data description files, and for sorting and merging files, data editing, checking of codes and consistencies, correcting, listing, subsetting, aggregating, and merging and transforming data, including the construction of new variables.

A data file can be created with a text editor (see '2j. Text editors'), but without built-in checks.

Data can also be entered in a spreadsheet (see '2f. Spreadsheets') for pasting into other programs.

2b. *Random numbers and random sampling*

Random numbers can be supplied by **Etcetera** (a **WinPepi** program) and by various programs in the 'Random number generators' sections of Pezzullo's lists. If an online program is wanted, then the choices include **SISA**, **OpenEpi**, **Research Randomizer**, and the **VassarStats** page.

Etcetera can select simple random samples and select from equally sized clusters. It can also provide a random 'yes' or 'no' decision (equivalent to tossing a coin) that may be of invaluable help to researchers who are faced with critical decisions in their lives.

Survey Toolbox, which is geared to veterinary epidemiological studies, can select simple random samples, select from differently sized clusters, and randomly select geographic coordinates.

2c. *Randomization*

Etcetera (a **WinPepi** program) can perform simple and balanced randomization (with or without stratification), balanced randomization of successive blocks of subjects, and random sequencing of treatments.

The Internet page **randomization.com** can randomize each subject to a single treatment by using the method of randomly permuted blocks, and can create random permutations of treatments for situations where subjects are to receive all of the treatments in random order.

Also on the Internet, **SISA** can randomize subjects to several groups.

2d. *Calculators*

There are a large number of free calculators, for downloading or online use; try http://_www.shambles.net/pages/learning/MathsP/Calcul. Many can evaluate expressions (e.g. '24/5677*10000' or 'ln(12.3)*2+ln(24.3)*2').

WinPepi's expression evaluator (**Whatis**) can save up to 24 values and 24 formulae, enabling them to be recalled (even in subsequent sessions) by entering labels (a, b, etc.) that represent them. This avoids repeated entry (e.g. of population denominators) and permits stage-wise calculations (by saving intermediate results) and the recomputation of stored formulae, using new data.

Google has a secret built-in expression evaluator. Just enter the expression in the search box. A guide is available at http://www.googleguide.com/help/calculator.html.

Instacalc, **Calcoolate** (which is downloadable), and **Calcr** are online expression evaluators.

2e. *P values*

Probabilities corresponding to given values of z (the standard normal deviate), t, *chi-square*, and F (and vice versa, i.e. quantiles) are provided by **Whatis** (a **WinPepi** program), and (on-line) by **SISA**, the **VassarStats** page, **Soper's Statistics Calculators,** and **StaTable** (which can also be downloaded).

PQRS and **Statistical Tables** provide probabilities and other statistics associated with the above and many other distributions.

StatCalc (version 2.0) computes one-tailed P values and other statistics based on numerous distributions (continuous, discrete, nonparametric, and other). Later versions are not free. A brief manual is available at http://www.ucs.louisiana.edu/~kxk4695/StatCalc_Cont.pdf

2f. Spreadsheets

Spreadsheet aficionados can find a number of free spreadsheets, including the one in the **Open Office** suite, which is slow to download and install, and the **Sphygmic Software spreadsheet**, which is faster.

Kyplot (version 2.0) provides a spreadsheet with elaborate statistical and graphing functions. Later versions are not free.

Free spreadsheets are also provided by Google, through its Docs & Spreadsheets service; your spreadsheets will be stored and available on the Web.

Episheet and Lamorte are easy-to-use spreadsheets that perform many procedures commonly used in epidemiological studies. **Episheet** provides useful graphs (survival curves, forest plots for meta-analyses, seasonal distribution).

2g. Graphs

RJSgraph and **SpectrumViewer** draw excellent data-plot graphs (*Y*-plots and *XY*-plots), with many optional trimmings; they can transform data, provide statistics, etc. **RJSgraph** can plot equations and provides a range of regression lines. Trepidation when using **SpectrumViewer** is unnecessary.[6]

The **Sphygmic Software** and **Open Office** spreadsheets draw pie, bar, line, scatter, 3-D, and other charts.

Dataplot is a multi-platform (Windows, Unix, VMS, Linux, etc.) software system for scientific visualization, statistical analysis, and nonlinear modelling. It supplies *X–Y* plots, distributional, time series, 3-D, multivariate, quality control, and numerous other plots. Downloading and installation are not simple.

Kyplot (version 2) is an elaborate program that draws line, scatter, bar, pie, 3-D and many other charts, as well as performing statistical analyses. Later versions are not free.

SBHisto draws simple histograms; it requires a text file with each value on a separate line. **VassarStats** draws simple histograms.

SSP (Smith's Statistical Package) draws simple histograms, bar charts, time-series graphs, scatterplots, and box-and-whiskers diagrams.

WinPepi draws time-series and box-and-whisker diagrams, forest plots, ROC curves, epidemic curves, and other diagrams.

Diagrams draws flowcharts and other diagrams.

EpiGram produces simple flowcharts and other diagrams.

Flowchart.com draws flowcharts online.

Diagrams can also be drawn by **Open Office**.

WinIDAMS draws scatterplots.

Episheet draws survival curves and forest plots.

2h. Epidemic curves

Describe (a **WinPepi** program) can plot epidemic curves based on data or models.

For a guide to the use of spreadsheets for drawing epidemic curves, see Torok (2006).[7]

2i. Card indexes

Scrapbook is a very simple program that creates a card index, with options for tagging and searching the individual records. **Treepad Lit**e is more elaborate; it can create a branching 'tree' of sets of the individual records,

Many other free personal information managers are available.

2j. Text editors

A large number of free text editors are available. For creating data files, **Crimson Editor** and **Notetab Light** are particularly useful, since they permit rectangular selections, i.e. rectangular blocks of data (e.g. selected groups of adjacent columns) can be copied and pasted into statistical programs.[8]

3. Analysis: General

3a. Online lists of free statistical programs

The most useful lists of free statistical programs are the following, especially the first two:

Pezzullo's 'Free Statistical Software' list, which is voluminous, at http://StatPages.org/javasta2.html

Pezzullo's 'Interactive Statistical Calculation Pages', which list '380 Calculating Pages – And Growing!' at http://statpages.org/

Statistical Science Web at http://www.statsci.org/free.html

Free Statistical Software at http://freestatistics.altervista.org/stat.php

Gene Shackman's list at http://gsociology.icaap.org/methods/soft.html

Freie wissenschaftliche software – List of free statistical software – at http://statistiksoftware.com/free_software.html

The Impoverished Social Scientist's Guide to Free Statistical Software and Resources at http://data.fas.harvard.edu/micah_altman/socsci.shtml.

3b. Selected multipurpose programs

WinPepi,[9] or Pepi-for-Windows, is a suite of Windows-based statistical programs for epidemiologists. It currently comprises seven programs, containing over 100 modules, each of which provides several and sometimes many statistical procedures – both commonly used ones and some that are less commonly used, and are difficult to find elsewhere. The programs give weight to measures of association and their confidence intervals, and do not concentrate on significance tests. Reviewers of the DOS-based set of **Pepi** programs[10] from which **WinPepi** developed repeatedly called it a 'Swiss army knife' of utilities for biomedical researchers. The programs have copious pop-up hints and on-screen help, and menus and buttons make them easy to use. They have comprehensive manuals, which explain the procedures and provide formulae or references. A desktop portal provides easy access to an alphabetical list of procedures and to the programs and manuals.

In general, **WinPepi** requires the entry of data that have already been counted or summarized, either manually or by using a program (e.g. **EpiData** – see above) that processes primary data. Data are entered at the keyboard, or (in the case of tables) can be pasted from a file or spreadsheet in which they are available. Some procedures (e.g. logistic and Poisson regression) can use data files.

OpenEpi is an interactive page produced by a project to create open source software for public health. It is compatible with PC, Mac and Linux browsers, and is downloadable. It provides statistics for counts and person-time rates in descriptive and analytic studies, stratified analysis with exact confidence limits, matched pair analysis, sample size calculations, random numbers, chi-square for dose–response trend, sensitivity, specificity and other evaluation statistics, and $R \times C$ tables. **OpenEpi** requires the entry (directly into the program) of data that have already been counted or summarized.

OS4 (previously OpenStat) was written as an aid to students and teachers for introductory and advanced statistics courses, primarily in the social sciences, and is said to perform nearly all of the analyses required in statistics courses. It is available in Windows and Linux versions, and sample data files and a 524-page manual[11] are offered. Raw data (up to a few thousand cases with up to 30 variables) can be entered into **OS4** to create a data file, or it can use data files created by other programs, e.g. **EpiData**.

WinIDAMS was developed by UNESCO to provide a reasonably comprehensive data management and statistical analysis software package. Its functions include regression analysis, analysis of variance, discriminant analysis, cluster analysis, and principal component analysis. Guides to its use and a manual are available.[12] Raw data can be entered into **WinIDAMS** to create a data set, or it can use data files created by other programs.

SISA (**Simple Interactive Statistical Analysis**) performs calculations online. Most of the modules are downloadable. It can display chi-square, normal and 20 other distributions, using Microsoft Excel or the freeware **Open Office**'s spreadsheet. **SISA** requires the entry of data that have already been counted or summarized.

The **VassarStats** website provides a number of small programs for the online analysis of proportions, ordinal, categorical, and numerical data, analysis of variance and covariance, and other procedures. Data may be entered at the keyboard or pasted.

MacAnova performs regression analysis, analysis of variance, multivariate analysis and time-series analysis, as well as more elementary analyses. There are Mac, Windows, DOS, Linux and Unix versions. MacAnova is not particularly user friendly, since it is primarily command driven (i.e. instructions must be typed in). A user's guide will be found hidden in the MacAnovaSharedsupportdocs folder.

Wessa.net performs calculations online. It has modules that provide descriptive statistics, multiple regression, hypothesis testing, plotting of mathematical equations, and other procedures. Data may be entered at the keyboard or pasted.

EasyReg is an extremely versatile program designed for econometric studies. It can manipulate and summarize data and perform linear and multiple regression and numerous involved analyses. 'Guided tours' are supplied. Downloading and installation are time consuming.

The **R Project for Statistical Computing** provides many procedures based on R (a language and environment for statistical computing and graphics: data handling and storage, tools for data analysis, and graphic facilities). There are Mac, Windows, DOS, Linux and Unix versions. Powerful and versatile, but not for the tyro (requires typing of instructions). The same applies to the procedures for survey analysis offered by **EpiTools**.[13] Numerous procedures are included in the **EpiCentre Package for R**. Other links to **R** will be found in Gene Shackman's list and the Impoverished Social Scientist's Guide (see '3a. Online lists of free statistical programs'). Introductory material on **R** is available.[14]

4. Analysis: Specific Tasks

4a. Descriptive statistics

Describe (a **WinPepi** program) provides procedures for use in descriptive epidemiology, including the appraisal of separate samples in comparative studies. It can handle categorical data (dichotomous, nominal or ordinal) and numerical data (including survival times and time trends). The **WinPepi** program **Etceter**a can analyse large and three-way contingency tables.

The **Episheet** and **LaMorte** spreadsheets provide procedures for use in descriptive epidemiology. **OS4** (OpenStat), **MacAnova**, and **LaMorte** analyse numerical data.

Wessa.net provides detailed descriptive statistics (with diagrams) for numerical data, online.

4b. Bivariate analyses

Compare2 (a **WinPepi** program) compares two independent groups or samples. It can handle both categorical data (dichotomous, nominal or ordinal; including clustered binomial data) and numerical data (including survival times). Compares person-time rates.

Pairsetc (a **WinPepi** program) compares matched observations (dichotomous, nominal, or numerical), appraising their differences and agreement. It does correlation and regression analysis.

OpenEpi compares two sets of dichotomous or numerical data. Compares person-time rates.

VassarStats (online) compares two sets of dichotomous, ordinal, or numerical data. It does correlation and regression analysis.

OS4 provides numerous tests, and does correlation and regression analysis.

WinIDAMS does correlation and regression analysis.

4c. Stratified analyses

Stratified data can be analysed by the following programs:

Compare2 and **Pairsetc** (two **WinPepi** programs), for categorical data (dichotomous, nominal or ordinal) and numerical data. **Pairsetc** handles matched observations.

Episheet and **VassarStat**, for dichotomous data.

4d. Multiple linear regression

WinIDAMS and **EasyReg** and (online) **Wessa.net**.

4e. Multiple logistic regression

Logistic (a **WinPepi** program) and **Epi Info** do logistic regression in Windows. In DOS, there are **MultLR** and another **Logistic** (unconditional logistic regression) and **Clogistic** (conditional).

Pezzulo and Sullivan's 'Logistic Regression' page does multiple logistic regression online.

4f. Cox regression analysis

OS4 (OpenStat), **Epi Info**, and **CoxSurv** (a DOS program).

Pezzullo and Sullivan's 'Cox Proportional Hazards Survival Regression' page does it online.

4g. Multiple Poisson regression

Poisson (a **WinPepi** program) performs multiple Poisson regression.

4h. Analysis of variance

OS4 (OpenStat), **VassarStats**, **OpenEpi** (one-way analysis of variance (ANOVA)), **WinIDAMS** (one-way ANOVA).
   Online: **Soper's Statistics Calculators** (one-way ANOVA).

4i. Misclassification

Effects of misclassification are controlled by **Describe** (for a single variable), **Compare2** (in comparisons of unpaired data) and **Pairsetc** (in comparisons of paired data). All three are **WinPepi** programs.

4j. Measuring the validity of screening/diagnostic tests or other measures

Describe (a **WinPepi** program) can provide a comprehensive assessment of the validity of tests or other measures that have 'yes–no' results, and also of those that have a range of values; it produces ROC curves, and can compare tests.
   On-line programs include:
   On-Line Clinical Calculator, which assesses 'yes–no' tests
   OpenEpi assesses 'yes–no' tests and tests with a range of values; produces a ROC curve
   ROC Analysis, which examines ROC curves in detail.

4k. Measuring the reliability of measures

Pairsetc (a **WinPepi** program) computes *kappa* and related measures of the reliability of categorical data, and also computes numerous coefficients that express the reliability of numerical measurements.
   DagStat computes *kappa* and related measures of the reliability of categorical data.
   Online, *kappa* for two or more categories is computed by **VassarStats** and **QuickCalcs**.

4l. Appraising synergism

Measures of synergism are computed by **Etcetera** (a **WinPepi** program) and by **Epinetcalculation.xls**, a spreadsheet.

4m. Assessing a scale

Composite scales made up of 'yes–no' items or items with Likert scores can be assessed by **Etcetera** (a WinPepi program), which computes Cronbach's *alpha* and Ferguson's *delta*, appraises conformity with a Guttman scale, and assesses the scale's discriminatory power.

4n. Multiple comparisons

Etcetera (a **WinPepi** program) and **Multi** adjust P values that are based on multiple tests. **Etcetera** uses three methods, **Multi** uses nine.

4o. Cluster samples

Cluster samples can be analysed by **Describe** (a **WinPepi** program) and **EpiInfo**. The required number of clusters can be computed by **Describe**.
   WinIDAMS does cluster analysis.

4p. Capture-recapture procedure

Describe (a **WinPepi** program) uses data from incomplete overlapping lists to estimate the number of cases of a disease in a population.

4q. Standardization (direct and indirect)

Describe (a **WinPepi** program) does direct and indirect standardization, including the standardization method that gives each year of age the same weight, and the computation of standardized morbidity or mortality ratios.
   Episheet and **LaMorte** can do standardization. **PamComp**, **OpenEpi**, and **LaMorte** calculate standardized mortality ratios.

4r. Regression to the mean

Pairsetc (a **WinPepi** program) can assess the effect of regression to the mean. It can also use analysis of covariance to avoid it, as can **OS4** and **VassarStats**.

4s. Survival analysis

Describe, **Compare2** (two **WinPepi** programs), **EpiInfo**, **OS4**, **Episheet**, and **LaMorte** perform Kaplan–Meier survival analysis, as does **KMsurv** in DOS.
   Hutchon's interactive page does survival analysis online.

4t. Meta-analysis

WinPepi programs: **Compare2** compares results (categorical or numerical) of studies of different kinds, computes overall tests and values and the fail-safe *N*, and performs tests for publication bias. **Pairsetc** compares and combines the results of studies using paired data. **Describe** can perform a meta-analysis of studies of screening or diagnostic tests.
   MIX ('**M**eta-analysis with **I**nteractive e**X**planations') performs meta-analyses of categorical or numerical data, using Microsoft Excel spreadsheets. The **Episheet** spreadsheet provides forest plots.
   DOS-based packages that perform meta-analysis include **Meta-analysis**, **EpiMeta**, and **EasyMA**.

4u. Multilevel studies

MLwiN analyses multilevel models. It is free if your e-mail address ends with *ac.uk*. A user's guide is available.[15] A review of multilevel software (including **MLwiN**)[16] provides insights into nesting behaviours in and of patients.
   MIXOR, **MIXREG**, **MIXNO**, and **MIXPREG** perform multilevel analysis for linear, logistic, probit, and Poisson regression and for survival analysis. Manuals are available at http://tigger.uic.edu/~hedeker/manuals.html
   Multilevel models can be modelled by **WinBugs**, using a Bayesian approach.

4v. Imputation

Programs that can perform multiple imputation of missing values (not for the faint of heart) include **Amelia**[17] and **NORM**.

4w. Bayesian analysis

The online lists in Section 3a (above) include a number of programs that use Bayesian statistics. **First Bayes**, which is intended as an aid to learning Bayesian statistics, performs most standard elementary Bayesian analyses; but its author says 'it does not claim or attempt to be for actually doing Bayesian analysis'. It is not easy to install or use. **WinBugs** is versatile, but requires prior understanding of Bayesian methods.[18]

4x. Appraisal of unmeasured confounders

Etcetera (a **WinPepi** program) appraises the possible effects of hypothetical unmeasured confounders.

5. Web Addresses (URLs)

Amelia	http://gking.harvard.edu/amelia
BiblioExpress	http://www.biblioscape.com/biblioexpress.htm
Clogistic	http://www.brixtonhealth.com/epiaddins.html
Calcoolate	http://www.calcoolate.com
Calcr	http://calcr.com
Compare2	http://www.brixtonhealth.com
CoxSurv	http/www.mcgill.ca/cancerepi/links/software
Crimson Editor	http://www.crimsoneditor.com
DagStat	http://www.mhri.edu.au/biostats/DAG%5FStat
Dataplot	http://www.itl.nist.gov/div898/software/ dataplot/ftp/homepage.htm
Describe	http://www.brixtonhealth.com
Diagrams	http://www.jansfreeware.com/jfgraphics. htm#diagrams
EasyMA	http://www.spc.univ-lyon1.fr/easyma
EasyReg	http://econ.la.psu.edu/~hbierens/ERIDOWNL. HTM
EpiCentre Package for R	http://epicentre.massey.ac.nz/Default.as-pxtabid=195
EpiData	http://www.epidata.dk
EpiGram	http://www.brixtonhealth.com
Epi Info	http://www.cdc.gov/EPIINFO/epiinfo.htm
EpiMeta	http://ftp.cdc.gov/pub/Software/epimeta
Epinetcalculation.xls	http://www.epinet.se/
Episheet	http://members.aol.com/krothman/episheet.xls
EpiSurveyor	http://www.datadyne.org/?q=episurveyor/about
EpiTools	http://faculty.washington.edu/tlumley/survey/
Etcetera	http://www.brixtonhealth.com
First Bayes	http://www.firstbayes.co.uk
Flowchart.com	http://www.flowchart.com
Hutchon's interactive page	http://www.hutchon.net/Kaplan-Meier.htm
Instacalc	http://instacalc.com
KMsurv	http://www.mcgill.ca/cancerepi/links/software
Kyplot	http://www.woundedmoon.org/win32/kyplot. html
LaMorte	http://www.bumc.bu.edu/www/Busm/Ome/ Images/LaMorte%20IP/LaMorte%20-%20stat%20tools.xls
Lenth's Java applets	http://www.stat.uiowa.edu/~rlenth/Power/index. html
LimeSurvey	http://www.limesurvey.org
Logistic (DOS program)	http://sagebrushpress.com/PEPI.html

Logistic (**WinPepi** program)	http://www.brixtonhealth.com
MacAnova	http://www.stat.umn.edu/macanova/download.html
Meta-analysis	http://web.fu-berlin.de/gesund/gesu_engl/meta_e.htm
MIX	http://www.mix-for-meta-analysis.info/index.html
MIXNO	http://tigger.uic.edu/~hedeker/mixwin.html
MIXOR	http://tigger.uic.edu/~hedeker/mixwin.html
MIXPREG	http://tigger.uic.edu/~hedeker/mixwin.html
MLwiN	http://www.cmm.bristol.ac.uk/MLwiN/download/index.shtml
Multi	http://biostatistics.mdanderson.org/Software-Download/SingleSoftware.aspxSoftware_Id=50
MultLR	http://www.mcgill.ca/cancerepi/links/software
NORM	http://www.stat.psu.edu/~jls/misoftwa.html
Notetab Light	http://www.notetab.com/ntl.php
On-Line Clinical Calculator	http://www.intmed.mcw.edu/clincalc/bayes.html
OpenEpi	http://www.openepi.com
Open Office	http://download.openoffice.org/
OS4 (OpenStat)	http://www.statpages.org/miller/openstat/.
Manual	http://www.statpages.org/miller/openstat/ATextBook.pdf
Pairsetc	http://www.brixtonhealth.com
PamComp	http://epi.klinikum.uni-muenster.de/pamcomp/pamcomp.html
Pezzullo and Sullivan's 'Cox Proportional Hazards Survival Regression' page	http://www.sph.emory.edu/~cdckms/CoxPH/prophaz2.html
Pezzulo and Sullivan's 'Logistic Regression' page	http://statpages.org/logistic.html
Poisson	http://www.brixtonhealth.com
PQRS	http://www.eco.rug.nl/~knypstra/pqrs.html
PS	http://biostat.mc.vanderbilt.edu/twiki/bin/view/Main/PowerSampleSize
QuickCalcs	http://graphpad.com/quickcalcs/kappa1.cfm
R	http://www.r-project.org/
Randomization.com	http://www.randomization.com
Research Randomizer	http://www.randomizer.org
RJSgraph	http://www.rjsweb.fsnet.co.uk/downloads.htm
ROC Analysis	http://www.rad.jhmi.edu/jeng/javarad/roc/main.html
Sampsize	www.abdn.ac.uk/hsru/epp/sampsize

SBHisto	http://www.freedownloadscenter.com/Authors/ SB_Software.html
School of Rural Public Health Free Web Survey Project	http://129.111.144.49:81/Research/cjcooper/ FreeSurvey/default.aspx
Scrapbook	http://enitzsche.home.comcast.net/scrapbook/ scrapbook.html
SISA	http://home.clara.net/sisa
Soper's Statistics Calculators	http://www.danielsoper.com/statcalc/
Sphygmic Software spreadsheet	http://www.ds.unifi.it/~stefanin/AGR_2001/SH/ sssheet.htm
SpectrumViewer	http://www.phys.tue.nl/people/etimmerman/ specview
SSP	http://www.economics.pomona.edu/StatSite/ SSP.html
StaTable	http://www.cytel.com/Products/StaTable/
StatCalc	http://www.ucs.louisiana.edu/~kxk4695/ StatCalc.htm
Statistical Tables	http://www.softpedia.com/progDownload/ Statistical-Tables-Download-40942.html
Survey Toolbox	http://www.ausvet.com.au/content. phppage=res_software#st
TreePad Lite	http://www.treepad.com/treepadfreeware
Trial Protocol Tool	http://www.practihc.org/toolindex.htm
VassarStats	http://faculty.vassar.edu/lowry/VassarStats.html
Web Survey Toolbox	http://sourceforge.net/projects/jspsurveylib/
Wessa.net	http://www.wessa.net
Whatis	http://www.brixtonhealth.com
WinAdams	To obtain the program, fill in a form at http:// www.unesco.org/webworld/portal/idams/ individual_request.html
WinBugs	http://www.mrc-bsu.cam.ac.uk/bugs/
WinPepi (programs and manuals)	http://www.brixtonhealth.com
Zotero	https://addons.mozilla.org/firefox/3504/

Notes and References

1. According to one website, **Zotero** is pronounced 'zoh-TAIR-oh'. According to another, the name is derived from the Shqip (Albanian) word 'zoteroj' (pronounced 'zote a roy'), which means 'to own or to master'.
2. 'How's Your Klingon? We're very interested in getting users to help us translate **Zotero** into other languages…' (http://www.zotero.org/blog/hows-your-klingon).
3. Campbell MK, Thomson S, Ramsay CR, MacLennan GS, Grimshaw JM. Sample size calculator for cluster randomized trials. Computers in Biology and Medicine 2004; 34: 113.

4. Treweek S, McCormack K, Abalos E, Campbell M, Ramsay C, Zwarenstein M. The Trial Protocol Tool: the PRACTIHC software tool that supported the writing of protocols for pragmatic controlled trials. Journal of Clinical Epidemiology 2006; 59: 1127.

5. Described by Cooper CJ, Cooper SP, del Junco DJ, Shipp EM, Whitworth R, Cooper SR (Web-based data collection: detailed methods of a questionnaire and data gathering tool. Epidemiological Perspectives and Innovations 2006; 3: 1) and available http://sp.srph.tamhsc.edu/dept/PHEB/Research/cjcooper/FreeSurvey/default.aspx

6. **SpectrumViewer**'s download page says 'If you download and use **Spectrum Viewer**, you're bringing all the pleasures and disasters that come with it on yourself... If, during usage, you die from ecstasy, your CPU explodes, your monitor melts, your hard drive is launched into space, an earthquake flattens your house, WW3 starts, or any other disaster strikes, I will not be responsible...'.

7. Torok M. Epidemic curves ahead. Focus on Field Epidemiology 2006; 1: 5. www2.sph.unc.edu/nccphp/|focus/vol1/issue5/

8. To make a rectangular selection, choose the 'Column mode' in **Crimson Editor**, and use the 'Modify|Block' command in **Notetab Light**.

9. Abramson, JH. WINPEPI (PEPI-for-Windows): computer programs for epidemiologists. Epidemiologic Perspectives & Innovations 2004; 1: 6. http://www.epi-perspectives.com/content/1/1/6.

10. Abramson JH, Gahlinger PM. Computer programs for epidemiologists: PEPI V.4.0. Salt Lake City, UT: Sagebrush Press; 2001.

11. Miller WG. Statistics and measurement using the free OpenStat packages; 2006. http://www.statpages.org/miller/openstat/ATextbook.pdf.

12. 'Self-teaching material' for **WinIDAMS** is available at http://www.unesco.org/webworld/idams/selfteaching/eng/eidams.htm.
    A manual is provided with the program. A guide is also available on the Internet: Nagpaul PS. Guide to Advanced Data Analysis using IDAMS Software (http://www.unesco.org/webworld/idams/advguide/TOC.htm).

13. A manual for **EpiTools** is available at http://www.epitools.net (Aragon T. Package 'epitools'; 2007).

14. See Hills H, Plummer P, Carstensen B (A short introduction to **R**; 2006. http://staff.pubhealth.ku.dk/~bxc/SPE/Rintro-spe.pdf), Aragon TJ, Enanoria WT (Applied epidemiology using **R**; 2007. http://www.medepi.net/epir/), and Myatt M (Open Source Solutions – **R**; 2005. http://brixtonhealth.com). A manual on the use of **R** in epidemiological studies (Aragon TJ, Enanoria WT. Applied epidemiology using R; 2007) is available at http://www.medepi.net/epir/. A list of **R** manuals is available at http://cran.r-project.org/manuals.html.

15. **MLwiN** requires considerable statistical know-how. Get a user's guide at http://www.cmm.bristol.ac.uk/MLwiN/download/manuals.shtml.

16. 'If a patient has multiple clinical visits to his doctor, multiple visit observations are nested within patients, who in turn are nested within doctors' (Zhou X-H, Perkins AJ, Hui SL. Comparisons of software for generalised linear multilevel models. American Statistician 1999; 53: 282).

17. This missing-value program is named after the missing aviatrix Amelia Earhart, the first woman to fly solo over the Atlantic, whose plane disappeared between the Nukumanu and Howland Islands in the Pacific in 1937.

18. The **WinBugs** software comes with a Health Warning stating that a knowledge of Bayesian statistics is assumed, that the methods are inherently less robust than the usual statistical methods, and that there is no in-built protection against misuse.

Index

Research Methods in Community Medicine: Surveys, Epidemiological Research, Programme Evaluation, Clinical Trials J. H. Abramson and Z. H. Abramson Copyright © 2008, John Wiley & Sons Ltd

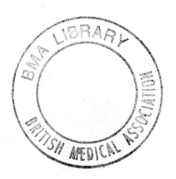